SLEEP DISORDERS

Dedication

To our wives and families,
who are the reasons for any of our accomplishments,
who have taught and aided us
in much of what we know and do

SLEEP DISORDERS
their impact on public health

Damien Léger MD PhD
Centre du Sommeill et de la Vigilance
Hôtel-Dieu de Paris
Publique Hôpitaux de Paris
Université de Paris 5
Paris
France

SR Pandi-Perumal MSc
Comprehensive Center for Sleep Medicine
Department of Pulmonary,
Critical Care and Sleep Medicine
Mount Sinai School of Medicine
New York, NY
USA

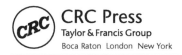
CRC Press
Taylor & Francis Group
Boca Raton London New York

CRC Press is an imprint of the
Taylor & Francis Group, an **informa** business

CRC Press
Taylor & Francis Group
6000 Broken Sound Parkway NW, Suite 300
Boca Raton, FL 33487-2742

First issued in paperback 2019

© 2010 by Taylor & Francis Group, LLC
CRC Press is an imprint of Taylor & Francis Group, an Informa business

No claim to original U.S. Government works

ISBN-13: 978-1-84184-535-7 (hbk)
ISBN-13: 978-0-367-38972-7 (pbk)

**Visit the Taylor & Francis Web site at
http://www.taylorandfrancis.com**

**and the CRC Press Web site at
http://www.crcpress.com**

Contents

List of contributors   vii

Preface   xi

Acknowledgments   xv

1.   Does the demography of sleep contribute to pre-existing health disparities?   1
     Lauren Hale, Paul E Peppard, and Terry Young

2.   Sleep in America: is race or culture an important factor?   19
     Girardin Jean-Louis, Ferdinand Zizi, Georges Casimir, and Jean Claude Compas

3.   Sleep-related problems in childhood   39
     Stephen H Sheldon

4.   Impact of sleep-disordered breathing on quality of life and school
     performance in children   49
     Nira A Goldstein

5.   Sleep in aging   59
     Andrew A Monjan

6.   Sleeping environments   67
     Alain Muzet

7.   Impact of sleeping environment on sleep quality   77
     Gaby Bader

8.   Interaction between sleep and stress in shift workers   101
     Torbjörn Åkerstedt

9.   Sleepiness, sleep disorders, and accidents   115
     Pierre Philip and Jaques Taillard

10. Medico-legal aspects of sleep disorders   123
     John Shneerson

11. Insomnia: impact on work, economics, and quality of life   137
    Damien Léger

12. Public health impact of insomnia and low-cost behavioral interventions   155
    Meagan Daley, Simon Beaulieu-Bonneau, and Charles M Morin

13. Economic impact of sleep loss, sleepiness, and sleep disorders   175
    Kin M Yuen and Clete Kushida

14. Pain and poor sleep   193
    Gilles Lavigne and Christiane Manzini

15. Sleep apnea and stroke   209
    Henry Yaggi and Vahid Mohsenin

16. Narcolepsy and idiopathic hypersomnia   225
    Michel Billiard

Index   235

Contributors

Torbjörn Åkerstedt, PhD
IPM and Karolinska Institute
Stockholm
Sweden

Gaby Bader, MD, PhD
Sleep Unit
Department of Clinical
  Neurophysiology
Institute of Clinical Neuroscience
University of Gothenburg
Sweden

Simon Beaulieu-Bonneau, MPs
École de psychologie
Université Laval
Québec
Canada

Michel Billiard, MD
School of Medicine
Guide Chauliac Hospital
Montpellier
France

Georges Casimir, MD
Department of Psychiatry
SUNY Downstate Medical Center
Brooklyn, NY
USA

Jean Claude Compas, MD
Multispecialty Clinic Maimonides
  Medical Center
Brooklyn, NY
USA

Meagan Daley, MA
École de psychologie
Université Laval
Québec
Canada

Nira A Goldstein, MD
Department of Otolaryngology
SUNY Downstate Medical Center
Brooklyn, NY
USA

Lauren Hale, PhD
State University of New York
Stony Brook, NY
USA

Girardin Jean-Louis, PhD
Department of Psychiatry
  and Brooklyn Center for
  Health Disparities
SUNY Downstate Medical Center
Brooklyn, NY
USA

Clete A Kushida, PhD
Stanford University Center of
    Excellence for Sleep Disorders
Stanford, CA
USA

Gilles Lavigne, DMD, PhD, FRCD(c) oral med
Faculté de Médecine Dentaire
Université de Montréal
Centre d'Etude sur le sommeil et les rythmes
    biologiques
Hôpital du Sacré Coeur de Montréal
Montréal, Québec
Canada

Damien Léger, MD, PhD
Center du Sommeil et de la Vigilance
Publique Hôpitaux de Paris
Université de Paris
Hôtel Dieu de Paris
Paris
France

Christiane Manzini, Cert Res
Faculté de Médecine Dentaire
Université de Montréal
Centre d'Etude sur le sommeil et les rythmes
    biologiques
Hôpital du Sacré Coeur de Montreal
Montréal, Québec
Canada

Vahid Mohsenin, MD
Yale Center for Sleep Medicine
Yale University School of Medicine
New Haven, CT
USA

Andrew A Monjan, PhD, MPH
Neurobiology of Aging Branch
Neuroscience and Neuropsychology
    of Aging Program
National Institute on Aging
Bethesda, MD
USA

Charles M Morin, PhD
Société Canadienne du Sommeil
École de psychologie
Université Laval
Sainte-Foy
Québec
Canada

Alain Muzet, MD
CEPA-CNRS
Strasbourg
France

S. R. Pandi-Perumal, MSc
Division of Pulmonary, Critical
    Care and Sleep Medicine
Mount Sinai School of Medicine
New York, NY
USA

Paul E Peppard, MD, PhD
Medical Sciences Center
Madison, WI
USA

Pierre Philip, MD, PhD
Clinique du Sommeil
Hôpital Pellegrin
Bordeaux
France

Stephen H Sheldon, DO, FAAP
Sleep Medicine Center
Children's Memorial Hospital
Northwestern University
Chicago, IL
USA

John Shneerson, MA, DM, FRCP
Respiratory Support and Sleep Centre
Papworth Hospital
Cambridge
UK

Jacques Taillard, PhD
Clinique de Sommeil
Hôpital Pellegrin
Bordeaux
France

Henry Yaggi, MD
Yale Center for Sleep Medicine
New Haven, CT
USA

Terry B Young, PhD
Medical Sciences Center
Madison, WI
USA

Kin Yuen, MD
Stanford University Center of
    Excellence for Sleep Disorders
Stanford, CA
USA

Ferdinand Zizi, BA
Brooklyn Center for Health Disparities
SUNY Downstate Medical Center
Brooklyn, NY
USA

Preface

Sleep is a universal biological phenomenon and in humans accounts for the way in which we spend a third of our lives. Although the exact mechanisms of its restorative function remain largely unelucidated, sleep's biological importance to life becomes obvious when humans or animals are prevented from sleeping, or when its normal activity is even slightly disrupted. Increasingly, the importance of studying sleep mechanisms is being recognized in government and scientific circles. Sleep disorders are now at the top of research and policy agendas in health care settings and in developed countries are recognized as significant public health challenges. Unfortunately, in the rest of the world, the public health consequences of sleep disorders remain largely under-recognized and poorly appreciated or treated.

In the last several decades, sleep research has seen enormous progress. Numerous discoveries in both basic and clinical research have been described in a wealth of papers of ever-increasing complexity. The purpose of this volume is to provide a forum for research that can improve our understanding of sleep disorders medicine from a global perspective. This volume is the first of its kind and focuses on the emerging challenges and public health consequence of sleep and wake dysfunctions.

Sleep as it relates to public health is a fascinating field of medical science. The significance of sleep and its disorders has generated a host of volumes, including this one, on its etiology, prognosis, diagnosis, pathophysiology, prevalence, prevention, treatment, and management. As the impact of sleep disorders on many facets of human health is becoming more apparent, the public health aspect of sleep disorders is similarly developing into an interdisciplinary field. We have striven to present comprehensive chapters that address issues related to the public health interventions for the prevention, treatment, and management of sleep disorders.

This volume is intended for sleep physicians, epidemiologists, population and public health researchers, and generalists alike. It can be useful for graduate students of biomedical and public health sciences, clinical researchers, and others who want to get an overall grasp of the public health ramifications of sleep disorders.

The contributions are from a wide range of authors many of whom are world-recognized authorities in their field. Chapters deal with a range of topics that have profound impact on the public health-related issues including the socioeconomic status and demographic factors that affect sleep, role of environmental factors, aging-related issues, effects of stress and shift work, and also sleep-related motor vehicle accidents. The volume also addresses the effects of other medical illnesses such as pain and effects of sleep apnea on stroke risk. The reader may feel confident that the information presented is based on the most recent literature.

It has been the intention of the editors to provide a comprehensive and up-to-date coverage of specialized topics on sleep and public health. It is our hope that we have succeeded in accomplishing this goal; nevertheless the editors and authors would appreciate feedback on the contents of the volume with particular regard to omissions and inaccuracies, which will be rectified in later editions. We would appreciate hearing from the readers about how we might continue to improve the coverage of topics. We also welcome your ideas and comments and constructive criticisms.

This is, to the best of our knowledge, the first look at the impact of sleep and alertness on public health.

A section of this volume has been dedicated to the effect of reduced alertness on child development and learning. It is obvious that sleep quality has a major impact on the ability of children to concentrate and memorize at school. Poor conditions of sleeping due to housing, environment, and security may negatively induce sleepiness at school and ultimately interfere with learning. Adolescent lifestyles often include late hours of going to bed and quite early awakenings for going to school. Sleep deprivation is thus very common in both age groups and the consequences of this chronic sleep deprivation are multiple: sleeping at school or while driving, anxiety, depression, social and familial problems. Lack of public awareness of the linkage between adequate sleep and efficient learning may have the effect of denying the full benefit of education to large segments of our population.

In the workplace, the relation between sleep and work ability is also an unexplored field despite the evidence of multiple interactions between the two domains. The desynchronization of biological timing mechanisms in millions of night-time shift workers around the world has significant public health implications. These workers are known to be severely sleep deprived and thus are more prone to accidents and cardiovascular or metabolic diseases. There remains, however, a lack of understanding about the contribution of sleep deprivation to occupational safety and personal health. One expression of this is the fact that shift work is a proliferating economic trend in the developing world. Other contributors to sleep deprivation are economic demands for rapid distribution of goods, which in turn encourage long distance driving among commercial vehicle operators. Leisure habits increasingly include late night television viewing which erodes the amount of time available for sleeping. Sleep-deprived workers have a higher risk of work and motorized vehicle accidents, decreased productivity, reduced attention spans, and increased irritability. At work, jet lag and early awakenings due to local work travel also negatively affect sleep and alertness.

The risk of accidents due to sleepiness and sleep disorders has been dramatically demonstrated by the American National Commission of Sleep Disorders in the cases of catastrophic events such as the Exxon Valdez oil spill, the Challenger space shuttle accident or the 'Bhopal' ecological disaster. In each of these events the people who may have had the power to reduce the impact of the catastrophe were severely sleep deprived at the time of the accident and were thus unable to react appropriately. About half of the fatal accidents in young drivers occur at night and are partially or directly due to an episode of sleepiness at the wheel. However, few educational efforts are directed toward alerting the public about the importance of sleep hygiene for accident prevention, especially in affected groups such as young drivers, truck drivers, or shift workers.

The influence of the environment on sleep quality and quantity is also an under-explored area. The reduction of noise, heat, and light in the bedroom is critical for optimizing sleep. Noise and sleep is a particular subject of concern in areas surrounding airports. The World Health Organization has provided recommendations based on the recognition that sleep disturbance is the most important health risk accruing from air transportation noise exposure. Airports and aircraft engineers have attempted to deal with this problem by reducing noise levels at their source. Local authorities sometimes regulate the schedule of flights at night. However, noise pollution appears to be one of the most important sources of sleep disruption and further efforts to educate pilots, airport administrators, and local officials are merited.

Sleep disorders have a major impact on the quality of life in affected individuals. Thus insomnia (which affects one adult in four), sleep apnea (which affects one in ten) and hypersomnia are shown to negatively impact the daytime functioning of millions of patients around the planet.

It is our hope that this volume improves the reader's understanding of the public health sequel of sleep disorders and that this knowledge will ultimately have an effect on public health policy. Sleep disturbance is unfortunately ignored in the public health plans of many countries around the world. The public health cost of disturbed sleep, however, is significant and merits whatever steps are required to reduce it.

Damien Léger
Paris, France
SR Pandi-Perumal
New York, USA

Acknowledgments

Creating a book which surveys a broadly interdisciplinary field such as sleep and public health involves the collaborative scholarship of many individuals. We express our profound gratitude to the many people who have helped and also to some who have contributed without realizing just how helpful they have been.

The editors wish to express their sincere appreciation and owe endless gratitude to all the authors for their scholarly contributions that facilitated the development of this volume.

Producing a volume such as this is a team effort and we acknowledge with gratitude the work of Informa Healthcare's editorial department. We are especially indebted to Mr Pete Stevenson, Commissioning Editor of Neurology and Psychiatry, who was an enthusiastic and instrumental supporter from the start. Our profound gratitude is offered also to Ms Rupal Malde whose equally dedicated efforts promoted a smooth transition and completion of our project following Pete Stevenson's unavoidable departure from Informa Healthcare. Despite our missed deadlines, both Pete and Rupal provided unflagging dedication, invaluable help, and encouragement. We appreciate their intellectual rigor and personal commitment to our project.

We also thank the Informa Healthcare production department. They all gave unstintingly of their time, energy, and enthusiasm. This talented and dedicated team of copy and production editors strengthened, polished, trimmed, and conscientiously checked the text for errors.

We also wish to thank the administrative and secretarial staffs at Centre du Sommeil, Hotel-Dieu de Paris, Paris, France and Comprehensive Center for Sleep Medicine Department of Pulmonary, Critical Care, and Sleep Medicine, Mount Sinai School of Medicine, for helping us to stay on task and for their attention to detail.

The editors would also like to acknowledge the close co-operation we have received from each other. We think we made a good team, even if we say it ourselves!

Finally, we are most grateful to our families, who provided love and support too valuable to measure. Their constant encouragement, understanding, and patience while the book was being developed are immeasurably appreciated. Being able to spend more time with them is our chief reward for finishing. They saw the work through from the conception of an idea to the completion of an interesting project with unwavering optimism and encouragement. They were the source of joy and inspiration for us, and we thank them for their continuing support, and for understanding the realities of academic life! For this, and for so much else, we are ever grateful.

Damien Léger
Paris
SR Pandi-Perumal
New York

CHAPTER 1

Does the demography of sleep contribute to health disparities?

Lauren Hale, Paul E Peppard, and Terry Young

The aim of this chapter is to incorporate the extensive and growing literature on health disparities into the discourse on sleep disorders and public health. The population health literature, quite distinct from the sleep research literature, describes the relationships between various sociodemographic characteristics and health. It describes how people with greater wealth exhibit, on average, greater health, and how this relationship persists even when controlling for health behaviors and pre-existing health conditions.[1-3] A life expectancy advantage is also observed for women over men, Whites over Blacks, highly educated people over less educated people, married people over unmarried people, and, of course, young people over old people.[1,4,5] The existence of these social and racial health differences has inspired a broad interdisciplinary research agenda that seeks to identify the sources of these health inequalities and ways to improve the health of the worse-off populations. Thus far, the research has discussed how factors such as early life conditions, health behaviors, wear and tear on the body (sometimes referred to as allostatic load), and health care utilization are relevant and active forces in determining the health of any given community or population.[4,6-8] In this chapter, we contribute to the population health discussion by

investigating whether sleep disorders and sleep behaviors are contributing to (or ameliorating) these health disparities.

We depict the conceptual framework for our research question in Figure 1.1 using a simple triangle in which the three circles, one at each vertex, represent the following clusters of variables: (1) health and well-being, (2) sleep disorders and sleep behaviors, and (3) social and demographic characteristics. The solid line between health and well-being and social and demographic characteristics depicts the documented association between social characteristics and a variety of health outcomes. On another side of the triangle, the solid line connecting sleep disorders and sleep behavior to health and well-being represents the relationship between sleep and health that is documented throughout the sleep literature and in other chapters of this book. The broken line drawn along the bottom of the triangle represents the relationship between social and demographic characteristics and sleep disorders and sleep behavior – what we are referring to as the demography of sleep. The line drawn here is broken because the demography of sleep is usually not studied as a topic in itself, and the relationships are much less understood. This part of the framework is the primary focus of our paper.

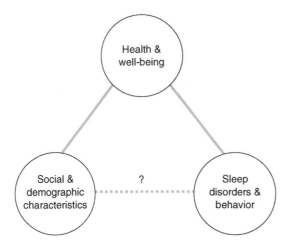

Figure 1.1 Conceptual framework for research question

We explore the hypothesis that getting adequate sleep is a function of endogenous and exogenous conditions, including health behavior, that contribute to (or ameliorate) pre-existing health disparities. This would occur if sleep disorders or health-related sleep behaviors were more common among the subpopulations that have greater (or lower) health risks. In this chapter, we focus on the primary demographic variables of gender, race, socioeconomic status/education, marital status, and age. In the first section 'Health disparities,' we briefly review the literature on health disparities for each of the above demographic characteristics. In the second section, 'What do we know about the demography of sleep?,' we investigate the demographic characteristics for three major sleep problems: unfavorable sleep duration, sleep apnea, and insomnia. For each subsection therein, we examine what is known about the relationship between each sleep condition and each of the five demographic dimensions listed above. We accomplish this through literature review and supplement it with results from our own analyses. We conclude with a summary of whether the sleep problems of various subsets of the population might contribute to health disparities.

HEALTH DISPARITIES

Gender

Gender disparities in mortality are observed throughout the developed world; they begin at infancy and last until very old age. Although, statistically, boys are born more frequently than girls, in industrialized countries their mortality rates are higher at every life stage.[9] This is not always true in developing countries, however.[9,10]

Despite the increased mortality risks for males over females, women report greater morbidities and poorer self-rated health than men over most of the life course.[11–13] Hypotheses for this paradox (i.e., that mortality is lower among women, but morbidity is higher) include the notions of gender inequality in paid and household work and differences in health behaviors and lifestyle.[13] For example, women are more likely than men both to go to the doctor and to report health problems.[12] Also, women may be more likely than men to suffer from health conditions (e.g., arthritis or headaches) that cause women to have poorer self-rated health, but do not necessarily cause increased mortality, and less likely to have cardiovascular disease and other morbidities that do cause increased mortality.[12] As described below, insomnia may be an example of a morbidity that is associated with worse health, but not necessarily with higher mortality.

Race

Historically, assessment of racial disparities in health often involved measuring differentials between Blacks and Whites in terms of mortality, heart disease, cancer, diabetes, and a variety of other morbidities.[4] While we acknowledge that additional races and ethnicities are important to investigate, we focus our discussion on differences between Blacks and Whites because this is where the majority of research has been. Increased health risks for Blacks begin early in life; Black children are more likely to be born of low birth weight and are more likely to grow up in a disadvantaged neighborhood.[4,14] The life expectancy at birth of Black men in the USA in 2002 was 68.8 years, whereas for White men it was 75.1, a difference of 6.3 years.[15] For Black women in the USA in 2002, life expectancy at birth was 75.6 compared to White women who had a life expectancy of 80.3, a difference of 4.7 years.[15] If the death rates between Blacks were the same as for Whites, there would be approximately 91 000 fewer Black deaths per year.[16] These large differences are to some extent attributable to health behaviors, such as diet and exercise, but even controlling for these characteristics, the health risk associated with being Black is much higher than it is for Whites. The residual effect may be due to stress, residential segregation, environmental factors, and medical care. The presence of chronic psychosocial stressors that alter physiological functioning may be a source of racial differences in health.[8,17] Residential segregation and neighborhood quality could be creating and reinforcing economic inequality by determining access to schools, employment opportunities, and social networks.[4,18] Limited health insurance coverage for Black Americans and differential access to, and utilization of, medical care may be relevant to differential mortality rates between Blacks and Whites. Black Americans are less likely than Whites to receive preventive, screening, diagnostic, treatment, and rehabilitation services for cancer.[15]

Socioeconomic status and education

The literature on health and socioeconomic status (SES) shows a positive relationship, sometimes referred to as the social gradient in health, between many measures of health (e.g., mortality, heart disease, self-reported health status) and SES (e.g., education, income, wealth, occupation).[17,19,20] For example, data from the Health and Retirement Survey show that respondents who self-report 'excellent health' have 2.5 times as much household income and 5 times as much household wealth

as respondents who report 'poor health.'[21] As with racial disparities, possible explanations for this relationship include differences in health behaviors, strategies for coping with stress, early life (prenatal and postnatal) conditions, and health care utilization practices along the SES spectrum. Social scientists have argued about whether the primary direction of this association goes from SES to health or vice versa.[19,20]

Marriage

On average, married people have a health advantage compared with unmarried people.[5,22–26] Approximately half of this advantage can be attributed to selection. That is, healthier people are the people who select into marriage.[22,27,28] Yet, evidence suggests that marriage itself confers a certain amount of health on its participants.[23,24] Not only does marriage improve health behaviors (reduced smoking, binge drinking, and increased visits to the doctor), it also provides social support and economic resources that are causally linked to better health.[24,29]

Age

The relationship between declining health and age is described in the gerontology literature.[30] Most chronic conditions are more prevalent in older age groups. Similarly, infectious diseases are more fatal among the elderly. In addition to the health concerns, aging individuals often face an increasing number of physical limitations, a lower quality of life, and a variety of psychosocial stressors associated with the aging process.[30,31]

WHAT DO WE KNOW ABOUT THE DEMOGRAPHY OF SLEEP?

We use the phrase 'demography of sleep' to refer to sociodemographic patterns of sleep quality, sleep quantity, and sleep disorders. Until recently, the demography of sleep had not been investigated as a line of inquiry of its own.

Rather, in the epidemiological and clinical studies that investigate sleep, demographic characteristics are typically listed in a descriptive table, and controlled for when known or appropriate. In contrast to a strategy that controls for various demographic characteristics, we aim to investigate how each of the usual sociodemographic control variables relates to sleep quantity, sleep apnea, and insomnia. We chose these three areas to investigate because they are well-studied topics in the sleep research field, and also have strong associations with health.

Sleep duration and health

The relationship between sleep duration and health is complicated, because there are numerous confounding factors and because causality is likely to flow in both directions. That is, inadequate or too much sleep may cause health problems *and* health problems may cause sleeping either too little or too much. Despite this complication, studies show that 6.5–7.5 hours of sleep on an average weeknight is associated with the lowest risk of all-cause mortality.[32–34] Controlling for demographic characteristics (e.g., age, race, education, occupation, marital status), health behaviors (e.g., exercise level, years of smoking, fat in diet), prior health conditions (e.g., body mass index, leg pain, and history of heart disease, hypertension, cancer, diabetes, stroke, bronchitis, emphysema, and kidney disease) and medication use, sleeping either a long or short amount increases the relative risk of all-cause mortality by up to 40%.[32] These studies indicate that both short sleeping and long sleeping durations are associated with higher mortality risk than mid-range sleeping, with the 7-hour night sleep being associated with the lowest mortality risk. In addition, in a nationally representative US sample, both short and long sleepers reported more sleep problems (i.e., wakening during the night, wakening too early, wakening unrefreshed, and daytime sleepiness) compared with the mid-range sleepers (7 or 8 hours).[35]

The adverse effect of sleep deprivation on health may be due to disruption of circadian rhythms and impaired glucose metabolism.[36–38] Whether the effects of someone *regularly* sleeping 5 versus 8 hours a night is physiologically similar to being sleep deprived is not well understood. Similarly, the causal relationship between sleeping for a long time and health is unclear.[32,38] Nonetheless, evidence suggests that having, on average, a long sleep duration is associated with as high, if not higher, a mortality risk factor than having mid-range or short sleep duration on a regular basis. However, interpretation of the findings of greater mortality with sleep durations of 8 hours after controlling for morbidity is controversial. It is important to note that these studies are based on self-reported sleep time. It is possible that some people, perhaps those with unrecognized health conditions, report sleep duration based on the hours they spend in bed, rather than actual sleep time. Long sleep duration may also be a marker for sleep apnea, a sleep disorder associated with breathing pauses that profoundly fragments sleep and causes daytime hypersomnolence.

Given this association between both short sleeping and long sleeping durations and high mortality risks, we are interested in looking at how the sociodemographic characteristics are associated with short, mid-range, or long sleep durations. There are only a few studies which have explicitly investigated the social and demographic characteristics of short, mid-range, and long sleepers.[39,40] Hale[39] uses time-use data from four cross-sectional data sets[41,42] and estimates a multinomial logistic regression equation on the amount of sleep reported for the 24-hour period of the time-use diary. The three outcome categories are short sleep, mid-range sleep, and long sleep. The definition of short sleep is less than 6.5 reported hours, whereas the definition of long sleep is greater than 8.5 reported hours and the mid-range sleep category refers to the intermediate duration (6.5–8.5 hours). The explanatory variables are dichotomous variables for calendar year, marital status, gender, educational status, employment, and minutes of television watched per day (in 1-hour intervals). Age and age-squared are also included as continuous variables. In a similar set of analyses, Hale and Do[40] use survey data from the National Health Interview Study (NHIS). In these models, they include additional variables to the ones above including race and neighborhood characteristics.

There are only a few other studies that investigate the relationships between social characteristics and sleep duration.[43–45] A major limitation of these other studies is that they only consider sleep as a continuous linear variable. As a result, they do not allow for the possibility of a non-linear relationship between sociodemographic characteristics and sleep duration by exploring both ends of the sleep duration distribution.

Sleep duration and gender

The two studies by Hale and colleagues[39,40] show that women are less likely than men to be short sleepers, by around 10–20% ($p < 0.01$). On the weekend, women are less likely to be short sleepers than men by as much as 40% ($p < 0.01$).[39] Given that short sleeping is associated with higher mortality risks, the fact that men are more likely to be short sleepers is consistent with the gender differential in mortality.

In the Hale studies,[39,40] there are no differences between men and women in terms of the risk of being a long sleeper. However, the National Sleep Foundation's Sleep in America Poll[46] found that male respondents are more likely than female respondents to report that they get more sleep than they need (49% vs. 37%). This may be because male respondents were more likely to report that they need less sleep than women to function at their best (6.2 hours vs. 6.8 hours).

Another study[45] found that women are significantly more likely to sleep longer than men in a sample of healthy adults. Whether this means

that women are less likely to be short sleepers (as found in both Hale studies) or if they are more likely to be long sleepers, or both, is not possible to ascertain from this analysis. A different study found that while women sleep more than men on average, after adjusting for hours in the labor force, men sleep more than women.[43]

Sleep duration and race

The small number of studies that have investigated the topic of race and sleep have revealed only marginal differences in sleep architecture by race.[47] While polysomnogram recordings show that Blacks have only about half as much slow-wave sleep as Whites,[48] rarely are these data collected with the intention of analyzing them for racial differences. Using survey data, Hale and Do[40] find that Black individuals have significantly increased risks of both short (<6.5 hours) and long (>8.5 hours) sleeping relative to Whites. Specifically, Blacks are more than 35% ($p < 0.001$) more likely to report being a short sleeper than Whites, and more than 75% ($p < 0.001$) more likely to report being a long sleeper than Whites. As described above, both short and long sleeping are associated with increased risks of mortality, supporting our hypothesis that sleep duration may contribute to mortality differences by race.

Sleep duration and socioeconomic status/education

Education is also associated with sleep duration as shown in the two studies by Hale's group.[39,40] Both studies find that people without a high school degree are more likely to be short sleepers than long sleepers. These results suggest that the relationship between education and short and long durations is in the hypothesized direction. That is, people with less education are sleeping in the higher-risk sleep duration categories.

In three studies that treat sleep duration as a linear characteristic, the results are more difficult to interpret. Jefferson et al.[45] find a positive relationship between self-report of sleep duration and education. However, when Biddle and Hamermesh[43] controlled for time in the labor force, there was a negative correlation between sleep duration and years of education. Moore et al.[44] did not find a correlation between education level and sleep quantity.

Sleep duration and marriage

Hale finds that marital status is correlated with sleep duration. On weekdays, relative to being married, separated/divorced (odds ratio [OR] = 1.29, $p < 0.05$), widowed (OR = 2.04, $p < 0.001$), and single people (OR = 1.61, $p < 0.001$) are more likely to be short sleepers compared with married people.[39] On the weekend, there is an increased risk of short sleeping for those who are separated/divorced (OR = 2.69, $p < 0.001$) and single (OR = 2.06, $p < 0.01$).[39] Single (but not separated/divorced or widowed) people also have an increased risk of long sleeping on weekdays (OR = 1.28, $p < 0.05$) and on weekends (OR = 1.51, $p < 0.05$) compared with married people.[39] Hale and Do[40] find similar relationships in the NHIS in which unmarried people are more likely to be short sleepers compared with married people, controlling for other social characteristics. They do not find that unmarried people are more likely to be long sleepers, however.

Neither Biddle and Hamermesh[43] nor Jefferson et al.[45] found a relationship between marriage and sleep duration. As described above, the treatment of sleep duration as a linear outcome makes interpretation difficult.

Sleep duration and age

In a meta-analysis of the quantitative sleep parameters across the life span, Ohayon et al.[49] found a linearly decreasing amount of total sleep time as people age. Sleep efficiency, percentage of slow-wave sleep (SWS), percentage of rapid eye movement (REM) sleep, and REM latency all decreased with age, while sleep latency, percentage of stage 1 sleep, percentage of stage 2 sleep and awakenings after sleep onset increased with age.[49] This is consistent with the findings by Hale that long sleeping decreases with age.[39,40] Short sleeping on the other hand is not associated with age.[39,40] In terms of duration alone, this suggests that as people age they move out of the high-risk sleep duration category of sleeping too long. Yet, since the Ohayon analysis showed that SWS and REM decrease with age, a decrease in quality of sleep with age might be associated with negative health outcomes.

In the studies that measured sleep duration linearly, such as those done by Biddle and Hamermesh[43] and Jefferson et al.,[45] there were no significant relationships between age and sleep duration.

Sleep apnea and health

Sleep apnea, a condition characterized by repeated episodes of apnea (breathing pauses) and hypopnea (reduced breathing) events during sleep, is highly prevalent among adults in North America, Australia, Europe, Japan, and Hong Kong.[50] The severity spectrum of sleep apnea is often described by the average number of apnea plus hypopnea events per hour of sleep (i.e., the apnea–hypopnea index or AHI), which can range from 0 to more than 100. Sleep apnea has well-established associations with multiple harmful health states[50] including hypertension,[51,52] cardiovascular and cerebrovascular morbidity,[53–55] metabolic syndrome and diabetes,[56] impaired daytime function,[57,58] excessive sleepiness and traffic accidents,[59,60] and poor health-related quality of life.[61,62] Few of these associations have been definitively established as causal; however, the evidence from recent prospective observational and randomized treatment studies has been generally concordant with the cross-sectional findings.

Here, we investigate the relationships between sleep apnea and social and demographic characteristics using the Wisconsin Sleep Cohort, a stratified random sample of four Wisconsin State agencies. Participants completed a four-page questionnaire on sleep

Table 1.1 Cross-sectional associations between sociodemographic variables (mutually adjusted[a]) and sleep apnea or insomnia assessed by logistic regressions using the Wisconsin Sleep Cohort

	Mild or worse sleep apnea (AHI ≥ 5 events/h) n = 1152		Moderate or worse sleep apnea (AHI ≥ 15 events/h) n = 1152		Insomnia (any of 4 symptoms[b]) n = 3717	
	Odds ratio (p-value)	Contribute to disparity?	Odds ratio (p-value)	Contribute to disparity?	Odds ratio (p-value)	Contribute to disparity?
Gender (male vs. female)	3.4 (<0.001)	Yes	6.1 (<0.001)	Yes	1.0 (0.74)	No (any symptoms); Yes (some symptoms)
Race (Black vs. White)	0.55 (0.44)	?	1.8 (0.46)	?	1.2 (0.19)	?
Education (no HS diploma vs. HS graduate)	3.6 (0.05)	Yes	5.7 (0.02)	Yes	2.2 (0.004)	Yes
Marital status (unmarried vs. married)	1.3 (0.18)	?	1.5 (0.14)	?	1.3 (<0.001)	Yes
Age (45–60 yr vs. 30–44 yr)	1.8 <0.001)	Yes	1.6 (0.05)	Yes	1.0 (0.52)	No (any symptoms); Yes (some symptoms)

[a]Predictor variables include: gender, age group, high school graduate (yes/no), currently married (yes/no), race (Black or White). Additionally, the sleep apnea models also include body mass index, and current smoker (yes/no).
[b]Self-report of often or always for any of the four symptoms: (1) difficulty initiating sleep; (2) waking too early; (3) waking repeatedly; (4) waking and having difficulty falling back to sleep; OR a self-report of often or always for use of pharmacologic sleep aids. HS, high school.

habits, health history, and demographic information, in addition to a baseline overnight protocol including assessments of physiologic characteristics of sleep. In Table 1.1, we present the results of logistic regression analyses in which the dependent variable is either mild or more severe (AHI ≥ 5 events/h) or moderate or worse (AHI ≥ 15 events/h) sleep apnea, and the various explanatory variables we consider are listed in each row. We discuss the results in more detail below.

Sleep apnea and gender

Sleep apnea was once thought to be a disease of men, but epidemiological studies beginning in

1993 have established that the prevalence of sleep apnea is high in women also.[63] Due to selection biases that favor referral of men for evaluation, the ratio of men : women (>5 : 1) with diagnosed sleep apnea is higher than the ratio (2 : 1) reported from population-based studies. In spite of indications that sleep apnea is more common and more severe in men compared with women, there is some evidence that women may have worse outcomes of sleep apnea.[64–66] Understanding the basis for gender differences in both the occurrence and outcomes of sleep apnea is of current interest. Several studies have shown that sleep apnea is more severe in men than women.[67,68]

In a community-based sample of the Cleveland Family Study, Patel et al.[69] found the AHI to be significantly higher among the men than women. For European-American men, the mean was 10.2 for the men compared to 5.2 for the women. The difference between the genders was smaller between African-American men and women at 9.3 and 5.7 events per hour. Cross-sectional results from Wisconsin Sleep Cohort data (Table 1.1), as expected, indicate that men are significantly more likely than are women to have sleep apnea, adjusting for age, education, race, and marital status, body mass index, and smoking habits.

Sleep apnea and race

The Wisconsin Sleep Cohort sample has very little variation in race, and the results in Table 1.1 show conflicting associations (none statistically significant) of sleep apnea with race, depending on the severity of sleep apnea. In an analysis of the Cleveland Family Study, which comprises both Black and White men and women, Patel[69] found that clear differences existed between the sexes, but not by race. On average, the AHI was lower for Black men compared with White men, whereas the AHI was higher for Black women compared with White women. In another analysis of this sample, Redline et al.[70] found among younger persons (≤25 years old) that

Blacks are more likely than Whites to have sleep apnea after controlling for obesity, race, and familial clustering. Among older adults (≥65 years old), Ancoli-Israel et al.[71] found that African-Americans are more than twice as likely as Caucasians to have an AHI of 30 or higher, controlling for body mass index and additional confounding factors. Yet, in an analysis of the Sleep Heart Health Study sample of 6000 adults, no statistically significant association between race and sleep apnea, after controlling for body mass index, age, and gender, was found.[72] The evidence on race and sleep apnea is thus inconclusive.

Sleep apnea and socioeconomic status/education

There have been few studies examining associations of socioeconomic variables such as education or social class with sleep apnea. One large study from Denmark found no association between social class (a derived variable combining educational attainment and occupation) and snoring (a sensitive but non-specific symptom of obstructive sleep apnea).[73] In contrast, in Table 1.1 we show that in the Wisconsin Sleep Cohort, persons with less than a high school education had 3.6 to 5.7 times the odds of having sleep apnea compared to persons with a high school education, adjusting for gender, race, marital status, and age group. If this finding is generalizable to wider populations of adults, then differences in sleep apnea occurrence among groups with different educational attainment levels may be partially responsible for education-related health disparities.

Sleep apnea and marriage

As with socioeconomic status, little research has been published examining the association of marital status and sleep apnea. The few available studies have measured correlations between marital status (e.g., married vs. not currently married) and survey-assessed symptoms of sleep apnea such as snoring or witnessed (e.g., by a bed-partner) apneas. One study found that married persons were almost twice as likely to report snoring than single persons;[74] another study found that married men, but not married women, were more likely to report snoring than unmarried persons;[75] and one study of only men found no association between marital status and questionnaire-assessed symptoms of sleep apnea.[76] Caution is advised in interpreting studies of subjectively assessed sleep apnea symptoms and marital status because the presence of a bed-partner (presumably more likely among married persons) increases the likelihood that symptoms of sleep apnea (such as snoring) will be observed and reported to afflicted persons. Thus an increased occurrence of reported symptoms among married persons may simply indicate better awareness of sleep apnea. In the Wisconsin Sleep Cohort, objectively assessed (by in-laboratory polysomnography – not susceptible to such a detection bias) sleep apnea was slightly more prevalent in unmarried persons, although the findings were not statistically significant (Table 1.1). It remains unclear whether sleep apnea might contribute to observed variations in the health of persons of different marital status.

Sleep apnea and age

The role of aging in sleep apnea is complex. While community studies show that sleep apnea prevalence increases with age, with some studies showing extremely high prevalence of sleep apnea in older adults, older patients are not common in sleep clinic settings.[77] Generally, sleep apnea prevalence appears to increase steadily with age in midlife, a consistent finding among many studies[50] and as seen, for example, in Table 1.1 showing a 60–80% greater prevalence of sleep apnea among adults aged 45–60 years compared to adults aged 30–45 years. However, age trends in younger (childhood and young adults) and older ages (>60 years) do not indicate a simple positive correlation of sleep apnea with age, possibly indicating distinct disease subtypes with different etiology and health sequelae at different life stages.[50] Thus it is likely that, like many other conditions, sleep apnea contributes to poorer health as persons pass from young adulthood to middle age. In addition, it is possible that older adults are less likely than younger adults to be referred for specialized sleep apnea diagnosis due to a clinical presumption of the 'normalcy' of increasing sleep problems in older persons. This would exacerbate disparities due to sleep problems such as sleep apnea between older and younger adults.

Insomnia and health

Chronic insomnia is estimated to affect between 9% and 24% of the general population.[78–80] The variation in the estimates occurs because the definition varies – with the lower bound referring to the population in which the disturbed sleep affects daytime functioning. Prevalence is also higher in clinical practices where approximately half of the population report sleep disruption symptoms. The health risks associated with insomnia include: depressed mood, difficulty with memory and concentration, a variety of comorbidities (e.g., cardiovascular, pulmonary, and gastrointestinal disorders, generalized anxiety, dementia), and possibly, increased mortality.[78] Separating the health effects of insomnia from its comorbidities is methodologically challenging. Some argue that insomnia *per se* is not directly related to mortality, but rather it is the comorbidities associated with insomnia that affect mortality.[81] While these relationships need to be disentangled, the public health costs of insomnia are large. For example, insomnia is associated with negative impacts on occupational, physical, and social performance. Overall, scientists have estimated that the economic cost of insomnia in the USA amounts to more than $77 billion per year.[82,83]

The National Institutes of Health (NIH) issued a State of the Science Consensus Report on the Manifestations and Management of Chronic Insomnia. This consensus statement[78] and a comprehensive literature review[79] addressed many of the issues that are relevant here. In the subsections below we present the results of this literature review, our own review of the literature, and supplement it with the results of a logistic regression analysis predicting insomnia in the Wisconsin Sleep Cohort (see column 3 of Table 1.1).

Insomnia and gender

Insomnia is more common among women than among men, as identified by the Buscemi et al.[79] review of the insomnia literature. There are more than 11 studies in which an association between gender and chronic insomnia revealed that women are more likely than men to suffer from chronic insomnia.[84–95] There were a handful of studies, however, that found no relationship between gender and insomnia.[96–100] The Wisconsin Sleep Cohort analysis shows that insomnia, defined as frequently experiencing *any* one of four insomnia symptoms (difficulty falling asleep; difficulty falling back to sleep upon waking during the night; waking repeatedly; or waking too early), is not more common among women than men (see Table 1.1). However, women were significantly more likely than men to have individual insomnia symptoms (data not shown). The explanation for this discrepancy is that the women tended to be more likely than men to have multiple insomnia symptoms, possibly indicating a tendency for more severe, if not more common, insomnia in women. Since insomnia is known to have comorbidities but not necessarily to cause mortality, this sex difference in insomnia may in part explain why women have more morbidities than men, but not necessarily more mortality.

Insomnia and race

Research on race and insomnia is limited and the results are mixed. Bixler et al.[84] found that chronic insomnia is more common among non-Caucasian minorities, while Riedel et al.[101] found that the reverse is true. Paine et al.[102] found that Maoris are more likely to have sleep problems than non-Maoris in New Zealand. However, a study based in a Brazilian population found no association between insomnia and race.[93,103] Similarly, Ancoli-Israel et al.[104] found no significant differences between Whites and non-Caucasians with regard to insomnia. The Wisconsin Sleep Cohort found no relationship between race and insomnia (see Table 1.1), although there was insufficient racial diversity for adequate statistical power. Given these varied results, this suggests that if a difference exists it may vary by study sample and may not be prevalent throughout the population.

Insomnia and socioeconomic status/education

Buscemi[79] reviewed several studies that found significant associations between socioeconomic status (SES) and insomnia.[88,93,94,100,103–108] All of those studies and several others[102,109] indicate that poorer, unemployed, or less educated individuals are more likely to have chronic insomnia than those with higher SES. Similarly, the Wisconsin Sleep Cohort data reveal a negative relationship between education and insomnia (Table 1.1): persons without a high school education were about twice as likely to report frequent experiences of any insomnia symptoms than persons with at least a high school education. However, some studies have found no evidence of an association between SES and insomnia.[97,99,105,110] These studies may vary in their results due to different definitions of insomnia, SES, sample bias, or sample power.

Insomnia and marriage

Some studies have found that chronic insomnia is higher among divorced/separated or widowed adults relative to married adults.[85,108]

Table 1.2 Current state of evidence for an association between sociodemographic factors and sleep problems or sleep disorders

	High risk sleep duration[a]	Sleep apnea	Insomnia
Gender	Yes	Yes	Yes
Race	Yes	?	?
Education	Yes	Yes	Yes
Marital status	Yes	?	?
Age	Yes	Yes	Yes

[a]Either short or long sleeping.

Léger,[88] on the other hand, found that never married singles have less insomnia than people with other marital status. There are also studies that do not show a relationship between insomnia and marriage.[103,105,110] The Wisconsin Sleep Cohort data show a modest negative relationship between insomnia and marriage (see Table 1.1) – unmarried persons were about 30% more likely to report frequent insomnia symptoms. Despite the conclusion of the Buscemi et al. study,[79] we found little evidence of a strong relationship between insomnia and marriage.

Insomnia and age

In the Buscemi et al.[79] literature review, 11 studies found an association between age and chronic insomnia[17,84,86,88–90,94,96,103,105–107,111] compared to eight studies where no relationship was found.[85,95,97,99,100,104,110,112] Of the studies that found a significant relationship between age and chronic insomnia, the direction of this relationship was positive in all but one of the studies, which found a negative relationship between age and chronic insomnia in female hospital nurses in Japan.[105]

The analysis of the Wisconsin Sleep Cohort data demonstrates a varying relationship between insomnia symptoms and age. Older adults were significantly more likely to report frequent problems with sleep maintenance (difficulty falling back to sleep upon waking during the night or waking repeatedly); however, younger adults were significantly more likely to report frequent problems initiating sleep (data not shown). Defining insomnia as having any of the four insomnia symptoms resulted in no significant association between insomnia and age (among middle-aged adults), reflecting a 'canceling' of the different directions of associations between sleep initiation and sleep maintenance with age (Table 1.1). The dependence of the direction of association on which specific insomnia symptoms are examined may, in part, explain the divergent results of the aforementioned studies.

SUMMARY AND DISCUSSION

In this section we summarize our results by demographic characteristic. The general findings are condensed into Table 1.2, which provides the three sleep characteristics as column headings and lists the five demographic characteristics. A 'YES' indicates that the research shows a noteworthy relationship between the demographic variable and the sleep characteristic. A question mark means that the results are inconclusive. In no case is 'NO' appropriate, for example, where the evidence convincingly shows, with adequate study power, that there is no relationship (positive or negative).

Does the demography of sleep contribute to gender disparities in health? Men and women have differing prevalence levels of sleep disorders and it is likely that this contributes in some way to the differences in health outcomes between the sexes. As stated above, women are more likely to have higher rates of morbidity of some chronic conditions, and women are also more likely to have insomnia (which is often observed with a host of comorbidities). However, age-adjusted mortality rates are higher in men compared with women. Accordingly, sleep apnea, which is more closely linked to mortality risk than insomnia, is more prevalent in men than women. If short and long sleeping are also associated with mortality, short or long sleeping among men may also contribute to the mortality differential by sex.

Does the demography of sleep contribute to higher health risks among African-Americans? The evidence with regard to sleep and racial disparities in health is very limited. The evidence that does exist leads us to cautiously conclude there is not a consistent or simple relationship with race for either sleep apnea or insomnia. However, based on limited results, we do find that Blacks are more likely than Whites to sleep for durations that are associated with higher risk.

Does the demography of sleep contribute to higher health risks among those of lower socioeconomic status and/or the less educated? Our review finds that unfavorable sleep duration (both long and short), insomnia, and perhaps, sleep apnea are more common among those with lower SES or lower education. This suggests that part of the relationship between health and SES may be due to differences in sleep disorders and sleep behaviors.

Does the demography of sleep contribute to higher health risks among the unmarried? Unmarried people are more likely to have worse sleep patterns with regard to both short sleeping and long sleeping. There is mixed evidence on the relationship between insomnia and marriage, and there are currently insufficient data to assess the association of marital status and sleep apnea. Whether the relationships that are observed are due to the selection into marriage, or due to the effect of marriage itself on sleep, is worth identifying. Yet for the purpose of this chapter, correlational evidence is sufficient to support the notion that sleep patterns of unmarried persons contribute to the pre-existing health disadvantage that already exists.

Does the demography of sleep contribute to the higher health risks among the elderly? Our data and review of the literature do not show a clear linear relationship between age and our three major sleep problems (unfavorable sleep duration, sleep apnea, and insomnia). These results are complicated due to variation in diagnosis, treatment, and the increased prevalence of comorbidities as one ages. In particular, insomnia may take different forms across the life course. While we cannot say that these sleep disorders contribute to higher health risks among the elderly, We do see age-related patterns in sleep disorders.

CONCLUSIONS AND RECOMMENDATIONS FOR FUTURE RESEARCH

Health disparities are a matter of political importance, social justice, and public health policy. Although data are sparse, we have presented evidence that supports our hypothesis that social and demographic differences in sleep disorders and sleep behaviors often reinforce pre-existing health disparities, especially by gender and socioeconomic status (SES). Here, we refer to this relationship as the 'social gradient in sleep-related disorders.'

Increasing awareness of sleep problems in primary care as well as diagnosis and treatment of sleep disorders is potentially an effective strategy to reduce health disparities. Ameliorating sleep disorders through social, behavioral, or policy changes may also have merit. A better understanding of the unmet needs of people with sleep disorders, especially among the elderly, is critically needed.

Future research is needed to investigate nearly all of the dimensions of the social gradient in sleep-related disorders described above, especially with regard to differences by age, race, and marital status. Aims for future research on this topic include an assessment of whether observed associations represent causality, and if so, causal direction, magnitude of the effect, and underlying mechanisms.

Careful attention must be paid to the causal direction that relates sleep behaviors to social and demographic characteristics, because the causal direction has implications for public health and social policy. For example, while there is overwhelming evidence that those with lower SES have greater insomnia, we do not know whether insomnia causes the low SES or if low SES causes the insomnia, or both. If low SES has a causal role in creating insomnia, then efforts aimed at increasing educational status and employment may reduce insomnia. On the other hand, if insomnia causes low SES, then effective treatment of insomnia may improve SES and health simultaneously.

If associations are causal, then illumination of underlying mechanisms is important. What is it about social and demographic characteristics that might relate them to various sleep problems? For example, Chen et al.[113] sought to determine whether social roles explain why women in Taiwan have more insomnia than men. Identifying the underlying mechanisms of the social gradient in sleep disorders (whether genetic, environmental, social, or some combination of these causes) is critical in devising a strategy to reduce the prevalence of these disorders and overall health disparities.

Finally, we must identify to what extent sleep patterns across the population contribute to health inequalities, if at all. Ongoing longitudinal studies that are providing information on demographic characteristics, sleep conditions, and health will enable us to better address these questions in the near future. It is crucial that well-formulated questions regarding sleep problems and health inequities stay in the forefront to be addressed when these data become available.

The aim of this chapter has been to provide an important starting point for understanding the linkage between health inequalities in the population and the prevalence of sleep disorders. With continued research and collaboration between sleep researchers, epidemiologists, population health scientists, policy makers, and public health practitioners, we will have a better understanding of how to reduce concurrently the burdens of both sleep disorders and health inequalities.

REFERENCES

1. Adler NE, Marmot M, McEwen BS, Stewart J. Socioeconomic Status and Health in Industrial Nations: Social, Psychological, and Biological Pathways, vol 896. New York: Annals of the New York Academy of Sciences, 1999.
2. Wilkinson RG. Unhealthy Societies: the Afflictions of Inequality. London: Routledge, 1996.
3. Williams DR. Socioeconomic differentials in health: a review and redirection. Social Psychology Quarterly 1990: 81–99.
4. Williams DR, Jackson PB. Social sources of racial disparities in health. Health Aff (Millwood) 2005; 24(2): 325–34.
5. Coombs R. Marital status and personal well-being: a literature review. Family Relations 1991; 40: 97–102.
6. Barker DJ. The fetal and infant origins of adult disease. Br Med J 1990; 301(6761): 1111.
7. McGinnis JM, Williams-Russo P, Knickman JR. The case for more active policy attention to health promotion. Health Aff (Millwood) 2002; 21(2): 78–93.
8. Szanton SL, Gill JM, Allen JK. Allostatic load: a mechanism of socioeconomic health disparities? Biol Res Nurs 2005; 7(1): 7–15.
9. Nathanson C. Sex differences in mortality. Ann Rev Sociol 1984; 10: 191–213.
10. Henry L. Men's and women's mortality in the past. Populations 1989; 44(1): 177–201.
11. Verbrugge LM, Wingard DL. Sex differentials in health and mortality. Women Health 1987; 12(2): 103–45.
12. Case A, Paxson C. Sex differences in morbidity and mortality. Demography 2005; 42(2): 189–214.
13. Ross CE, Bird CE. Sex stratification and health life-style – consequences for men's and women's perceived health. J Health Soc Behavior 1994; 35(2): 161–78.
14. Conley D, Strully K, Bennett N. Starting Gate: Birth Weight and Life Chances. Berkeley: University of California Press, 2003.
15. Making Cancer Health Disparities History. Department of Health and Human Services

(DHHS), Trans-HHS Cancer Health Disparities Progress Review Group, 2004. http://www.chdprg.omhrc.gov/pdf/chdprg.pdf.

16. Levine RS, Foster JE, Fullilove RE, et al. Black-White inequalities in mortality and life expectancy, 1933–1999: implications for healthy people 2010. Public Health Rep 2001; 116(5): 474–83.

17. Taylor DJ. A Cross-Sectional Analysis of Depression, Anxiety, and Insomnia. Memphis, TN: University of Memphis, 2003.

18. Diez Roux AV, Merkin SS, Arnett D, et al. Neighborhood of residence and incidence of coronary heart disease. N Engl J Med 2001; 345(2): 99–106.

19. Williams DR, Collins C. US socioeconomic and racial differences in health: patterns and explanations. Annual Review of Sociology 1995; 21: 349–86.

20. Smith JP. Socioeconomic status and health. American Economic Review 1998; 88(2): 192–6.

21. Smith JP, Kington R. Race, socioeconomic status and health in late life. In: Martin L, Soldo B, eds. Racial and Ethnic Differences in the Health of Older Americans. Washington, DC: National Academy Press, 1997: 106–62.

22. Goldman N, Korenman S, Weinstein R. Marital status and health among the elderly. Social Science and Medicine 1995; 40: 1717–30.

23. Gove WR. Sex, marital status, and suicide. Journal of Health and Social Behavior 1972; 13: 204–13.

24. Kobrin FE, Hendershot GE. Do family ties reduce mortality? Evidence from the United States, 1966–1968. Journal of Marriage and the Family 1977; 39: 737–44.

25. Cheung YB. Marital status and mortality in British women: a longitudinal study. Int J Epidemiol 2000; 29(1): 93–9.

26. Pienta AM, Hayward MD, Jenkins KR. Health consequences for marriage for the retirement years. Journal of Family Issues 2000; 21(5): 559–86.

27. Goldman N. Marriage selection and mortality patterns – inferences and fallacies. Demography 1993; 30(2): 189–208.

28. Murray JE. Marital protection and marital selection: evidence from a historical-prospective sample of American men. Demography 2000; 37(4): 511–21.

29. Umberson D. Family status and health behaviors: social control as a dimension of social integration. Journal of Health and Social Behavior 1987; 28: 306–19.

30. Aldwin CM, Gilmer DF. Health, Illness, and Optimal Aging: Biological and Psychosocial Perspectives. Thousand Oaks, CA: Sage Publications, 2004.

31. Miller ME, Rejeski WJ, Reboussin BA, Ten Have TR, Ettinger WH. Physical activity, functional limitations, and disability in older adults. J Am Geriatr Soc 2000; 48(10): 1264–72.

32. Kripke DF, Garfinkel L, Wingard DL, Klauber MR, Marler MR. Mortality associated with sleep duration and insomnia. Arch Gen Psychiatry 2002; 59(2): 131–6.

33. Tamakoshi A, Ohno Y. Self-reported sleep duration as a predictor of all-cause mortality: results from the JACC study, Japan. Sleep 2004; 27(1): 51–4.

34. Wingard DL, Berkman LF. Mortality risk associated with sleeping patterns among adults. Sleep 1983; 6(2): 102–7.

35. Grandner MA, Kripke DF. Self-reported sleep complaints with long and short sleep: a nationally representative sample. Psychosom Med 2004; 66(2): 239–41.

36. Ayas NT, White DP, Manson JE, et al. A prospective study of sleep duration and coronary heart disease in women. Arch Intern Med 2003; 163(2): 205–9.

37. Van Cauter E, Spiegel K. Sleep as a mediator of the relationship between socioeconomic status and health. In: Adler N, Marmot M, McEwen B, eds. Socioeconomic Status and Health in Industrial Nations: Social, Psychological, and Biological Pathways, vol 896. New York: Annals of the New York Academy of Sciences, 1999.

38. Redwine L, Hauger RL, Gillin JC, Irwin M. Effects of sleep and sleep deprivation on interleukin-6, growth hormone, cortisol, and melatonin levels in humans. J Clin Endocrinol Metab 2000; 85(10): 3597–603.

39. Hale L. Who has time to sleep? J Public Health (Oxf) 2005; 27(2): 205–11.

40. Hale L, Do DP. Sleep and the city: an analysis of sleep duration, race, and neighborhood context in the NHIS. Presented at the Annual Meetings of the Population Association of America 2006, Los Angeles, April 1st 2006.

41. Robinson J, Bianchi S, Presser S. Family Interaction, Social Capital, and Trends in Time

Use. University of Maryland Survey Research Center. Ann Arbor, MI: Inter University Consortium for Political and Social Research, 2001.

42. Robinson J, Godbey G. Time for Life: the Surprising Ways Americans Use Their Time. University Park: Pennsyvania State University, 1999.

43. Biddle JE, Hamermesh DS. Sleep and the allocation of time. Journal of Political Economy 1990; 98(5): 922–43.

44. Moore PJ, Adler NE, Williams DR, Jackson JS. Socioeconomic status and health: the role of sleep. Psychosom Med 2002; 64(2): 337–44.

45. Jefferson CD, Drake CL, Roehrs T, Roth T. Sleep Habits in Healthy Normals. Poster Presentation at the Annual Meeting of the Associated Professional Sleep Society, 2005.

46. Sleep in America Poll, 2005, National Sleep Foundation. http://www.sleepfoundation.org/_content/hottopics/2005_summary-of-findings.pdf.

47. Rao U, Poland RE, Lutchmansingh P, et al. Relationship between ethnicity and sleep patterns in normal controls: implications for psychopathology and treatment. J Psychiatr Res 1999; 33(5): 419–26.

48. Van Dongen HP, Vitellaro KM, Dinges DF. Individual differences in adult human sleep and wakefulness: Leitmotif for a research agenda. Sleep 2005; 28(4): 479–96.

49. Ohayon MM, Carskadon MA, Guilleminault C, Vitiello MV. Meta-analysis of quantitative sleep parameters from childhood to old age in healthy individuals: developing normative sleep values across the human lifespan. Sleep 2004; 27(7): 1255–73.

50. Young T, Peppard PE, Gottlieb DJ. Epidemiology of obstructive sleep apnea: a population health perspective. Am J Respir Crit Care Med 2002; 165(9): 1217–39.

51. Peppard PE, Young T, Palta M, Skatrud J. Prospective study of the association between sleep-disordered breathing and hypertension. N Engl J Med 2000; 342(19): 1378–84.

52. Nieto FJ, Young TB, Lind BK, et al. Association of sleep-disordered breathing, sleep apnea, and hypertension in a large community-based study. Sleep Heart Health Study. J Am Med Assoc 2000; 283(14): 1829–36.

53. Shahar E, Whitney CW, Redline S, et al. Sleep-disordered breathing and cardiovascular disease: cross-sectional results of the Sleep Heart Health Study. Am J Respir Crit Care Med 2001; 163(1): 19–25.

54. Hu FB, Willett WC, Manson JE, et al. Snoring and risk of cardiovascular disease in women. J Am Coll Cardiol 2000; 35(2): 308–13.

55. Arzt M, Young T, Finn L, Skatrud JB, Bradley TD. Association of sleep-disordered breathing and the occurrence of stroke. Am J Respir Crit Care Med 2005; 172(11): 1447–51.

56. Vgontzas AN, Bixler EO, Chrousos GP. Sleep apnea is a manifestation of the metabolic syndrome. Sleep Med Rev 2005; 9(3): 211–24.

57. Kim HC, Young T, Matthews CG, et al. Sleep-disordered breathing and neuropsychological deficits. A population-based study. Am J Respir Crit Care Med 1997; 156(6): 1813–19.

58. Redline S, Strauss ME, Adams N, et al. Neuropsychological function in mild sleep-disordered breathing. Sleep 1997; 20(2): 160–7.

59. Teran-Santos J, Jimenez-Gomez A, Cordero-Guevara J. The association between sleep apnea and the risk of traffic accidents. Cooperative Group Burgos-Santander. N Engl J Med 1999; 340(11): 847–51.

60. Young T, Blustein J, Finn L, Palta M. Sleep-disordered breathing and motor vehicle accidents in a population-based sample of employed adults. Sleep 1997; 20(8): 608–13.

61. Finn L, Young T, Palta M, Fryback DG. Sleep-disordered breathing and self-reported general health status in the Wisconsin Sleep Cohort Study. Sleep 1998; 21(7): 701–6.

62. Baldwin CM, Griffith KA, Nieto FJ, et al. The association of sleep-disordered breathing and sleep symptoms with quality of life in the Sleep Heart Health Study. Sleep 2001; 24(1): 96–105.

63. Young T, Palta M, Dempsey J, et al. The occurrence of sleep-disordered breathing among middle-aged adults. N Engl J Med 1993; 328(17): 1230–5.

64. Faulx MD, Larkin EK, Hoit BD, et al. Sex influences endothelial function in sleep-disordered breathing. Sleep 2004; 27(6): 1113–20.

65. Shepertycky MR, Banno K, Kryger MH. Differences between men and women in the clinical presentation of patients diagnosed with obstructive sleep apnea syndrome. Sleep 2005; 28(3): 309–14.

66. Young T, Peppard PE. Clinical presentation of OSAS: gender does matter. Sleep 2005; 28(3): 293–5.

67. Young T, Hutton R, Finn L, Badr S, Palta M. The gender bias in sleep apnea diagnosis. Are women missed because they have different symptoms? Arch Intern Med 1996; 156(21): 2445–51.

68. Tishler PV, Larkin EK, Schluchter MD, Redline S. Incidence of sleep-disordered breathing in an urban adult population: the relative importance of risk factors in the development of sleep-disordered breathing. J Am Med Assoc 2003; 289(17): 2230–7.

69. Patel SR, Palmer LJ, Larkin EK, et al. Relationship between obstructive sleep apnea and diurnal leptin rhythms. Sleep 2004; 27(2): 235–9.

70. Redline S, Tishler PV, Hans MG, et al. Racial differences in sleep-disordered breathing in African-Americans and Caucasians. Am J Respir Crit Care Med 1997; 155(1): 186–92.

71. Ancoli-Israel S, Klauber MR, Stepnowsky C, Estline E, Chinn A, Fell R. Sleep-disordered breathing in African-American elderly. Am J Respir Crit Care Med 1995; 152(6 Pt 1): 1946–9.

72. Young T, Peppard P, Palta M, et al. Population-based study of sleep-disordered breathing as a risk factor for hypertension. Arch Intern Med 1997; 157(15): 1746–52.

73. Jennum P, Hein HO, Suadicani P, Gyntelberg F. Cardiovascular risk factors in snorers. A cross-sectional study of 3323 men aged 54 to 74 years: the Copenhagen Male Study. Chest 1992; 102(5): 1371–6.

74. Ohayon MM, Guilleminault C, Priest RG, Caulet M. Snoring and breathing pauses during sleep: telephone interview survey of a United Kingdom population sample. Br Med J 1997; 314(7084): 860–3.

75. Enright PL, Newman AB, Wahl PW, et al. Prevalence and correlates of snoring and observed apneas in 5201 older adults. Sleep 1996; 19(7): 531–8.

76. Teculescu D, Hannhart B, Virion JM, Montaut-Verient B, Michaely JP. Marital status and sleep-disordered breathing in a sample of middle-aged French men. Lung 2004; 182(6): 355–62.

77. Bixler EO, Vgontzas AN, Ten Have T, Tyson K, Kales A. Effects of age on sleep apnea in men: I. Prevalence and severity. Am J Respir Crit Care Med 1998; 157(1): 144–8.

78. State-of-Science Conference Statement: National Institutes of Health; 2005. http://consensus.nih.gov/2005/2005insominaSOS026PDF.pdf.

79. Buscemi N, Vandermeer B, Friesen C, et al. Manifestations and management of chronic insomnia in adults. Evid Rep Technol Assess (Summ) 2005; (125): 1–10.

80. Chesson AL, Jr., Anderson WM, Littner M, et al. Practice parameters for the nonpharmacologic treatment of chronic insomnia. An American Academy of Sleep Medicine report. Standards of Practice Committee of the American Academy of Sleep Medicine. Sleep 1999; 22(8): 1128–33.

81. Phillips B, Mannino D. Does Insomnia Kill? Annual Meetings of the Associated Professional Sleep Societies. Denver, 2005.

82. Léger D. Public health and insomnia: economic impact. Sleep 2000; 23 (Suppl 3): S69–76.

83. Walsh JK, Engelhardt CL. The direct economic costs of insomnia in the United States for 1995. Sleep 1999; 22 Suppl 2: S386–93.

84. Bixler EO, Vgontzas AN, Lin HM, Vela-Bueno A, Kales A. Insomnia in central Pennsylvania. J Psychosom Res 2002; 53(1): 589–92.

85. Hajak G. Epidemiology of severe insomnia and its consequences in Germany. Eur Arch Psychiatry Clin Neurosci 2001; 251(2): 49–56.

86. Ishigooka J, Suzuki M, Isawa S, et al. Epidemiological study on sleep habits and insomnia of new outpatients visiting general hospitals in Japan. Psychiatry Clin Neurosci 1999; 53(4): 515–22.

87. Hohagen F, Kappler C, Schramm E, et al. Sleep onset insomnia, sleep maintaining insomnia and insomnia with early morning awakening – temporal stability of subtypes in a longitudinal study on general practice attenders. Sleep 1994; 17(6): 551–4.

88. Léger D, Guilleminault C, Dreyfus JP, Delahaye C, Paillard M. Prevalence of insomnia in a survey of 12778 adults in France. J Sleep Res 2000; 9(1): 35–42.

89. Leppavuori A, Pohjasvaara T, Vataja R, Kaste M, Erkinjuntti T. Insomnia in ischemic stroke patients. Cerebrovasc Dis 2002; 14(2): 90–7.

90. Ohayon MM, Partinen M. Insomnia and global sleep dissatisfaction in Finland. J Sleep Res 2002; 11(4): 339–46.

91. Ohayon MM, Roth T. What are the contributing factors for insomnia in the general population? J Psychosom Res 2001; 51(6): 745–55.

92. Ohayon MM, Roth T. Place of chronic insomnia in the course of depressive and anxiety disorders. J Psychiatr Res 2003; 37(1): 9–15.

93. Rocha FL, Uchoa E, Guerra HL, et al. Prevalence of sleep complaints and associated factors in community-dwelling older people in Brazil: the Bambuí Health and Ageing Study (BHAS). Sleep Med 2002; 3(3): 231–8.

94. Terzano MG, Parrino L, Cirignotta F, et al. Studio Morfeo: insomnia in primary care, a survey conducted on the Italian population. Sleep Med 2004; 5(1): 67–75.

95. Yeo BK, Perera IS, Kok LP, Tsoi WF. Insomnia in the community. Singapore Med J 1996; 37(3): 282–4.

96. Bixler EO, Kales A, Soldatos CR, Kales JD, Healey S. Prevalence of sleep disorders in the Los Angeles metropolitan area. Am J Psychiatry 1979; 136(10): 1257–62.

97. Han SY, Yoon JW, Jo SK, et al. Insomnia in diabetic hemodialysis patients. Prevalence and risk factors by a multicenter study. Nephron 2002; 92(1): 127–32.

98. Hidalgo MP, Caumo W. Sleep disturbances associated with minor psychiatric disorders in medical students. Neurol Sci 2002; 23(1): 35–9.

99. Lichstein KL, Durrence HH, Bayen UJ, Riedel BW. Primary versus secondary insomnia in older adults: subjective sleep and daytime functioning. Psychol Aging 2001; 16(2): 264–71.

100. Pallesen S, Nordhus IH, Kvale G, et al. Psychological characteristics of elderly insomniacs. Scand J Psychol 2002; 43(5): 425–32.

101. Riedel BW, Durrence HH, Lichstein KL, Taylor DJ, Bush AJ. The relation between smoking and sleep: the influence of smoking level, health, and psychological variables. Behav Sleep Med 2004; 2(1): 63–78.

102. Paine SJ, Gander PH, Harris RB, Reid P. Prevalence and consequences of insomnia in New Zealand: disparities between Maori and non-Maori. Aust NZ J Public Health 2005; 29(1): 22–8.

103. Rocha FL, Guerra HL, Lima-Costa MF. Prevalence of insomnia and associated sociodemographic factors in a Brazilian community: the Bambuí study. Sleep Med 2002; 3(2): 121–6.

104. Ancoli-Israel S, Roth T. Characteristics of insomnia in the United States: results of the 1991 National Sleep Foundation Survey. I. Sleep 1999; 22 Suppl 2: S347–53.

105. Kageyama T, Nishikido N, Kobayashi T, Oga J, Kawashima M. Cross-sectional survey on risk factors for insomnia in Japanese female hospital nurses working rapidly rotating shift systems. J Hum Ergol (Tokyo) 2001; 30(1–2): 149–54.

106. Kappler C, Hohagen F. Psychosocial aspects of insomnia. Results of a study in general practice. Eur Arch Psychiatry Clin Neurosci 2003; 253(1): 49–52.

107. Martikainen K, Partinen M, Hasan J, et al. The impact of somatic health problems on insomnia in middle age. Sleep Med 2003; 4(3): 201–6.

108. Savard J, Simard S, Blanchet J, Ivers H, Morin CM. Prevalence, clinical characteristics, and risk factors for insomnia in the context of breast cancer. Sleep 2001; 24(5): 583–90.

109. Gellis LA, Lichstein KL, Scarinci IC, et al. Socioeconomic status and insomnia. J Abnorm Psychol 2005; 114(1): 111–18.

110. Kawada T, Yosiaki S, Yasuo K, Suzuki S. Population study on the prevalence of insomnia and insomnia-related factors among Japanese women. Sleep Med 2003; 4(6): 563–7.

111. Kageyama T, Kabuto M, Nitta H, et al. A population study on risk factors for insomnia among adult Japanese women: a possible effect of road traffic volume. Sleep 1997; 20(11): 963–71.

112. Harvey AG, Greenall E. Catastrophic worry in primary insomnia. J Behav Ther Exp Psychiatry 2003; 34(1): 11–23.

113. Chen YY, Kawachi I, Subramanian SV, Acevedo-Garcia D, Lee YJ. Can social factors explain sex differences in insomnia? Findings from a national survey in Taiwan. J Epidemiol Community Health 2005; 59(6): 488–94.

CHAPTER 2

Sleep in America: is race or culture an important factor?

Girardin Jean-Louis, Ferdinand Zizi, Georges Casimir, and Jean Claude Compas

While the exact functions of sleep have yet to be elucidated, its importance in our life is 'unquestionable. Phenomenologically, philosophers and mythologists, artists and poets, and scientists alike have all pondered the mystery of sleep. Sleep is observed in myriad species and across cultures, although appreciable differences have been observed in its ontogeny and phylogeny. Inadequate sleep endangers personal distress and can have adverse effects on society at large. This chapter presents results of epidemiologic research on sleep duration and complaints and focuses on racial disparities in the experience of sleep.

DECLINE IN SLEEP DURATION

Commensurate with the recognition of the importance of sleep and sleep disorders is the realization that the average American has been sleeping less and less. The alarming decline in sleep duration has been gradual, rather than abrupt as might have been thought. Empirical evidence indicates that the modal sleep duration was ≥8 hours about four decades ago.[1,2] Hence, the proverbial requirement that we should all sleep 8 hours at night to foster optimal daytime alertness. The first indication of an apparent reduction in sleep time was evident in a 1974 landmark study using polysomnographic recordings. That study showed that volunteers were sleeping an average of 7 hours at night.[3] It is worth noting that sleep length recorded in that study may have been affected by restricted time in bed, as is typical in scheduled laboratory studies; individuals are not always able to maintain their sleep habits.

A decade later, the National Health Interview Survey, which studied Alameda County residents (≥18 years old), suggested that Americans were probably sleeping 7–8 hours at night.[4] After another decade had elapsed, the 1995 Gallup Survey interviewing American adults through random telephone dialing found that the modal sleep duration may have in fact decreased to 7 hours.[5] Remarkably, three years later the Sleep in America Poll, sponsored by the National Sleep Foundation, found that the estimated average sleep duration was reportedly 6.57 hours.[6]

One would be right to point out that most of the studies reviewed used subjective sleep estimates, which are often discordant from objective findings, even among healthy sleepers.[7] This point would raise some doubt as to the veracity of the claim that Americans are sleeping less if in fact one could not rely on subjective data.

One could also reason that the landmark polysomnographic study, mentioned earlier, could have shown longer sleep times had the volunteers been allowed to sleep *ad lib*.[3] However, this argument is counterbalanced by more recent evidence from a home-based actigraphic study finding a similar pattern of sleep reduction.[8] That study, which was conducted contemporaneously with the 1998 Sleep in America Poll, showed that adults (40–64 years old) were sleeping only an average of 6.22 hours at night. We should emphasize that volunteers in that study were allowed to follow their individual routines, including bedtime and daytime behavior.

It is worth noting that with each successive poll sanctioned by the National Sleep Foundation a downward trend is observed in the amount of sleep reported by adult men and women. In 2001, the proportion of Americans sleeping 8 hours or more on week nights was 38%; in 2002, it was 30%, and in 2005, it is 26%.[9] It is likely that we are sleeping 25% less than our forefathers did 100 years ago, argues an article in *Sleep Medicine*.[10]

The causes of sleep loss are an important topic to discuss, but are not addressed in this chapter. We simply remark that since sleep plays a vital role in our lives its daily restriction will inevitably bring about undesired consequences. It is, therefore, explicable why sleep investigators have undertaken so many laboratory and epidemiologic studies to understand fully the impact of sleep loss on the individual as well as on public health.

CONSEQUENCES OF SLEEP LOSS

In light of the reductions in sleep time, be it actual or perceived, it is not surprising that rates of sleep complaints reported by Americans have dramatically increased. According to the most recent Sleep in America Poll surveying insomnia complaints, 21% of respondents reported they had difficulty initiating sleep (DIS) a few nights a week, 32% had difficulty maintaining sleep (DMS), and 21% reported experiencing early morning awakening (EMA).[9] These rates are considerably greater than those noted in a pioneering epidemiologic study conducted in Los Angeles in 1972.[11] In that study, the proportion of residents (≥18 years old) reporting DIS was 14.4%; for DMS, the proportion was 22.9%, and for EMA, 13.8%.

Sleep researchers are particularly concerned with increases in the rate of residual daytime sleepiness, which is estimated to be 37% according to the National Sleep Foundation.[12] A Sleep in America Poll found that 50% of individuals surveyed reported feeling tired or fatigued at least one day a week.[13] Fifty-seven per cent of Americans reported that sleepiness interfered with their ability to drive; of those, 23% admitted falling asleep at the wheel.[5] This trend in fatigue level is consistent with a report comparing questionnaire responses from the Minnesota Multiphasic Personality Inventory obtained in the 1930s and 1980, which found increased fatigue among contemporary men.[14] Estimates from the National Highway Traffic Safety Administration indicate that drowsing driving is probably responsible for 100 000 accidents, 71 000 injuries, 1550 fatalities, and $12.5 billion in monetary losses yearly. Such trends have led advocates concerned with the impact of curtailed sleep durations on public health to decry increased sleepiness as an important public health risk.[5,6,15–27]

On balance, restricted sleep, which might augur a medical/psychiatric problem or simply a personal decision to pursue one's aspirations, does not necessarily connote a diminished quality of life. A recent study conducted among San Diego adults found that greater sleep quality, rather than longer sleep duration, measured objectively or subjectively, is a predictor of a more satisfying life.[28] We should emphasize that this observation does not discount the importance of habitual sleep duration itself. Sleep duration is a key factor in the comprehensive assessment of overall health and functioning.

As discussed below, it is a strong correlate of comorbidities and a predictor of mortality.

It is noteworthy that the amount of sleep essential for optimal daytime functioning, the most satisfying sense of well-being, or the greatest longevity has not been established. We do know, however, that sleeping too little or too much is predictive of increased mortality according to two sets of data from the American Cancer Society Cancer Prevention Study.[1,29-31] Based on the most recent report by investigators at the University of California at San Diego, which sampled over 1 million men and women aged 30–102 years, the greatest longevity was observed among individuals sleeping 7 hours per night. Those who slept 8 hours or more experienced significantly increased mortality risks, as did participants who reported sleeping 6 hours or less. The increased risk of mortality exceeded 15% for individuals who reportedly slept more than 8.5 hours or less than 3.5 or 4.5 hours. This does not in any way imply that increasing or decreasing one's sleep time will necessary change one's mortality risks. However, one might consider whether the amount of time spent sleeping habitually is adequate for one's overall functioning or whether one's sleep duration is affected by a medical or a psychiatric problem, in which case the cause, rather than the symptom, should be addressed.

These results are in tandem with more recent data collected among women who participated in the Nurses Health Study, which showed that sleeping less than 6 hours or more than 7 hours was associated with an increased risk of death. Specifically, the relative mortality risk for sleeping ≤ 5 hours was 1.15; for 6 hours, it was 1.01, for 7 hours, 1.00; for 8 hours, 1.12; and for ≥ 9 hours 1.42.[32] The Japan Collaborative Cohort Study on Evaluation of Cancer Risk, which monitored a sample of 104 010 men and women, found that sleep duration of shorter or longer than 7 hours was associated with a significantly elevated risk of mortality from all causes. While results of these studies might be slightly discrepant, which in some respect reflects differences in statistical analysis, they nevertheless yield similar trends. These findings support the suggestion that sleep duration should be considered as one of the indices of mortality in vital statistics. This line of research also underlines that sleep duration above the population mode[33] correlates with poor health and morbidity,[29,34-36] and that sleep complaints may not always relate to sleeping less than the mode.[1,37-40]

FACTORS AFFECTING SLEEP

A literature review following the model of Zepelin's work on sleep across species lists several factors that affect sleep duration. Ranked in order of importance, they include: body weight, metabolic rate, brain weight, encephalization, and body temperature.[41,42] In humans, physical health, anxiety, and depression are all significant correlates of sleep.[34-36,40,43,44] Individuals experiencing sleep problems are often characterized by worse functioning and well-being, more work-related problems, and a greater likelihood of comorbid physical and mental health conditions than those without sleep disorders.[34] Both anxiety and depression correlate positively with insomnia and negatively with sleep duration.[44]

Age effects on sleep duration are not unequivocal and must be interpreted within the context of disparate study designs.[45,46] Whereas polysomnographic data showed that adults 25 years old sleep 7.17 hours and those aged 75 years old 6.90 hours,[3] the National Health Interview Survey and the American Cancer Society data showed increased sleep durations among older adults (> 74 years old).[1,4] It may be that sleep duration decreases between the ages of 20 and 50 years and increases after reaching the age of 60.[47] Combining results of the Sleep in America polls conducted in 2002 and in 2003, it is noted that the average American aged 18–54 years reported sleeping 6.7 hours on weeknights.[12] For those aged 55–64 years, the average sleep duration was 6.9 hours, and those between 65 and 84 years old averaged 7.1 hours. These results by no means offer definitive evidence that older adults sleep longer than do younger individuals, but they argue against the notion that sleep duration naturally decreases as we get older. The observation that most polysomnographic studies show an age-related decline in sleep duration[48] might be explained in part by the fact that sleep in the laboratory is often restricted by imposed scheduling.

With regard to sex differences in sleep, research has shown that women generally sleep longer than do men, although the former disproportionately report more sleep complaints.[8,43,45,49] A population-based actigraphic study found that the average man and woman (age range 40–64 years) living in San Diego sleep 5.96 hours and 6.43 hours, respectively.[8] The sex disparity is much less evident when comparing older men and older women. In effect, in the 2003 Sleep in America Poll men and women (55–84 years old) reported sleeping 7 hours on week nights. Other factors that might affect sleep include ambient temperature, body heating, carbohydrate consumption, exercise, noise, and the phase of the endogenous pacemaker.[50–56] Effects of race on sleep are not as clearly delineated and, in some respects, have received much less attention. In fact, none of the reports from the National Sleep Foundation considers race as a factor that might influence response rates. Based on the available evidence, race effects on sleep have been mixed, thus warranting further investigations.

Race/culture and sleep

In the social science literature, race is often considered a proxy for socioeconomic constructs. In the context of sleep medicine, it remains unclear whether race has unique influences on sleep patterns. At least within the purview of culture, which is often inextricably linked to one's race, accumulating evidence suggests that sleep profiles might differ among individuals from different countries. Focusing on the two

most commonly reported sleep complaints for instance, epidemiologic evidence shows that 32.2% of Americans ≥ 18 years old reported either difficulty initiating sleep or difficulty maintaining sleep.[11] These rates are much lower in Canada and Mexico: among Canadians of comparable ages, 10.95% reported these complaints;[57] in Mexico, 16.4% reported being bothered by either DIS or DMS.[58] In France, 20% reported DIS or DMS,[59] and in the United Kingdom, only 8.7% reported experiencing DIS or DMS.[60]

The possibility that the sleep experience might differ as a function of one's country of origin was further explored in a study investigating the concept of nonrestorative sleep.[61] Aside from the obvious fact that the variable of interest in that study was different from the aforementioned studies, it sampled individuals from the general population representative of seven European countries: France, the United Kingdom, Germany, Italy, Portugal, Spain, and Finland. Using the Sleep-EVAL system, which allowed telephone interviews, it was found that nonrestorative sleep is a frequent symptom among European men and women (10.8%), but prevalence rates differed among countries. The United Kingdom, for instance, had the highest prevalence rate of nonrestorative sleep (16.1%), whereas Spain had the lowest rate (2.4%). These divergences in national incidence rates suggest that sleep experience may be a response to various environmental factors.

Despite the inherent methodological differences in the aforementioned studies, which preclude a direct comparison between them, the substantial discrepancies in the reported incidence of nonrestorative sleep might reflect unique sociocultural influences on sleep experience. It is of interest to determine whether trends in sleep profiles observed among American adults are observable among individuals from other countries. We are not aware of any data that permit a valid assessment of a decline in sleep durations among Europeans, but data obtained from a study involving seven European countries suggest few differences in sleep duration exist between European and American men and women.[62] Specifically, using the Sleep-EVAL system to interview a total of 8091 volunteers (55–101 years old) regarding sleep habits and sleep disorders, it was observed that the older European adult slept an average of 6.57 hours; British citizens showed the shortest sleep durations (~6.58 hours), and Spanish citizens, the longest (~7.65 hours). While a cogent argument cannot be offered to suggest a comparable decline in sleep duration among Europeans, their sleep durations are more or less equivalent to those reported by Americans.

Equally interesting is the idea that downward trends in sleep duration or increases in sleep complaints may not have affected each ethnic group in America proportionately. Unfortunately, this could not be assessed, as we aren't aware of any published data permitting such analyses. Whether sociocultural differences, in their own right, might explain differences observed between individuals of European descent and those of African descent remains an important question. The idea that sociocultural differences can influence sleep patterns is supported by a prevalence study conducted among New Zealanders. According to that study, surveying 4000 New Zealand adults (20–59 years old), greater rates of insomnia symptoms were found among Maori respondents relative to non-Maoris,[63] who don't share similar cultural attitudes and spiritual beliefs.

INSOMNIA COMPLAINTS: BLACKS VERSUS WHITES

Conflicting observations have been made regarding racial differences in sleep complaints. About four decades ago, prevalence data from residents (≥18 years old) of Alachua, an urban county in Florida, indicated that 40% of Black[a] respondents experienced difficulty sleeping compared to 33% of their White counterparts.[64] However, according to the Cardiovascular Health Study, a more recent study of non-institutionalized Medicare enrollees (≥65 years old) in four American counties (Forsyth, Sacramento, Washington, and Pittsburgh), nocturnal awakenings were reported by 68% of Whites and by 62% of Blacks.[65]

Evidently, the age disparity in these two samples precludes a direct comparison of the two studies, and in effect it might explain differences in the overall frequency of reported sleeping difficulty in the two studies. Nonetheless, it is important to note that Blacks in the latter sample reported less sleeping difficulty than did Whites, suggesting that the frequency of sleeping difficulty reported by Blacks in Florida might be influenced by greater incidence of sleep problems among younger Blacks relative to younger Whites. Unfortunately, this could not be verified in the Florida report because no age-by-race contrasts were available, but the suggestion is supported by survey data obtained from college students, showing better sleep for White students.[66–68]

The finding of fewer sleep complaints among Blacks relative to Whites is supported by data from the Duke Established Populations for Epidemiologic Studies of the Elderly, a longitudinal study of adults ≥65 years old selected from urban and rural counties of North Carolina.[69] In the initial report of Duke's data, 24% of the respondents complaining of wakeful sleep were Blacks and 76% were Whites. However, when Duke's data on incidence rates for insomnia were compiled, Blacks showed an incidence rate of 16%, and Whites 14%.[70]

These results would seem contradictory if we did not consider that the criteria used for incident insomnia included only trouble falling

[a]Throughout the text, we use the term Black in lieu of African American for there are instances where we refer to individuals who self-state their race/ethnicity as Black, African American, African, or Caribbean American; the term White is used to denote individuals of European descent.

asleep and early morning awakening, but not difficulty maintaining sleep. Furthermore, the overall incidence rates noted for Blacks were influenced by the greater frequency of complaints of incident insomnia among Black women (19%) compared to Black men (12%). The investigators reasoned that higher rates of insomnia among Blacks might be due to higher incidence of morbidity, but cohort differences are also suspected.[71] Indeed, according to one report the percentages of Blacks and Whites reporting physical disability and poor health were 19% vs. 14% and 31% vs. 22%, respectively.[70] One might expect that higher rates of incident insomnia among Blacks would be attributable to greater depressive symptomatology, but interpretations of such findings are complicated by the fact that depressed mood is also predictive of incident insomnia.[70,71] Although the absence of depression is suggestive of remission,[70] the Duke study found virtually no racial differences in the frequency of depressive symptoms when controlling for education, income, cognitive impairment, chronic health problems, and disability.[72] These findings thus point to the possibility that factors other than mood were responsible for the incidence of insomnia among Blacks.

The hypothesis that the high frequency of reported insomnia among Blacks may have been due to a co-occurring medical condition was considered. The findings of the Duke study for instance showed that among Blacks the relative risk for sleep-disordered breathing, a condition characterized by respiratory arrests disrupting sleep, was twice that of age-matched Whites.[73] One population-based study of American adults (40–60 years old), found that rates of sleep-disordered breathing were much higher among members of minority groups, with estimates indicating that 16.3% of ethnic minorities have ≥ 20 respiratory events per hour as compared to 4.9% of non-Hispanic Whites.[74]

This finding is very important and has been supported by other prevalence studies. One such study compared community-dwelling older Blacks and Whites, finding that Blacks were experiencing severe sleep-disordered breathing with a relative risk twofold as great (relative risk = 2.13) as that of their counterparts.[73] The mean respiratory disturbance index (RDI)[b] for Blacks with severe sleep-disordered breathing was significantly higher than that for Whites (72.1 vs. 43.3).

It is noteworthy that race is associated with the presence of sleep-disordered breathing (RDI ≥ 30) independently of age, sex, and body mass index, three of the main risk factors for sleep-disordered breathing.[75,76] This race disparity is not solely observable among adults who are 40 years old or older. In a case–control family study of sleep-disordered breathing comparing 225 Blacks and 622 Whites (2–86 years old), 31% of Blacks vs. 10% of Whites had RDI > 10.[77] Also important in that study was the observation that young Blacks may be at increased risk for sleep-disordered breathing than age-matched Whites. This age difference in the occurrence of sleep-disordered breathing along with notable anatomic risk factors has suggested possible racial differences in the genetic underpinnings of this condition. Emerging evidence based on studies using whole genome scans and segregation analysis has strengthened the hypothesis that sleep-disordered breathing may be the result of genetic influences.[78–81] Evidence of the existence of a codominant gene among Blacks with an allele frequency of 0.14,[78] which is possibly linked to breathing disorders, has tended to support this inference.

Available data suggest that findings of greater sleep complaints among young Blacks might be indicative of the presence of undiagnosed sleep disorders, causing unnecessary distress. The National Commission on Sleep Disorders Research estimates that sleep-disordered

---

[b]RDI is defined as the number of apneas plus hypopneas per hour of sleep. RDI is often categorized into four groups (<5, 5 to <15, 15 to <30, ≥ 30),

breathing is probably responsible for 38 000 cardiovascular deaths yearly, with an associated 42 million dollars spent on related hospitalizations.[82] Available data suggest that Blacks are at higher risk for sleep-disordered breathing than Whites and suffer from associated medical and psychosocial complications, in part because of delayed diagnosis[83] and limited access to health care, either because of economic barriers or cultural barriers.[84,85] Of note is the fact that, compared to Whites, African Americans are not as likely to receive screening or satisfactory care, even when we consider those who are Medicare beneficiaries and have access to health care.[82,83] Thus, other factors influencing the likelihood of seeking medical care should be considered in any campaign geared towards reducing sleep problems among Blacks.

Typically, the public health literature has tended to list being male, overweight, and over the age of 40 years as risk factors for sleep-disordered breathing. However, recent data strongly suggest that race should also be considered as an important risk factor. Indeed, hypertension and cardiovascular diseases (e.g., myocardial infarction, angina, heart failure, and stroke), which are two of the most important comorbid conditions of sleep-disordered breathing, are more prevalent among Blacks.[86] Moreover, based on results of several multivariate analytical models, sleep-disordered breathing represents an independent risk factor for hypertension,[87–89] and hypertension constitutes a significant predictor of cardiopulmonary deaths among patients with sleep-disordered breathing.[87] More recently, we reported that Black hypertensives with a positive family history exhibited a significantly greater number of oxygen desaturations and apnea-hypopnea indices than hypertensives without a positive family history.[90] Notwithstanding these alarming data, the vast majority of suspected cases in minority communities remain undiagnosed and therefore untreated because of the lack of awareness by the public and health care professionals.

These observations demonstrate that race/ethnic factors affecting disease states[91,92] or genetic factors predisposing people to express different diseases[93] might differentially influence sleep regulatory processes. In addition to sleep-disordered breathing, there are data showing race differences in sleep regulation among patients with depression, who generally show characteristically different sleep architecture than do healthy sleepers.[94–96] In one study, Black patients with depression had less total sleep time, less slow-wave sleep, more stage 2 sleep, longer rapid eye movement (REM) sleep latency, less REM sleep, and lower REM density than their White counterparts.[95] We note that these two groups did not differ in symptom severity, age of onset, number of episodes, socioeconomic status, or sex. We are reminded that no such race differences have been found among Black healthy sleepers.[94,97]

Important race differences are also observed when studying the phenomenology of sleep paralysis, which is believed to vary as a function of the culture being investigated. A recent study on recurrent sleep paralysis found that 59% of Blacks with panic disorder experienced this condition, compared to 7% among their White counterparts.[98] Among individuals in the community at large reporting recurrent sleep paralysis, 23% were Blacks and 6% were Whites.

SLEEP DURATION: BLACKS VERSUS WHITES

Insomnia complaints among Blacks might not result necessarily from reduced sleep length. Data reported in 1997 from the National Health and Nutrition Examination Survey, which used a nationally representative probability sample of noninstitutionalized adults, revealed that a greater proportion of Blacks (11%) compared to Whites (8%) slept more than 8 hours,[29] the recommended sleep time according to reports from the National Sleep Foundation.[6,99] Interestingly, although Blacks slept more than did Whites, the survey showed that 19% of Blacks, compared to

16% of Whites, complained of daytime somnolence. About a decade earlier, estimates of sleep length greater than 8 hours were 11% for Whites and 18% for Blacks, based on the National Health Interview Survey of Alameda County residents.[4]

These data are important, since sleeping greater than 8 hours is a correlate of observed comorbidities[35,36] and is predictive of mortality.[1,29–31] Perhaps, the fact that a greater proportion of Blacks slept longer than 8 hours should not be viewed as conferring any adaptive advantage. Rather, it may be suggestive of greater comorbidities,[70,92] as has been documented in this racial group. Determining the nature of the relationships between sleep duration and mortality specifically among Blacks would be enlightening. It is not certain whether the general pattern observed in the Cancer Prevention data – sleeping longer than 8 hours is predictive of excess mortality – would prevail. It would also be important to ascertain whether, based on the available epidemiologic data, Blacks were experiencing better or worse sleep quality compared to Whites. Ultimately, if one is primarily concerned with living a satisfying life, one might be more concerned with the quality of one's sleep, rather than with the amount of sleep one experiences habitually.

Considering the extant literature on self-reported data, the finding of better sleep for Blacks is by no means universal. Several factors should be considered when interpreting available data. First, differing sampling strategies and lack of parity in the cohorts investigated might help explain discrepant findings. Second, one might consider the nuances in the outcome measures reported in those studies. Questions about sleep problems are not always formulated and coded the same way. Third, at the time those epidemiologic studies were being conducted, differing definitions for insomnia were used, which no doubt influenced the selection of outcome measures from one study to the next. Considering further the issue of the influence of race or culture on sleep, we analyzed two sets of data recently obtained from older adults living in Brooklyn, New York. These individuals participated in two multifactorial population-based studies conducted between 1999 and 2004.[100,101]

Sleep among older adults living in Brooklyn, New York

In our population-based study of older adults living in Brooklyn, New York, we re-examined race differences in sleep complaints. We also investigated whether within a specific racial group sleep complaints might differ as a function of ethnic grouping. Specifically, we contrasted Blacks with Whites broadly defined (see Table 2.1). Furthermore, since the Black stratum included both US-born and immigrant (Caribbean) Blacks and the White stratum included both US-born and immigrant Whites, we also explored whether differences in sleep complaints existed within ethnic subgroups.

Based on data obtained from 1118 respondents who participated in face-to-face interviews, we used regression modeling to assess which factor from the available set (i.e., age, sex, race, education, income, marital status, physical health, depression, stress, body mass index, smoking status, drinking status, social support, emotion, and religion) was the best predictor of sleep disturbances. Our analysis showed that of the factors considered, race was the most significant predictor of sleep problems, accounting for 20% of the variance in sleep disturbance.

Although the cohort we examined differed in many respects from those reported previously, sleep complaints of older Blacks in our sample showed some similarities to previous studies regarding the three main indices of insomnia: difficulty initiating sleep, difficulty maintaining sleep, and early morning awakenings (see Table 2.2). By contrast, a greater number of Whites reported these complaints, relative to Blacks in the same sample or both Whites and Blacks in previous samples. Except for the Florida sample, which does not permit direct examination of race differences in sleep complaints of older

Table 2.1 Characteristics of participating older adults in the Brooklyn study

| Variable | Black (60%) | | White (40%) | |
	US-born (n=236)	Caribbean (n=435)	Immigrant (n=173)	US-born (n=274)
Mean age (SD)	74 (6)	73 (6)	73 (6)	76 (6)
Mean household income, K (SD)	16 (14)	19 (18)	16 (17)	23 (24)
Mean body mass index (SD)	30 (12)	28 (5)	27 (5)	27 (4)
% Female	64	60	65	60
% Married	23	37	57	31
% No high school degree	59	68	38	31

Table 2.2 Rate of sleep-related complaints by race

Variable	Black	White	χ^2
Difficulty initiating sleep (%)	14	41	98**
Difficulty maintaining sleep (%)	37	75	162**
Early morning awakening (%)	17	46	116**
Daytime sleep (%)	12	12	0.07
Sleep medicine (%)	3	17	72**

**indicates significant differences using chi square test at alpha = 0.01.

adults, the finding of fewer sleep complaints among Blacks was constant across studies, having been observed in different geographic locations and with differing cohorts. It is important to note, however, that compared to previous data, complaints of daytime sleep did not differ between Black and White respondents. Indeed, race was not the most likely predictor of daytime sleep.

In the first study, we could only compare sleep complaints between races, as the number of sleep measures was limited. Although the second study sampled only women participants, it expanded on the first study design in several ways, one of which was the addition of global sleep measures. As predicted by the first study, analysis of those data showed that, compared to White women, Black women reported greater sleep satisfaction (r_s=0.20, $p<0.001$). They also experienced earlier rise times (r_s=0.18, $p<0.001$) and bedtime (r_s=0.17, $p<0.001$), relative to their White counterparts. Trends suggested longer sleep duration and better sleep quality for Blacks as well (r_s=−0.10, $p=0.04$; r_s=−0.11, $p=0.02$, respectively). Thus, Blacks living in Brooklyn, NY, tended to report fewer sleep complaints, and therefore seem to be more satisfied with their sleep.

RESPONSE BIAS AND INSOMNIA COMPLAINTS

The finding of similar proportions of sleep complaints among Blacks, as found in mixed samples, is important and suggests in some respect that Whites in our sample were probably reporting substantially greater complaints overall (see Table 2.1). It is also possible, however, that Blacks may be underreporting sleep complaints to some degree, although we could not assume that Blacks in our sample might have experienced greater sleeping difficulty without objective sleep recordings. Objective studies have tended to show that Blacks are likely to have sleep patterns that are more disturbed than those of Whites.[73] In the population-based actigraphic study of San Diegans, we found that White men and women slept an average of 6.32 hours, whereas Blacks averaged 5.9 hours a night.[8]

The possibility of a bias in reporting among Blacks is consistent with the finding that they also reported significantly fewer self-perceived health problems than did Whites, whereas converging epidemiologic and vital statistics data demonstrate quite the contrary.[85,92] Indeed, according to the National Center for Health Statistics, the age-adjusted proportion of Blacks with fair or poor health status was 76% greater than for Whites, and prevalence rates for the leading causes of death (e.g., heart disease and cancer) were much higher among Blacks than among Whites.[92]

The notion of a reporting bias among older Blacks is also supported by studies comparing Black and White caregivers, finding that Blacks used more positive reappraisal than did Whites.[102] Relative to Whites, Black caregivers often appraised patients' problems as being less stressful and reported fewer depressed moods and higher self-efficacy in managing caregiving problems.[103] Based on appraisal and coping research, several hypotheses have been advanced suggesting that older Blacks might have developed effective strategies to deal with hardships due to poverty, racism, segregation, and other life stresses. These strategies over time would have fostered effective reframing of difficult life experiences that could not be easily changed.[103] While this may be true for Blacks, positive reframing among Whites is not believed to be protective; rather, it may lead to increased psychophysiological distress.[102]

REPRESSIVE COPING AND INSOMNIA

Using the second data set on sleep and psychosocial factors, we specifically explored whether coping strategy mediated the likelihood of reporting sleep complaints. As in the previous study, we obtained physical health characteristics and sociodemographic data. In addition, we acquired data on repressive coping assessed with the index of self-regulation of emotion (ISE), which constitutes a modified version of Weinberger's conceptual model of repression.[104] The model purports to explain how dispositional repressors distance themselves from emotional experiences that threaten their self-concept.[105–107] ISE scores were derived following Mendolia's conceptualization, which amalgamates the defensive scale from the Social Desirability Scale and the anxiety subscale from the State-Trait Anxiety Inventory; high scores represented greater defensiveness/repressive coping.

Preliminary analysis of those data showed that women with high self-regulation scores reported fewer insomnia complaints and greater sleep satisfaction than those categorized as low regulators.[101] Those women tended to sleep longer and had better sleep quality as well. Within-group analysis indicated that Black women classified as high regulators reported significantly lower rates of insomnia compared to low regulators (28% vs. 70%; $\chi^2 = 163.71$, $p < 0.0001$). Within the White race, high regulators also reported significantly lower rates of insomnia (54% vs. 77%; $\chi^2 = 10.64$, $p < 0.001$); thus, race differences in insomnia rates are more striking among high regulators.

In a separate analysis, we used partial correlations to examine whether repressive coping represented a mediating factor relative to racial differences in insomnia complaints. These analyses showed that the magnitude of the relationship of race to insomnia and sleep satisfaction was significantly reduced. Controlling for effects of age, income, education, marital status, and body mass index did not result in significantly lower correlations of race to insomnia or sleep satisfaction. We surmise that the relationships of race to insomnia complaints and to sleep satisfaction are jointly dependent on the degree of repressive coping. This implies that

Blacks report fewer insomnia complaints because they seem to have a greater ability to regulate their emotions. It may be that Blacks cope with sleep problems within a positive self-regulatory framework, which allows them to deal more effectively with sleep-interfering psychological processes to stressful life events and to curtail dysfunctional sleep-interpreting processes. Whether self-reported and physiologically monitored sleep patterns differ greatly among individuals showing divergent repressive coping styles remains to be determined.

Conceivably, lower rates of sleep complaints among Black elders may be explained by an acceptance of sleep disturbance as part of the aging process, as they might for health problems as well. Except for hypertension, rates for other medical illnesses were lower for Black respondents. Accepting sleep disturbances in old age constitutes one of the cornerstones of cognitive behavior therapy, at least in its adaptation by sleep clinicians. Cognitive behavior therapy has been successfully employed to treat late-life insomnia.[108] In essence, this therapeutic technique attempts to promote acceptance of sleep, when deemed in the normal range, by specifically targeting dysfunctional sleep-related beliefs or negative cognitions about sleep.

It is believed that a reduction in dysfunctional beliefs (or self-perceived stress) obviates sleep complaints, even among those with severe sleeping difficulty.[108,109] This belief is based on the finding that highly stressed older adults with insomnia symptoms exhibit anxious, depressed, negative cognitive-affective dispositions, whereas older poor sleepers with less self-perceived stress cope well with age-related sleep changes and display similar psychological adjustment as do good sleepers.[40] It would be enlightening to ascertain whether Blacks reporting fewer sleep complaints are in fact characterized by relatively greater positive reappraisal than their counterparts or whether they experience verifiably fewer sleep problems. There is a body of research showing that some self-described normal sleepers may endure significant sleeping difficulty with no corresponding reports of sleep complaints, and others, even when admitting sleeping difficulty, may yet fail to report sleep-related dissatisfaction.[40,57]

Whereas Blacks with insomnia may benefit from this unique ability to cope with challenges posed by sleep disturbances, this may be maladaptive among those suffering from sleep apnea or other medical conditions causing insomnia. This might explain in part why sleep-disordered breathing, for instance, is regarded as a major public health problem in the Black population.[77] In fact, our own data collected at a sleep clinic in Brooklyn, NY, suggest that only 35% of Blacks are likely to comply with a doctor's recommendation to undergo a polysomnographic evaluation. This is quite alarming since 61% of Black patients in our clinic who consented to be evaluated received a diagnosis of sleep-disordered breathing.[110]

It is estimated that more than half of Blacks with sleep-disordered breathing may be unaware of it. This is compounded by the fact that timely assessment and treatment are often hampered by a lack of recognition of sleep-disordered breathing in primary care.[83] Results of the Sleep in America Poll reveal that while most respondents (89%) agree that doctors should discuss sleep issues with their patients, only 29% of doctors actually inquired about sleep problems.[9] This might explain why a review of approximately a million patient records by the National Commission on Sleep Disorders Research found only 17 positive diagnoses for sleep disorders.[111] Yet, most of the risk factors (e.g., age, sex, race/ethnicity, body habitus, familial predisposition, alcohol consumption, and chronic rhinitis) for sleep-disordered breathing can be recognized with appropriate training and education.

Another important observation from the study we conducted in Brooklyn relates to the relatively low proportion of Blacks (3%) reporting reliance on sleep medicine. It is not clear whether this finding could be due to lower sleep complaints *per se* in that stratum. It might have been assumed that differences in socioeconomic

Table 2.3   Within-group rate of reliance on medicine to treat sleep problems

Variable	Black		White	
	US-born	Caribbean	US-born	Immigrant
Difficulty initiating sleep (%)	21	16	48	28
Difficulty maintaining sleep (%)	7	6	29	13
Early morning awakening (%)	6	13	35	19

status, as found in the Brooklyn study (see Table 2.1), could predict the likelihood of sleep medicine consumption, but income or education were not independent predictors of sleep disturbance. Blacks in general are less inclined to use prescription or over-the-counter medications than are Whites,[112-114] although consumption of certain medications tends to be more prevalent in one stratum than in the other, as disease expressions vary.[91-93] Restricted access to health care, because of either economic barriers or cultural barriers, has also been hypothesized to be a likely cause for lower medication use.[84] One might surmise, therefore, that such restrictions could have influenced the Brooklyn data as well. Unfortunately, this view remains speculative, as issues involving access to health were beyond the scope of that study.

Sleep complaints: within-group differences

Besides the confirmation of existing data showing that Blacks reported fewer sleep complaints, analysis of the Brooklyn data has allowed the recognition of within-group heterogeneity in sleep complaints. Population-based sleep studies reported up till now in the literature have not addressed this possibility, although it might have been suggested by the multitude of studies showing ethnic disparities in physical health.[84,85,92] Indeed, even within a specific ethnic group homogeneity of disease expressions cannot be assumed as lifestyle, cultural, economic, and environmental factors enhancing or attenuating the incidence or the prevalence of diseases may vary.

Similarly, analysis of the Brooklyn data showed no within-group homogeneity in sleep complaints; 49.2% of US-born Blacks reported either difficulty initiating sleep, difficulty maintaining sleep, or early morning awakenings compared to 41.8% of Caribbean Americans. Eighty-seven per cent of immigrant Whites indicated at least one of those sleep complaints compared to 82.1% of US-born Whites. We also found that compared with Caribbean Americans (8%), a greater proportion of US-born Blacks (19%) experienced daytime sleep, suggesting further ethnocultural heterogeneity. Of note, although within-group disparities were found, seemingly they did not disproportionately influence (negatively or positively) the rate of sleep complaints of each ethnic group overall.

It is noteworthy that a larger percentage of Caribbean Americans in the Brooklyn study did not obtain a high school degree, but they reported higher income and were more likely to be married compared to US-born Blacks (see Table 2.1). However, these subgroups did not differ substantially in terms of reliance on sleep medicine nor in difficulty initiating or maintaining sleep, but twice as many Caribbean Americans were dependent on sleep medicine to prevent early morning awakenings (see Table 2.3). There was a greater likelihood for immigrant Whites to be married compared with US-born Whites, but the latter reported higher educational attainment and greater household income. The higher economic status of US-born

Whites might explain why they were more likely to rely on sleep medicine than their Black counterparts, despite the fact that immigrant Whites expressed more sleep complaints. The average household income for immigrant Whites was comparable to that of US-born Blacks; indeed, it was lower than that of Caribbean Americans. Nonetheless, a greater proportion of immigrant Whites depended on sleep medicine relative to US-born Blacks and Whites or Caribbean Blacks. Thus, income by itself may not account for the differences in the likelihood of sleep medicine consumption by elders in these ethnic groups.

Analysis of the socioeconomic variables within race/ethnic group led to an important observation, which to some degree might constitute the basis for another plausible explanation of the lower rates of insomnia complaints among Blacks. The finding that Caribbean Americans had greater household incomes was surprising at first. We would have assumed the opposite to be true, since older Caribbean Americans generally report much less education. In our experience, many Caribbean American men and women often have financial obligations that require holding a job even in old age; moreover, some have to hold more than one job. One such obligation relates directly to the desire to own a home, as a sign of having realized the 'American dream,' which at times may stretch their financial resources.

One wonders, therefore, whether this might have an influence on their perception of sleep or their own sleep need. It is possible that their sense of obligation to their families prevails over their own personal interests or desires. The need to sleep, although vital, too often takes a back seat by comparison to what they regard as their ultimate purpose: to provide for their family. It is plausible that by restricting their sleep time in the pursuit of their familial and financial obligations these individuals might forego their 'optional sleep.'[115] If it is the case that their perceived 'core sleep' needs are met, it might explain their reticence to express

dissatisfaction with sleep. An experimental study would have to bear this out before any solid claim could be made. At this juncture, we simply remark that these individuals may be practicing sleep restriction, a proven therapeutic modality for insomnia, without prescription. When older adults spend too much time in bed, they often experience daytime lethargy, which may lead to sleep fragmentation, thus culminating in a vicious cycle of more time spent in bed and greater sleep fragmentation. If one also assumes that shorter sleep prolongs survival, Caribbean Americans and, perhaps, Blacks in general should be living longer lives, especially if no significant morbidities are expressed.

CONCLUDING REMARKS

Some investigators have questioned whether Americans are sleeping less than observed four decades ago.[116] This stems from a single finding of no statistical difference between sleep durations reported then and current estimates. As presented in this chapter, the preponderance of evidence suggests that total sleep time has been declining gradually, at least in the USA. Be that as it may, care must be exercised before recommending that the population as a whole sleep more, as no convincing evidence has been brought forth to support such a recommendation. Targeting individuals at risk for adverse effects of sleep loss seems a prudent practice. There is much less debate regarding staggering increases in daytime sleepiness, which as discussed before constitutes a major public health risk.

Public health advocates are concerned about the likelihood that different segments of the US population may be at greater risk of succumbing to the adverse impact of sleep loss. A cursory view of the available evidence within the context of race would have suggested that Blacks might be at a lower risk than Whites. Most of the epidemiologic studies reviewed in this chapter offer data suggesting that Whites have a greater frequency of sleep complaints, although based on objective evidence they often sleep longer than Blacks. With regard to subjective data, however, trends favor longer sleep times for Blacks. We note that no objective population-based sleep recordings have been reported to support such differences. Clearly, when studying individuals with a diagnosis of sleep-disordered breathing, Blacks often experience less sleep than their White counterparts.

We cannot affirm with certainty why Blacks tend to report fewer sleep complaints overall. It does not appear that differences in reported sleep or health complaints are explainable solely on the basis of socioeconomic factors or immigration status. Across age groups, socioeconomic factors have played an important role in influencing sleep patterns of Blacks. In the analysis of the Brooklyn data, such factors did not prove to be significant independent predictors of sleep disturbance. Arguably, racial disparities in the utilization of health services are an important explanatory factor when examining health-related data,[84,92,117] but we could not ascertain their influence on the present data since it was not included in the initial interview. One might also consider differences in religious or cultural beliefs, which might hinder participation in recommended health care practices.[117] In the Brooklyn data, we observed significant within-group heterogeneity in the religious identifications of the respondents, but religion itself was not a significant independent predictor of sleep disturbance.

One cannot discount, however, the possibility that specific ethnocultural factors may have differentially influenced the response styles of Black and White respondents. Similarly, one would not be surprised if it were shown that Caribbean respondents differed from US-born Blacks in their response styles, considering their divergent ethnocultural origin. Unfortunately, these important hypotheses could not be tested with the Brooklyn data. Such hypotheses should be explored in future investigations, as analyses of those data showed both between-group and within-group ethnic differences in sleep complaints.

Conceivably, Blacks (US-born or Caribbean) may benefit from a unique cultural background, which provides a positive context for reframing the perceived need for sleep, as they would for other life challenges that are not easily resolvable. Likewise, a predilection for traditional medicine might account for so little reliance on sleep medicine in that racial group. Evidence suggests that some Caribbean Americans might resort to an elder family member, to a pastor, or to a folk practitioner to deal with health-related issues.[118] In sum, while economic and cultural barriers limiting access to health care might prevent adequate medical care where morbidities are expressed, paradoxically these may set in motion the processes leading to decreased somatic and sleep complaints among Blacks.

There are virtually no population-based data suggesting greater reductions in sleep duration or increased sleepiness among Blacks in contradistinction to Whites. Perhaps, the decline in sleep duration observed among Americans affects each racial grouping to the same degree. It seems clear, on the one hand, that the ability of older Blacks to cope more effectively with insomnia challenges, if proven, would constitute an important asset. On the other hand, minimizing the effects of sleep disturbances when accompanied by evidence of comorbidity represents a liability for Blacks.

This liability is most notable when we consider the consequences of untreated sleep-disordered breathing, which might include increased odds of involvement in a motor vehicle accident and vulnerability to hypertension or cardiovascular diseases.[75,88,89,119–121] Since individuals belonging to the Black race are at greater risk, they would benefit from increased efforts to improve awareness of the importance of early detection of sleep-disordered breathing and the necessity to comply with treatment recommendations. Whereas there is no direct evidence to encourage Blacks to sleep more than the current population mode, it seems a prudent practice that they avoid acute sleep loss as they are at greater risk for adverse events.

Acknowledgment

We thank Dr Carol Magai, the director of the Intercultural Institute at Long Island University, for providing access to the Brooklyn data on sleep complaints reviewed in this chapter.

REFERENCES

1. Kripke DF, Simons RN, Garfinkel L, Hammond EC. Short and long sleep and sleeping pills. Is increased mortality associated? Arch Gen Psychiatry 1979; 36: 103–16.
2. Gallup. The Gallup Study of Sleeping Habits. The Gallup Organization, 1979; 1–60.
3. Williams RL, Karacan I, Hursch CJ. Normal sleep. In: Karacan I, Hursch CJ, eds. Electroencephalography (EEG) of human sleep: clinical applications. New York: John Wiley & Sons, 1974: 26–68.
4. Schoenborn CA. Health habits of US adults, 1985: the 'Alameda 7' revisited. Public Health Rep 1986; 101: 571–80.
5. Sleep in America. The Gallup Organization, 1995; 1–78.
6. Omnibus Sleep in America Poll. The Gallup Organization, 1998: 1–70.
7. Baker FC, Maloney S, Driver HS. A comparison of subjective estimates of sleep with objective polysomnographic data in healthy men and women. J Psychosom Res 1999; 47: 335–41.
8. Jean-Louis G, Kripke DF, Ancoli-Israel S, Klauber M, Sepulveda RS. Sleep duration, illumination, and activity patterns in a population sample: effects of gender and ethnicity. Biol Psychiatry 2000; 47: 921–7.
9. Omnibus Sleep in America Poll. Washington, DC: National Sleep Foundation, 2005.
10. Mahowald M. Assessing excessive daytime sleepiness: a complaint to be taken seriously. Sleep Medicine Alert 1999; 4: 1–4.
11. Bixler EO, Kales A, Soldatos CR, Kales JD, Healey S. Prevalence of sleep disorders in the Los Angeles metropolitan area. Am J Psychiatry 1979; 136: 1257–62.
12. Omnibus Sleep in America Poll. Washington, DC: National Sleep Foundation, 2003.
13. Strakowski SM, Stoll AL, Tohen M, Faedda GL, Goodwin DC. The Tridimensional Personality Questionnaire as a predictor of six-month outcome in first episode mania. Psychiatry Res 1993; 48: 1–8.
14. Bliwise DL. Historical change in the report of daytime fatigue. Sleep 1996; 19: 462–4.
15. Mullaney DJ, Kripke DF, Fleck PA, Johnson LC. Sleep loss and nap effects on sustained continuous performance. Psychophysiology 1983; 20: 643–51.
16. Pack AI, Pack AM, Rodgman E, Cucchiara A, Dinges DF, Schwab CW. Characteristics of crashes attributed to the driver having fallen asleep. Accid Anal Prev 1995; 27: 769–75.
17. McCartt AT, Ribner SA, Pack AI, Hammer MC. The scope and nature of the drowsy driving problem in New York State. Accid Anal Prev 1996; 28: 511–17.
18. Horne JA, Reyner LA. Sleep related vehicle accidents. Br Med J 1995; 310: 565–7.
19. Reyner LA, Horne JA. Falling asleep whilst driving: are drivers aware of prior sleepiness? Int J Legal Med 1998; 111: 120–3.
20. Mitler MM, Miller JC, Lipsitz JJ, Walsh JK, Wylie CD. The sleep of long-haul truck drivers. N Engl J Med 1997; 337: 755–61.
21. Mitler MM, Carskadon MA, Czeisler CA et al. Catastrophes, sleep, and public policy: consensus report. Sleep 1988; ii: 100–9.
22. Marcus CL, Loughlin GM. Effect of sleep deprivation on driving safety in housestaff. Sleep 1996; 19: 763–6.
23. Carskadon MA. Patterns of sleep and sleepiness in adolescents. Pediatrician 1990; 17: 5–12.
24. Summala H, Mikkola T. Fatal accidents among car and truck drivers: effects of fatigue, age, and alcohol consumption. Hum Factors 1994; 36: 315–26.
25. Lyznicki JM, Doege TC, Davis RM, Williams MA. Sleepiness, driving, and motor vehicle crashes. Council on Scientific Affairs, American Medical Association. J Am Med Assoc 1998; 279: 1908–13.
26. Webb WB. The cost of sleep-related accidents: a reanalysis. Sleep 1995; 18: 276–80.
27. Briones B, Adams N, Strauss M et al. Relationship between sleepiness and general health status. Sleep 1996; 19: 583–8.
28. Jean-Louis G, Kripke D.F, Ancoli-Israel S. Sleep and quality of well-being. Sleep 2000; 23: 1115–21.
29. Qureshi AI, Giles WH, Croft JB, Bliwise DL. Habitual sleep patterns and risk for stroke and coronary heart disease: a 10-year follow-up from NHANES I. Neurology 1997; 48: 904–11.

30. Wingard DL, Berkman LF. Mortality risk associated with sleeping patterns among adults. Sleep 1983; 6: 102–7.

31. Kripke DF, Assmus JD. A duration ≥ 8 hours for sleep is not safer! Sleep Research Online 1999; 2: 144.

32. Patel SR, Ayas NT, Malhotra MR, et al. A prospective study of sleep duration and mortality risk in women. Sleep 2004; 27: 440–4.

33. Johnson EO. Sleep in America: 1999. Washington, DC: National Sleep Foundation, 1999: 1–122.

34. Kuppermann M, Lubeck DP, Mazonson PD, et al. Sleep problems and their correlates in a working population. J Gen Intern Med 1995; 10: 25–32.

35. Habte-Gabr E, Wallace RB, Colsher PL. Sleep patterns in rural elders: demographic, health, and psychobehavioral correlates. J Clin Epidemiol 1991; 44: 5–13.

36. Bliwise DL, King AC, Harris RB. Habitual sleep durations and health in a 50–65 year old population. J Clin Epidemiol 1994; 47: 35–41.

37. Carskadon MA, Dement WC, Mitler MM, et al. Self-reports versus sleep laboratory findings in 122 drug-free subjects. Am J Psychiatry 1976; 133: 1382–8.

38. Frankel BL, Coursey RD, Buchbinder R, Snyder F. Recorded and reported sleep in chronic primary insomnia. Arch Gen Psychiatry 1976; 33: 615–23.

39. Morin CM, Gramling SE. Sleep patterns and aging: comparison of older adults with and without insomnia complaints. Psychol Aging 1989; 4: 290–4.

40. Fichten CS, Creti L, Amsel R, et al. Poor sleepers who do not complain of insomnia: myths and realities about psychological and lifestyle characteristics of older good and poor sleepers. J Behav Med 1995; 18: 189–223.

41. Zepelin H. Mammalian sleep. In: Kryger MH, Roth T, Dement WC, eds. Principles and Practice of Sleep Medicine. Philadelphia, PA: WB Saunders Company, 1994: 69–80.

42. Rechtschaffen A. Current perspectives on the function of sleep. Perspect Biol Med 1998; 41: 359–90.

43. Lindberg E, Janson C, Gislason T et al. Sleep disturbances in a young adult population: can gender differences be explained by differences in psychological status? Sleep 1997; 20: 381–7.

44. Beullens J. Determinants of insomnia in relatively healthy elderly. A literature review. Tijdschr Gerontol Geriatr 1999; 30: 31–8.

45. Bliwise D. Sleep and circadian rhythm disorders in aging and dementia. In: Turek FW, Zee PC, eds. Regulation of Sleep and Circadian Rhythms. New York: Prentice Hall, 1999: 487–525.

46. Bliwise DL. Sleep in normal aging and dementia. Sleep 1993; 16: 40–81.

47. Johns MW, Egan P, Gay TJ, Masterton JP. Sleep habits and symptoms in male medical and surgical patients. Br Med J 1970; 2: 509–12.

48. Ohayon MM, Carskadon MA, Guilleminault C, Vitiello MV. Meta-analysis of quantitative sleep parameters from childhood to old age in healthy individuals: developing normative sleep values across the human lifespan. Sleep 2004; 27: 1255–73.

49. Hoch CC, Reynolds CF, Kupfer DJ et al. Empirical note: self-report versus recorded sleep in healthy seniors. Sleep 1988; 11: 521–7.

50. Czeisler CA, Weitzman E, Moore-Ede MC, Zimmerman JC, Knauer RS. Human sleep: its duration and organization depend on its circadian phase. Psychiatry Res 1990; 32: 221–7.

51. Garcia-Garcia F, Drucker-Colin R. Endogenous and exogenous factors on sleep-wake cycle regulation. Prog Neurobiol 1999; 58: 297–314.

52. Horne JA, Staff LH. Exercise and sleep: body-heating effects. Sleep 1983; 6: 36–46.

53. Zammit GK, Kolevzon A, Fauci M, Shindledecker R, Ackerman S. Postprandial sleep in healthy men. Sleep 1995; 18: 229–31.

54. Hauri P. The influence of evening activity on the onset of sleep. Psychophysiology 1969; 5: 426–30.

55. Libert JP, Bach V, Johnson LC et al. Relative and combined effects of heat and noise exposure on sleep in humans. Sleep 1991; 14: 24–31.

56. Saletu B, Frey R, Grunberger J. Street noise and sleep: whole night somnopolygraphic, psychometric and psychophysiologic studies in comparison with normal data. Wien Med Wochenschr 1989; 139: 257–63.

57. Ohayon MM, Caulet M, Guilleminault C. How a general population perceives its sleep and how this relates to the complaint of insomnia. Sleep 1997; 20: 715–23.

58. Tellez-Lopez A, Sanchez E, Torres FG. Habitos y transtornos del dormir en residentes del area metropolitana de Monterrey. Salud Mental 1995; 18: 14–22.

59. Ohayon M, Caulet M, Lemoine P. The elderly, sleep habits and use of psychotropic drugs by the French population. Encephale 1996; 22: 337–50.

60. Ohayon MM, Guilleminault C, Priest RG, Caulet M. Snoring and breathing pauses during sleep: telephone interview survey of a United Kingdom population sample. Br Med J 1997; 314: 860–3.

61. Ohayon MM. Prevalence and correlates of non-restorative sleep complaints. Arch Intern Med 2005; 165: 35–41.

62. Ohayon MM. Interactions between sleep normative data and sociocultural characteristics in the elderly. J Psychosom Res 2004; 56: 479–86.

63. Paine SJ, Gander PH, Harris R, Reid P. Who reports insomnia? Relationships with age, sex, ethnicity, and socioeconomic deprivation. Sleep 2004; 27: 1163–9.

64. Karacan I, Thornby JI, Anch M et al. Prevalence of sleep disturbance in a primarily urban Florida County. Soc Sci Med 1976; 10: 239–44.

65. Whitney CW, Enright PL, Newman AB et al. Correlates of daytime sleepiness in 4578 elderly persons: the Cardiovascular Health Study. Sleep 1998; 21: 27–36.

66. Hicks RA, Lucero-Gorman K, Bautista J, Hicks GJ. Ethnicity, sleep hygiene knowledge, and sleep hygiene practices. Percept Mot Skills 1999; 88: 1095–6.

67. Hicks RA, Lucero-Gorman K, Bautista J, Hicks GJ. Ethnicity, sleep duration, and sleep satisfaction. Percept Mot Skills 1999; 88: 234–5.

68. DiPalma J, Jean-Louis G, Zizi F et al. Self-reported sleep duration among college students: consideration of ethnic differences. Sleep 2001: 24; 430–1.

69. Blazer DG, Hays JC, Foley DJ. Sleep complaints in older adults: a racial comparison. J Gerontol A Biol Sci Med Sci 1995; 50: M280–4.

70. Foley D, Monjan AA, Izmirlian G, Hays JC, Blazer D. Incidence and remission of insomnia among elderly adults in a biracial cohort. Sleep 1999; 22: S377–8.

71. Foley DJ, Monjan AA, Wallace RB, Blazer D. Incidence and remission of insomnia among elderly adults: an epidemiologic study of 6800 persons over three years. Sleep 1999; 22: S366–72.

72. Blazer DG, Landerman LR, Hays JC, Simonsick EM, Saunders WB. Symptoms of depression among community-dwelling elderly African-American and white older adults. Psychol Med 1998; 28: 1311–20.

73. Ancoli-Israel S, Klauber MR, Stepnowsky C et al. Sleep-disordered breathing in African-American elderly. J Gerontol 1989; 44: M18–21.

74. Kripke DF, Ancoli-Israel S, Klauber MR et al. Prevalence of sleep disordered breathing in ages 40–64 years: a population-based survey. Sleep 1997; 20: 65–76.

75. Gottlieb DJ, Whitney CW, Bonekat WH et al. Relation of sleepiness to respiratory disturbance index: the Sleep Heart Health Study. Am J Respir Crit Care Med 1999; 159: 502–7.

76. Young T, Finn L. Epidemiological insights into the public health burden of sleep disordered breathing: sex differences in survival among sleep clinic patients. Thorax 1998; 53 Suppl 3: S16–19.

77. Redline S, Tishler P, Hans M et al. Racial differences in sleep-disordered breathing in African-Americans and Caucasians. Am J Respir Crit Care Med 1997; 155: 186–92.

78. Buxbaum SG, Elston RC, Tishler PV, Redline S. Genetics of the apnea hypopnea index in Caucasians and African Americans: I. Segregation analysis. Genet Epidemiol 2002; 22: 243–53.

79. Colilla S, Rotimi C, Cooper R, Goldberg J, Cox N. Genetic inheritance of body mass index in African-American and African families. Genet Epidemiol 2000; 18: 360–76.

80. Palmer LJ, Buxbaum SG, Larkin E et al. A whole-genome scan for obstructive sleep apnea and obesity. Am J Hum Genet 2003; 72: 340–50.

81. Palmer LJ, Buxbaum SG, Larkin EK et al. Whole genome scan for obstructive sleep apnea and obesity in African-American families. Am J Respir Crit Care Med 2004; 169: 1314–21.

82. The National Commission on Sleep Disorders Research. Wake Up America: A National Sleep Alert. Executive Summary and Executive Report Washington DC: US Government Printing Office 1993.

83. Rosen RC, Zozula R, Jahn EG, Carson JL. Low rates of recognition of sleep disorders in primary care: comparison of a community-based versus clinical academic setting. Sleep Med 2001; 2: 47–55.

84. Penn NE, Kar S, Kramer J, Skinner J, Zambrana RE. Ethnic minorities, health care systems, and behavior. Health Psychol 1995; 14: 641–6.

85. Mayberry RM, Mili F, Ofili E. Racial and ethnic differences in access to medical care. Med Care Res Rev 2000; 57 Suppl 1: 108–45.

86. Silverberg DS, Oksenberg A, Iaina A. Sleep-related breathing disorders as a major cause of essential hypertension: fact or fiction? Curr Opin Nephrol Hypertens 1998; 7: 353–7.

87. Lavie P, Herer P, Hoffstein V. Obstructive sleep apnoea syndrome as a risk factor for hypertension: population study. BMJ 2000; 320: 479–82.

88. Ohayon MM, Guilleminault C, Priest RG, Zulley J, Smirne S. Is sleep-disordered breathing an independent risk factor for hypertension in the general population (13 057 subjects)? J Psychosom Res 2000; 48: 593–601.

89. Young T, Peppard P, Palta M et al. Population-based study of sleep-disordered breathing as a risk factor for hypertension. Arch Intern Med 1997; 157: 1746–52.

90. Jean-Louis G, Zizi F, Casimir G, DiPalma J, Mukherji R. Sleep-disordered breathing and hypertension among African Americans. J Hum Hypertens 2005; 19: 485–90.

91. Kleinman A. Culture and patient care: psychiatry among the Chinese. Drug Therapy 1981; 11: 134–40.

92. Flack JM, Amaro H, Jenkins W, Kunitz S, Levy J, Mixon M, Yu E. Epidemiology of minority health. Health Psychol 1995; 14: 592–600.

93. Partinen M, Kaprio J, Koskenvuo M, Putkonen P, Langinvainio H. Genetic and environmental determination of human sleep. Sleep 1983; 6: 179–85.

94. Mendlewicz J, Kerkhofs M. Sleep electroencephalography in depressive illness. A collaborative study by the World Health Organization. Br J Psychiatry 1991; 159: 505–9.

95. Giles DE, Perlis ML, Reynolds CF, Kupfer DJ. EEG sleep in African-American patients with major depression: a historical case control study. Depress Anxiety 1998; 8: 58–64.

96. Poland RE, Rao U, Lutchmansingh P et al. REM sleep in depression is influenced by ethnicity. Psychiatry Res 1999; 88: 95–105.

97. Rao U, Poland RE, Lutchmansingh P et al. Relationship between ethnicity and sleep patterns in normal controls: implications for psychopathology and treatment. J Psychiatr Res 1999; 33: 419–26.

98. Paradis CM, Friedman S. Sleep paralysis in African Americans with panic disorder. Transcult Psychiatry 2005; 42: 123–34.

99. Omnibus Sleep in America Poll. National Sleep Foundation 2000; 1–19.

100. Jean-Louis G, Magai C, Cohen CI et al. Ethnic differences in reported sleep problems in older adults. Sleep 2001; 24: 926–33.

101. Jean-Louis G, Magai C, Pierre-Louis J et al. Insomnia complaints and repressive coping among Black and White Americans. Sleep 2005; 28: 23.

102. Knight BG, McCallum TJ. Heart rate reactivity and depression in African-American and white dementia caregivers: reporting bias or positive coping? Aging and Mental Health 1998; 2: 212–21.

103. Haley WE, Roth DL, Coleton MI et al. Appraisal, coping, and social support as mediators of well-being in black and white family caregivers of patients with Alzheimer's disease. J Consult Clin Psychol 1996; 64: 121–9.

104. Weinberger DA, Schwartz GE, Davidson RJ. Low-anxious, high-anxious, and repressive coping styles: psychometric patterns and behavioral and physiological responses to stress. J Abnorm Psychol 1979; 88: 369–80.

105. Mendolia M. An index of self-regulation of emotion and the study of repression in social contexts that threaten or do not threaten self-concept. Emotion 2002; 2: 215–32.

106. Mendolia M, Moore J, Tesser A. Dispositional and situational determinants of repression. J Pers Soc Psychol 1996; 70: 856–67.

107. Mendolia M. Repressors' appraisals of emotional stimuli in threatening and nonthreatening positive emotional contexts. Journal of Research in Personality 1999; 33: 1–26.

108. Morin CM, Kowatch RA, Barry T, Walton E. Cognitive-behavior therapy for late-life insomnia. J Consult Clin Psychol 1993; 61: 137–46.

109. Edinger JD, Fins AI, Glenn DM et al. Insomnia and the eye of the beholder: are there clinical markers of objective sleep disturbances among adults with and without insomnia complaints? J Consult Clin Psychol 2000; 68: 586-93.

110. DiPalma J, Jean-Louis G, Zizi F et al. Screening and treatment of obstructive sleep apnea in a Brooklyn-based minority sample. Sleep 25: 2002.

111. The National Comission on Sleep Disorders Research. http://www.stanford.edu/~dement/overview-ncsdr.html. Accessed 20 Feb 2002.

112. Hanlon JT, Fillenbaum GG, Burchett B et al. Drug-use patterns among black and nonblack community-dwelling elderly. Ann Pharmacother 1992; 26: 679–85.

113. Salber EJ, Greene SB, Gagnon P, Jones B. Black/white drug use patterns in rural North Carolina. Comtemp Pharm Pract 1979; 2: 4–11.

114. Blazer D, Hybels C, Simonsick E, Hanlon JT. Sedative, hypnotic, and antianxiety medication

use in an aging cohort over ten years: a racial comparison. J Am Geriatr Soc 2000; 48: 1073–9.

115. Horne J. Why We Sleep: The Functions of Sleep in Humans and Other Mammals. New York: Oxford University Press, 1988.

116. Groeger JA, Zijlstra FR, Dijk DJ. Sleep quantity, sleep difficulties and their perceived consequences in a representative sample of some 2000 British adults. J Sleep Res 2004; 13: 359–71.

117. Curtis S, Lawson K. Gender, ethnicity and self-reported health: the case of African-Caribbean populations in London. Soc Sci Med 2000; 50: 365–85.

118. Brice J. West-Indian families. In: McGoldrick J, Pearce J, Giordano J. eds. Ethnicity and Family Therapy. New York: Guilford Press, 1982: 123–33.

119. Shahar E, Whitney CW, Redline S et al. Sleep-disordered breathing and cardiovascular disease: cross-sectional results of the Sleep Heart Health Study. Am J Respir Crit Care Med 2001; 163: 19–25.

120. Young T, Peppard P. Sleep-disordered breathing and cardiovascular disease: epidemiologic evidence for a relationship. Sleep 2000; 23 Suppl 4: S122–6.

121. Young T, Blustein J, Finn L, Palta M. Sleep-disordered breathing and motor vehicle accidents in a population-based sample of employed adults. Sleep 1997; 20: 608–13.

CHAPTER 3

Sleep-related problems in childhood

Stephen H Sheldon

Sleep is not a unitary event. Identification of specific transition into sleep is often problematic. Sleep onset can be correlated with behavioral and biological changes that occur over a short period of time. However, behaviors typically associated with transitional sleep seen in adults (e.g., eye lids closed, recumbence, quiescence) are often paradoxical during childhood. Behavioral changes also consist of modulation in responsiveness to auditory and visual stimuli, decrease in the ability to perform and complete simple tasks, motor restlessness, mood changes, impulsivity, and varying degrees of attention problems. Although biological changes in electrocardiography (EEG) activity commonly associated with transitional sleep may be recorded, they are typically perceived by the child as sleepiness.[1]

Sleep is heralded by two major electrophysiological events: normal alpha activity on EEG is replaced by a *relatively* low voltage, mixed frequency (RLVMF) pattern; and the appearance of slow, rolling eye movements. There is typically a gradual fall in skeletal muscle tone below that of waking. Engagement with the environment often continues, automatic behaviors can occur, and many children do not perceive stage 1 sleep and will report that they are not sleeping during this period of transition.[2]

A number of groups have examined sleep during adolescence in laboratory studies.[3–7]

When such studies are performed, laboratory constraints may affect outcomes and certainly need to be accounted for when interpreting findings. Early studies used participants' habitual schedules to set bedtimes and rise times, whereas others included a scheduled time in bed (10 p.m. to 8 a.m.) for laboratory sleep. Some studies use a longitudinal approach whereas others use a cross-sectional design. In laboratory studies where sleep schedule varied, total sleep time decreased as puberty advanced. This may be expected due to sleep habits on school nights combined with additional social requirements and responsibilities. Despite differences in methodology, consistent changes in sleep/wake architecture have been reported, including a decrease in slow-wave sleep by nearly 40% from prepubertal to late pubertal adolescents, an increase in the amount of stage 2 sleep and a reduction in the latency to the first episode of rapid eye movement (REM) sleep.[8]

In these studies REM sleep time typically changes according to total sleep time. When total sleep time is reduced, REM sleep as a percentage of the total sleep time is also reduced. On the other hand, REM sleep time was maintained across adolescence when time in bed was held constant.[8] Although total sleep time in the laboratory across ages in this study of 'fixed time in bed' was approximately 9.2 to 9.4 hours, the less mature children (Tanner stages 1 or 2) were more likely to wake sponta-neously before 0800, whereas the more mature adolescents (Tanner stages 3–5) were never spontaneously awake at 0800.[9]

DAYTIME SLEEPINESS

The multiple sleep latency test (MSLT) has become the 'gold standard' of assessment of daytime sleepiness. Rapid sleep onset indicates a greater sleepiness. Increased number of sleep onsets during multiple tests is also consistent with excessive daytime sleepiness. In a lon-gitudinal study using the MSLT, Carskadon assessed developmental changes in daytime sleepiness, and demonstrated a change in the pattern of daytime alertness occurring at mid-puberty.[9] The pre-/early pubertal adolescents did not fall asleep on most of the tests of the MSLT (average latency across all the naps was about 19.5 out of a maximum of 20 minutes), whereas mid-/late pubertal adolescents were more likely to fall asleep during the mid-afternoon tests, and the average sleep latency across all the naps was reduced to about 15 min-utes. Reduction in sleep propensity occurred even though more mature adolescents were sleeping as much as those who were less mature. This finding suggests either adolescents need more sleep than prepubertal children, or that the pattern of symptoms of sleepiness that is similar to adult sleepiness is reorganized during adolescent development.[9]

CHILDREN OF 2 TO 5 YEARS OLD

Normative data and controlled studies of chil-dren in the preschool age group and in the early school years are surprisingly few. In contrast to the dramatic changes that take place during the first year of life, transformations during this period are more gradual. Growth and develop-ment continue in a steady manner. Sleep becomes consolidated into a long nocturnal period of approximately 10 hours.[10–13] During the first 2–3 years, daytime sleep continues, but in discrete, short, daytime naps. The first nap is usually mid-morning, the second occurring early in the afternoon. Gradually, the morning nap is given up, and by 3–5 years of age, sleep is completely consolidated into a single nocturnal period.

During the latter half of the first year of life, REM sleep averages about 30% of the total sleep time. Small and large body movements associ-ated with REM sleep during infancy become less frequent. Periods of REM are approximately uniform in length, despite daytime naps. As the child continues to develop, a gradual change is seen in the uniformity and duration of these REM periods. The first REM period of the night becomes quite short, while succeeding periods tend to become longer and more intense as morning approaches. There is also a slight lengthening of the overall cycle length.[14] Two-to three-year-old children still show a cycle length of about 60 minutes, with the first REM period occurring 1 hour after sleep onset. By 4–5 years of age, the cycle lengthens gradually to 60–90 minutes. The first REM period, how-ever, may be missed in the younger age groups. In these patients, after lightening of the EEG tracing occurs, it again deepens without an intervening REM period. It is only after another cycle of about 60–90 minutes that the first REM period can be actually documented.

Between 2 and 5 years of age, REM percent-age gradually decreases from 30% of the total sleep time to the adult level of 20–25%. There appears to be a close relationship between these changes and the augmented periods of wake-fulness during the daytime. Diminution of REM volume progresses until about 3–4.5 years, when daytime napping has terminated. By this age distinct differences between early and late portions of the sleep period have emerged.[14]

Typically, children in this age range have approximately seven cycles during each noctur-nal sleep period.[13] Sleep onset latency averages about 15 minutes in the younger children, but lengthens to between 15 and 30 minutes in the older children in this developmental grouping. Slow-wave sleep predominantly occurs during the first third of the night[12] and as much as 2 hours may be spent in stage 3 and stage 4; EEG voltage is also very high during this period. Stage 2 first appears from 3 to 4 minutes after the child falls to sleep, stage 3 appears about 11 minutes after sleep onset, and stage 4 first appears about 4 minutes later.[13]

Unique characteristics of sleep occur in this age range which may signify stabilization and balancing of this state. A relatively small number of sleep stage changes is a striking feature.[11] Approximately 3.5 stage shifts per hour occur, which significantly differs from that of the young adult, EEG voltage is consistently higher, and non-REM stage 4 is consistently longer. Another outstanding difference of sleep in this age group is the smooth progression of stages, whether moving deeper (toward stage 4) or moving lighter (toward wake). Transition is regular and consistent, in contrast to the adult pattern where abrupt movements often occur across several stages at a time, with the EEG progressing toward lighter or deeper sleep.[11,12]

CHILDREN OF 5 TO 10 YEARS OLD

Growth and development again are constant, steady, and gradual during middle childhood. This time, however, is not a latent period. It is characterized by activation and change, searching, exploration, and increasingly sophisticated decision making. It is a period of preparation and rehearsal, trials and errors.[15]

Sleep continues to coalesce into an adult pattern. Sleep patterns of children during middle childhood resemble those of older individuals but show considerable individual variability; however, there is an orderly sequence of sleep stages, spontaneously shifting from one stage to another. There is a certain stability of the pattern for a given individual and a fairly consistent amount of time spent in each sleep stage and the number of sleep stages from night to night.[12] When compared with adult sleep patterns, total sleep time in middle childhood is approximately 2.5 hours longer, with unequal distribution of the time added to each of the sleep stages. Stages in children of this age group tend to be of longer duration than in adults, but the sleep architecture seems to be as stable.

Middle childhood is also a time of transition. After an initially long NREM period, some children will exhibit regularly spaced REM periods of quite similar duration (the pattern seen in infancy), while others will reveal a more mature pattern of progressively longer REM periods as sleep progresses.[14] The volume of REM sleep approximates the adult level, which is a considerable decrease in the number of minutes spent in REM sleep when compared to infants and younger children.

Though body movements during sleep decrease in frequency, they are generally more often seen in this age group than in adolescents and young adults. Stage 4 volume decreases from approximately 2 hours in the preschool child to 75–80 minutes in the latter portion of middle childhood.[14] There does appear, however, to be a gender-related difference in slow-wave sleep. Males tend to exhibit a significantly greater volume of slow-wave sleep than females of comparable age.[4,12,16]

Naps during this period of development are very rare. The tendency to sleep during the day seems to be lowest in this age group, and consistent daytime napping during middle childhood often represents a pathological process. Prepubescent children are generally very alert throughout the entire day. Carskadon and coworkers have shown mean sleep onset latencies of pre-adolescent (Tanner stage 1) children to be greater than 15 minutes,[9,15] which is an extremely alert and vigilant level.

In contrast to the sleepless child, the sleepy child often goes undetected. One major factor for delays in seeking medical attention rests in the uncertainty of what constitutes normal sleep.[1] Though normative data are available for many age-related laboratory values, observations of normal amounts of sleep and wakefulness at various ages during childhood are still sparse. Little information is available regarding what constitutes normal daytime alertness and sleepiness during early childhood.

Sleep/wake schedules are usually well established by 6 months of age; daytime napping occurs between 3 and 5 years of age. Nonetheless, acceptable intervals of napping depend to a large extent on social and cultural factors. What is normal for one child may be considered abnormal for another.

The sleepy child is frequently ignored by both parents and health care professionals. Identification is difficult because behaviors associated with sleepiness may be attributed to a variety of other factors. Excessively sleepy children are more commonly recognized after entering school. They may have difficulty participating in normal classroom activities, and can manifest impaired learning.[17] Indeed, symptoms are often first recognized by teachers or other school personnel who pressure parents into obtaining an evaluation because of attention-span problems, learning difficulties, or repeated daytime naps during class. Delays in seeking medical attention have been reported to range from 7 months to 7 years, with an average of 28 months.[1]

Daytime sleepiness and hypersomnia may be caused by a variety of conditions. These include, but are not limited to: narcolepsy, obstructive sleep apnea, idiopathic central nervous system hypersomnia, neurological disorders, seizure disorders, environmental, toxic, and medical problems. They may also be behavioral or conditioned. Only recently have data been collected that assess the effect of primary and/or secondary sleep-related problems as a cause for daytime sleepiness and attention deficits. Sleepiness in both children and adults can be mild, presenting with subtle signs and symptoms, or can be severe. Symptoms may range from brief lapses in concentration, decreased motivation, easy distractibility, frustration, and aggressiveness, to more overt signs of somnolence such as slow speech, bland facial expression, droopy eyelids, and increased effort in movements.

Despite objective signs of sleepiness, the way a child feels or appears may be misleading. The degree of sleepiness is related to a number of factors including: circadian influences; time since the last sleep period; previous quantity, quality, and continuity of sleep; and the level of central nervous system (CNS) stimulation at a given time. **Physiological sleep tendency** refers to the degree to which an individual's CNS is compatible with sleep. The degree of CNS stimulation interacts with this physiological state to determine the degree of subjective sleepiness. **Manifest sleep tendency** is the degree to which sleepiness is experienced or is evident in behavior. Clearly, different individuals with the same physiological sleep tendency may manifest different levels of sleepiness and present with a variety of symptoms.

It should be pointed out that a report of sleepiness is not necessarily the same as high physiological sleep tendency. Frequently, lethargy, malaise, muscular exhaustion, or fatigue may be described as sleepiness. Clearly, being tired and being sleepy are not the same. Given soporific conditions, sleepy patients will manifest their sleepiness; patients who are tired but have a low physiological sleep tendency will not. In general, daytime sleepiness should be considered excessive if subjective symptoms or signs *interfere with normal waking function, social responsibilities, or quality of life.*

Symptoms of sleepiness and drowsiness in children are often confusing. They may overlap and be mistaken for signs and symptoms of other conditions which do not, on the surface, appear to be linked with sleepiness. For example, Weinberg and Brumback[18] have described a **primary disorder of vigilance**, where vigilance is considered to be the state of being watchful, awake, and alert. When vigilance is lost, difficulty sustaining attention occurs, followed by manifestations of motor restlessness (fidgeting and moving about), yawning and stretching, talkativeness, or a combination of symptoms. Motor restlessness has been ascribed to attempts to improve alertness when sitting or standing still, or when involved in tasks requiring continuous mental performance. When prevented from being active, youngsters may stare off, daydream, exhibit motor restlessness, fidget extensively, express decreased attention to current activities, avoid or lose interest in structured repetitive activities, but may not fall asleep.

These symptoms are remarkably similar to those of other described syndromes, such as attention deficit hyperactivity disorder (ADHD). Easy distractibility, difficulty concentrating on school work or other tasks requiring sustained attention, shifting excessively from one activity to another, fidgeting excessively, moving about excessively during sleep, and always 'on the go' are characteristics of ADHD. Extensive data are not available delineating the relationship of objective sleepiness with this symptom complex. However, some evidence is available. Kahn and coworkers[19] have shown that school achievement difficulties are encountered significantly more often among pre-adolescent children who are considered poor sleepers than among children without sleep problems. Their preliminary study suggested the need for more systematic attention by the pediatric practitioner to the possible presence of chronic sleep problems in apparently normal pre-adolescents.

SLEEP–WAKE PATTERNS, SCHOOL PERFORMANCE, AND ADHD

When assessing sleep during childhood and adolescence, focus cannot only be placed on daytime or night-time behavior. Lack of sleep due to imposed sleep restriction can have very significant effects on performance and behavior. Nonetheless, it is now clearly understood that intrinsic sleep disorders (e.g., obstructive sleep apnea syndrome and periodic limb movement disorder) occur during childhood and present with daytime performance problems that are often mistaken for behavioral and/or learning disorders. Effects of primary sleep disorders differ from those seen in adults. Adults often manifest excessive daytime sleepiness by symptoms that are known to be associated with sleepiness. Unintentional sleep episodes during times that are soporific often occur. On the other hand, children are more likely to present with cognitive and behavioral problems, rather than overt symptoms that are associated with sleepiness in adults. Some children show inattentive and hyperactive behavior that leads to a diagnosis of ADHD and treatment with stimulants before the underlying sleep problem is recognized.

Children diagnosed with ADHD commonly exhibit disturbed and restless sleep.[20,21] These sleep abnormalities are typically attributed to stimulant medications, or to persistence of hyperactivity into nocturnal hours. Monitoring of movement in children with ADHD does not demonstrate nocturnal hyperactivity, but does reveal a lack of stability of sleep onset and total sleep time when compared to children without the diagnosis of ADHD.[22] Nocturnal polysomnographic studies of children with diagnosis of ADHD have not identified specific primary sleep disorders related to the diagnosis.[23–25] A review of polysomnographic studies of ADHD,[26] as well as a subsequent video-polysomnographic study,[27] both failed to identify consistent abnormalities. However, these investigations did identify increased movement during sleep. A possibility that primary sleep disorders may underlie or contribute to symptoms of ADHD is rarely considered.[28,29] Nonetheless, increasing evidence suggests that primary sleep disorders might result in inattentive and hyperactive behavior as a manifestation of daytime sleepiness or other underlying processes.

More than 60 years ago, Bradley & Bower[30] showed that stimulants rather than sedatives provide effective treatment for hyperactivity. Sedative medications often worsen hyperactive behaviors. Children with ADHD show lower levels of arousal rather than increased arousal.[31] Multiple sleep latency tests (MSLTs) among 26 children diagnosed with ADHD and 21 matched control children showed increased daytime sleepiness in the ADHD patients.[32] A survey of parents of more than 800 children at general pediatrics clinics suggested a substantial association between sleepiness and behavior that characterizes ADHD.[33]

ADHD symptoms may be due to cognitive changes that occur with disrupted nocturnal sleep and/or excessive sleepiness.[34] One study of 16 children randomized to receive either 5 or 11 hours in bed for one night revealed impairment of verbal creativity and abstract thinking in those with restricted sleep.[35] A larger investigation of 82 children randomized to either 4 or 10 hours of sleep for one night revealed increased inattentive behaviors when they were sleep deprived, but not hyperactive–impulsive behavior or impaired performance on tests of response inhibition and sustained attention.

EVALUATION OF EXCESSIVE DAYTIME SOMNOLENCE (EDS)

Of significant importance is determination of whether a child's presenting symptoms might be related to excessive sleepiness. This is often difficult: extreme degrees of sleepiness may be obvious, but milder degrees are typically harder to detect with clinical evaluation alone.

Discriminating normal from abnormal total sleep requirements is sometimes problematic. During a typical 24-hour period, there should be some cause for concern if the usual total sleep time is 2 hours greater than the average for the child's age. However, this does not always mean the child is pathologically sleepy. A child who sleeps up to 2 hours longer than the average total 24-hour sleep time, but is active and alert during the day, is most likely normal but has a long sleep requirement.[36] Daytime napping decreases significantly after the age of

3 years. By 6 years of age, the need for daytime naps is uncommon. Therefore, continued napping by children during middle childhood is another clue that EDS may be present.

Unlike disorders of initiating and maintaining sleep, behavioral and psychosocial etiologies are less common than biological factors. Evaluation of the child with excessive sleepiness should begin with a comprehensive history and physical examination. Historical information regarding the child's normal sleep–wake pattern should include the following.[37]

- The child's normal bedtime.
- The length of time it takes the child to fall asleep. A truly sleepy child will fall asleep quickly. If the sleep onset latency is prolonged, it may suggest the problem is not due to hypersomnolence, but may be caused by a circadian rhythm disorder or insufficient sleep.
- Total sleep time, which should be compared to the mean volume for the child's age. Nocturnal sleep patterns should be well documented and a sleep diary maintained for a period of 2 weeks will provide more objective information regarding the child's actual sleep–wake pattern.
- Presence of sleep disruptions, interruptions, and snoring. These may indicate a lack of continuity or deprivation of various stages of sleep.
- Daytime behavior and degree of alertness. Symptoms of EDS may include over-activity, attention-span problems, aggressiveness with other children, daydreaming, learning problems, sleep attacks, or frequent napping. Focus should be placed on the length, frequency, time of day, and activities interrupted by naps. The child's behavior and subjective feeling upon waking from naps should also be recorded.

In order to adequately assess the patient with possible EDS, polysomnographic studies are often necessary. Polysomnography can provide information regarding progression of sleep stages across the night, volume of sleep stages, disruptions of architecture by arousals, presence of obstructive sleep-disordered breathing, and/or EEG abnormalities which may suggest seizures or other intracranial pathology. Since it is often difficult to determine whether a child is sleepy just by the way she or he looks or acts, MSLTs may be required to objectively assess the degree of sleepiness.

Several normative studies of sleep in the pre-adolescent child have been published, and Carskadon and colleagues[6] have performed studies on patients during middle childhood similar to those performed on adolescent patients. The most notable feature of the MSLT data was that during middle childhood, patients rarely fell asleep. *Sleep was seen within the 20-minute test period on fewer than one-fourth of the tests.* In those tests where sleep was noted, the children never fell asleep in less than 15 minutes. These data appear to document the extreme level of alertness of children during this developmental period. Children during middle childhood who do have significant sleep tendency on MSLT most likely are indeed excessively sleepy during the daytime, regardless of daytime symptomatology.

During late childhood and early adolescence, bedtimes are commonly delayed and morning wakings are later than those of younger children.[38,39] Social activities, academic responsibilities, and after-school work contribute to this delay in timing of sleep. Biological factors also contribute to later bedtimes and wake times for teens.

Traditionally school starts early in the morning throughout the USA.[41] About half of middle schools and high schools begin at 7:30 a.m. or earlier. This early start seems to be a significant factor contributing to sleeplessness at night and problem sleepiness during the day. Other factors such as late night social activities, work requirements, and early morning school schedules significantly restrict hours available for sleep. Several surveys of high school students found that youngsters who begin class at 7:30a.m. or earlier obtain less total sleep on school nights due to earlier rise times.[40]

Carskadon and colleagues demonstrated significant problems that occur when the school day begins early. A 65-minute advance in school start time was required of 9th grade school children moving into 10th grade.[42] Their findings demonstrated that only 62% of the students in 9th grade and fewer than half the students in 10th grade obtained 7 hours of sleep on school nights. Students woke earlier on school days in 10th grade than in 9th grade; they had shorter sleep latencies on MSLT in 10th than in 9th grade, particularly on the 8:30 a.m. assessment; and 16% of participants experienced two REM episodes on MSLT in 10th grade (one REM episode occurred in 48%). These results strongly suggest that early start times at school may require impractical and infeasible bedtimes for adequate sleep to be obtained. These data have been supported and replicated by other investigations.

SUMMARY AND FUTURE DIRECTIONS FOR RESEARCH

There are clear gaps in knowledge related to the affect of sleep and underlying sleep disorders. More research is required to ascertain the relationship between restricted sleep in otherwise normal children and those children with underlying sleep and/or circadian rhythm disorders. Health outcomes may be significantly affected by disordered sleep. Susceptibility to infection may increase, accidents may become more frequent, school performance can clearly suffer, and mood may be adversely affected by inadequate sleep and/or primary sleep disorders during childhood and adolescence.

The etiology of ADHD and associated sleep disturbances in childhood may be multifactorial and can vary among individuals and groups. In addition to medication-related sleep disturbance and the influence of comorbidity that may be secondary to, or associated with, the sleep disorder, there is considerable evidence that obstructive sleep-disordered breathing in childhood is strongly associated with inattention, hyperactivity, and impaired cognitive function, which results in disruptive behaviors. Treatment of the sleep-related breathing disorder results in significant improvement or complete resolution of the symptoms. Other primary sleep disorders (e.g., periodic limb movement disorder, circadian rhythm disorders, narcolepsy syndrome) may present with identical symptoms. It is clear that a relationship exists and future investigation into similarities and differences in sleep patterns and architecture in these youngsters is imperative. Symptoms of inattention and hyperactivity may result from a final common pathway that intimately involves sleep-related pathophysiology.

REFERENCES

1. Agnew HW, Webb WB. Measurement of sleep onset by EEG criteria. Am J EEG Technol 1972; 12: 127.

2. Carskadon MA, Dement WC. Normal human sleep: an overview. In: Kryger MH, Roth T, Dement WC, eds. Principles and Practice of Sleep Medicine. Philadelphia, PA: WB Saunders, 1989.

3. Karacan I, Anch M, Thornby JI, Okawa M, Williams RL. Longitudinal sleep patterns during pubertal growth: four-year follow up. Pediatr Res 1975; 9: 842–6.

4. Coble PA, Kupfer DJ, Taska LS, Kane J. EEG sleep of normal healthy children. Part I: findings using standard measurement methods. Sleep 1984; 7: 289–303.

5. Carskadon MA. The second decade. In: Guilleminault C, ed. Sleeping and Waking Disorders: Indications and Techniques. Menlo Park, CA: Addison-Wesley, 1982: 99–125.

6. Carskadon MA, Orav EJ, Dement WC. Evolution of sleep and daytime sleepiness in adolescents. In: Guilleminault C, Lugaresi E, eds. Sleep/ Wake Disorders: Natural History, Epidemiology, and Long-term Evolution. New York, NY: Raven Press, 1983: 201–16.

7. Gaudreau H, Carrier J, Montplasier J. Age-related modifications of NREM sleep EEG: from childhood to middle age. J Sleep Res 2001; 10: 165–72.

8. Carskadon MA, Acebo C, Fallone G. Morningness/ eveningness (M/E), phase angle, sleep restriction, and MSLT: a pilot study in adolescents [Abstract]. Sleep 2002; 25(Suppl): A127–8.

9. Carskadon MA, Harvey K, Duke F, et al. Pubertal changes in daytime sleepiness 1980. Sleep 2002; 25: 453–60.

10. Mattison RE, Handford HA, Vela-Bueno A. Sleep disorders in children. Psychiatr Med 1987; 4: 149.

11. Kohler WC, Coddington D, Agnew HW. Sleep patterns in 2-year-old children. J Pediatr 1968; 72: 228.

12. Ross JJ, Agnew HW Jr, Williams RL, Webb WB. Sleep patterns in pre-adolescent children: An EEG-EOG study. Pediatrics 1968; 42: 324.

13. Williams RL, Karacan I, Hursch CJ. Electroencephalography (EEG) of Human Sleep: Clinical Applications. New York: John Wiley & Sons, 1975.

14. Roffwarg HP, Dement WC, Fisher C. Preliminary observations of the sleep-dream pattern in neonates, infants, children, and adults. In: Harms E, ed. Problems of Sleep and Dreams in Children. New York: Macmillan, 1964: 000–000.

15. Levine ME: Middle childhood. In: Levine ME, Carey WB, Crocker AC, Gross RT eds. Developmental-Behavioral Pediatrics. Philadelphia, PA: WB Saunders, 1983.

16. Carskadon MA, Keenan S, Dement WC. Nighttime sleep and daytime sleep tendency in preadolescents. In: Guilleminault C, ed. Sleep and its Disorders in Children. New York: Raven Press, 1987: 000–000.

17. Carskadon MA, Dement WC. Normal human sleep: an overview. In: Kryger MH, Roth T, Dement WC, eds. Principles and Practice of Sleep Medicine. Philadelphia, PA: WB Saunders, 1989: 000–000.

18. Weinberg WA, Brumback RA. Primary disorder of vigilance: a novel explanation of inattentiveness, daydreaming, boredom, restlessness, and sleepiness. J Pediatr 1990; 116: 720–5.

19. Kahn A, Van de Merckt C, Rebuffat E, et al. Sleep problems in healthy preadolescents. Pediatrics 1989; 84: 542–46.

20. Ring A, Stein D, Barak Y, et al. Sleep disturbances in children with attention-deficit/ hyperactivity disorder: a comparative study with healthy siblings. J Learn Disab 1998; 31: 572–8.

21. Marcotte AC, Thacher PV, Butters M, et al. Parental report of sleep problems in children with attentional and learning disorders. J Devel Behav Pediatr 1998; 19: 178–86.

22. Gruber R, Sadeh A, Raviv A. Instability of sleep patterns in children with attention-deficit/hyperactivity disorder. J Am Acad Child Adolescent Psychiatry 2000; 39: 495–501.

23. Greenhill L, Puig-Antich J, Goetz R, Hanlon C, Davies M. Sleep architecture and REM sleep measures in prepubertal children with attention deficit disorder with hyperactivity. Sleep 1983; 6: 91–101.

24. Small A, Hibi S, Feinberg I. Effects of dextroamphetamine sulfate on EEG sleep patterns of hyperactive children. Arch Gen Psychiatry 1971; 25: 369–80.

25. Platon MJR, Bueno AV, Sierra JE, Kales S. Hypnopolygraphic alterations in attention deficit disorder (ADD) children. Intern J Neurosci 1990; 53: 87–101.

26. Corkum P, Tannock R, Moldofsky H. Sleep disturbances in children with attention-deficit/hyperactivity disorder. J Am Acad Child Adolescent Psychiatry 1998; 37: 637–46.

27. Konofal E, Lecendreux M, Bouvard M, Mouren-Simeoni MC. High levels of nocturnal activity in children with attention-deficit hyperactivity disorder: a video analysis. Psychiat Clin Neurosci 2001; 55: 97–103.

28. Chervin RD. Attention-deficit–hyperactivity disorder: Letter to the Editor. N Engl J Med 1999; 340: 1766–6.

29. Yuen KM, Pelayo R. Sleep disorders and attention-deficit/hyperactivity disorder. J Am Med Assoc 1999; 281: 797.

30. Bradley C, Bowen M. Amphetamine (benzedrine) therapy of children's behavior disorders. Am J Orthopsychiat 1941; 11: 92–103.

31. Satterfield JH, Cantwell DP, Satterfield BT. Pathophysiology of the hyperactive child syndrome. Arch Gen Psychiatry 1974; 31: 839–44.

32. Lecendreux M, Konofal E, Bouvard M, Falissard B, Mouren-Simeoni MC. Sleep and alertness in children with ADHD. J Child Psychol Psychiatry 2000; 41: 803–12.

33. Chervin RD, Archbold KH, Dillon JE, et al. Inattention, hyperactivity, and symptoms of sleep-disordered breathing. Pediatrics 2002; 109: 449–56.

34. Barkley RA. Genetics of childhood disorders: XVII. ADHD, part 1: the executive functions and ADHD. J Am Acad Child Adolescent Psychiatry 2000; 39: 1064–8.

35. Randazzo AC, Muehlbach MJ, Schweitzer PK, Walsh JK. Cognitive function following acute sleep restriction in children ages 10–14. Sleep 1998; 21: 861–8.

36. Ferber, R. Solve Your Child's Sleep Problems. New York: Simon and Schuster, 1985: 214–32.

37. Sheldon SH. Disorders of initiating and maintaining sleep. In: Sheldon SH, Ferber R, Kryger MH, eds. Principles and Practices of Pediatric Sleep Medicine. Philadelphia, PA: Elsevier/Saunders, 2005: 127–60.

38. Millman RP. Working Group on Sleepiness in Adolescents/Young Adults, AAP Committee on Adolescence. Excessive sleepiness in adolescents and young adults: causes, consequences, and treatment strategies. Pediatrics 2005; 115: 1774–86.

39. Wolfson AR, Carskadon MA. Sleep schedules and daytime functioning in adolescents. Child Devel 1998; 69: 875–87.

40. Carskadon MA. Factors influencing sleep patterns of adolescents. In: Adolescent Sleep Patterns: Biological, Social, and Psychological Influences. Cambridge: Cambridge University Press, 2002: 4–26.

41. Nudel M. The schedule dilemma. Am School B J 1993; 180: 37–40.

42. Carskadon MA, Wolfson AR, Acebo C, Tzischinsky O, Seifer R. Adolescent sleep patterns, circadian timing, and sleepiness at a transition to early school days. Sleep 1998; 21: 871–81.

CHAPTER 4

Impact of sleep-disordered breathing on quality of life and school performance in children

Nira A Goldstein

Pediatric sleep-disordered breathing (SDB) is viewed as a continuum of severity from partial obstruction of the upper airway producing snoring, to increased upper airway resistance to continuous episodes of complete upper airway obstruction or obstructive sleep apnea (OSA). Although the prevalence of primary snoring in children is 12%, the prevalence of OSA is 1–3%.[1] Children with SDB are usually brought to medical attention because of snoring and night-time breathing difficulties. Over the past decade, there has been an increasing awareness of the quality of life impact of pediatric SDB as well as its impact on daytime function. This chapter reviews the published studies that have evaluated the quality of life and school performance of children with SDB.

HEALTH-RELATED QUALITY OF LIFE

Outcomes research utilizes patient-based assessments to evaluate health-related quality of life (HRQL). An HRQL survey focuses on the physical problems, functional limitations, and emotional consequences of a disease. Surveys are self-administered questionnaires composed of items grouped into domains that reflect a particular focus of attention. A survey is designed to

discriminate among individuals who have a better quality of life from those who have a worse quality of life, and/or to evaluate how much quality of life has changed after a particular intervention. Two disease-specific HRLQ surveys, the Obstructive Sleep Apnea-18 (OSA-18) and the Obstructive Sleep Disorders-6 (OSD-6), have been found to be psychometrically reliable, valid, and responsive to longitudinal change.[2–6] The OSA-18 has been validated against nap polysomnography and has been widely used and accepted by other investigators.

Change scores of < 0.5 indicate trivial change, ≥ 0.5 to 0.9 indicate small change, 1.0 to 1.4 indicate moderate change, and ≥ 1.5 indicate large change. The OSA-18 consists of 18 items divided into five domains: sleep disturbance, physical suffering, emotional distress, daytime problems, and caregiver concerns. The OSD-6 consists of six domains represented by a single question designed to reflect the global impact of the symptom cluster: physical suffering, sleep disturbance, speech and swallowing difficulties, emotional distress, activity limitations, and caregiver concern. Another disease-specific HRLQ survey, the Tonsil and Adenoid Health Status Instrument, is also fully validated and is divided into subscales based on different types of problems caused by tonsil and adenoid disease: infection, airway and breathing, behavior, swallowing, health care utilization, and cost of care.[7]

Eleven outcomes studies evaluated disease-specific quality of life in children with SDB (Table 4.1). In five studies, the diagnosis of SDB was made clinically,[2,3,6,14,15] while in six studies the children were diagnosed by polysomnography (PSG).[4,8,9,11–13] In general, the impact of the children's SDB was moderate or large for 70% of the children. The domains most affected were sleep disturbance, physical symptoms, and caregiver concerns.

Eight studies have evaluated disease-specific improvements in the quality of life of children with SDB after adenotonsillectomy (T&A) using the OSA-18 or the OSD-6. A large improvement in quality of life was found in seven studies, while a moderate improvement was found in one study. Significant improvements were found for the total score and all the individual domains. In seven of the studies, the improvements were demonstrated in the short term, 6 months or less. Mitchell et al.[11] found that the improvements persisted at 12-month follow-up although some symptoms recurred. Stewart et al.[9] administered the Tonsil and Adenoid Health Status Instrument to 47 children, 31 of whom had positive PSG at enrollment and 6 months later. There was a significant improvement in the airway and breathing subscale in the 24 children who underwent T&A as compared to the five children whose parents refused surgery. There were also significant improvements in the infection, swallowing, and behavior subscales.

There have been four studies evaluating global quality of life in children with SDB. McLaughlin Crabtree et al.[10] administered the PedsQL™ 4.0 and the Children's Depressive Inventory to 85 children referred to the sleep laboratory for suspected SDB, 44 of whom were obese (body mass index ≥95th percentile for age) and 35 controls. The children with SDB, both obese and non-obese, had significantly lower scores on both the parent- and child-reported total PedsQL scores

and all the individual subscales (physical health, emotional functioning, social functioning, and school functioning) compared to controls. Depressive symptoms were also significantly higher in both SDB groups than the control group. The children with suspected SDB were divided into primary snorers and SDB based on overnight PSG. There were no significant differences in the PedsQL and depressive inventory scores between the primary snorers and the children with SDB, indicating that snoring alone may not be completely benign.

Rosen et al.[16] administered the Child Health Questionnaire (CHQ-PF50) and performed overnight home sleep studies on 298 children of index families identified because one member had laboratory-confirmed sleep apnea and community control families. Significant differences were found in overall physical health and complaints of bodily pain in children with generally mild levels of SDB as compared to control children. Flanary[14] evaluated global quality of life using the Children's Health Questionnaire Parent Form-28 (CHQ-PF28) before and after T&A. Although there were significant improvements in the physical summary parameter, there was no significant improvement in the psychosocial scores. Stewart et al.[9] also administered the CHQ-PF28 in their study. There were significant improvements in the behavior and parental impact-emotional subscales in the T&A children as compared to the control children, but there were no significant improvements in the physical functioning subscale or the remainder of the psychosocial scores.

None of the studies were randomized to T&A versus no surgery, as ethical considerations precluded the performance of such a study. Only Stewart et al.[9] had a control group of children with SDB who did not undergo T&A, but the numbers were small. Tran et al.[8] included a control group of children without a history of snoring or SDB who were undergoing unrelated elective surgery, and the improvements in the OSA-18 survey scores were significant

Table 4.1 Impact of tonsillectomy and adenoidectomy (T&A) on quality of life in children with sleep-disordered breathing (SDB)

Author	Year	Design	n	Mean age in years (SD or range)	Instrument	Mean follow-up in months (SD or range)	Initial survey score, mean (SD or CI)[a]	Change score, mean (SD or CI)[b]	p-value for change
Tran et al.[8]	2005	Prospective cohort, control group underwent unrelated surgery	42 study 41 control	5.8 (2.5) 7.3 (3.8)	OSA-18	5.4 (1.9) 5.3 (1.4)	4.0 (1.2) 1.5 (0.5)	2.5 (1.2) −0.07 (0.62)	<0.001
Stewart et al.[9]	2005	Prospective cohort, control group of children whose parents refused T&A	24 study 5 control	8.1 6–12	T&A Health Status – airway subscale[c]	6.0	58.8 (23.4) for all patients	51.9 study −3.8 control	0.002
					CHQ-PF28[d]	—	92.8 (18.3) for all patients	5.6 study −8.0 control	0.10
McLaughlin Crabtree et al.[10]	2004	Prospective cohort	44 SDB Obese 41 SDB 31 control	10.1 (1.5) 10.2 (1.4) 9.6 (0.9)	PedsQL™ 4.0[e]	—	55.93 (16.5) 63.62 (19.1) 86.43 (11.2)	—	—
Mitchell et al.[11]	2004	Prospective cohort	34	6.7 (3.0–16.8)	OSA-18	12.4	4.3 (2.5–4.6)	2.3 (2.0–2.6)	<0.001
Mitchell et al.[13]	2004	Prospective cohort	60	7.1 (3–12)	OSA-18	4.2	4.0	2.0 (1.6–2.4)	<0.002
Mitchell & Kelly[12]	2004	Prospective cohort	29	7.1 (1.4–17.0)	OSA-18	1.8	4.3 (4.0–5.3)	2.5	<0.0001
Flanary[14]	2003	Prospective cohort	55	6 (1–16)	CHQ-PF28[f] OSA-18	6.0	41.7 (13.9) 4.22 (0.95)	9.4 2.14	0.002 <0.001

(continued)

Table 4.1 (Continued)

Author	Year	Design	n	Mean age in years (SD or range)	Instrument	Mean follow-up in months (SD or range)	Initial survey score, mean (SD or CI)[a]	Change score, mean (SD or CI)[b]	p-value for change
Sohn & Rosenfeld[6]	2003	Prospective cohort	69	6.1 (0.6–13)	OSA-18	1.0	3.1(0.9)	1.14 (0.71)	<0.001
Goldstein et al.[15]	2002	Prospective cohort	64	5.8 (3.1)	OSA-18	3.0	3.9 (1.5)	2.3 (1.9–2.7)	<0.001
de Serres et al.[3]	2002	Prospective cohort	101	6.2 (2.5)	OSD-6	1.2 (0.49)	3.6 (1.0)	2.3 (2.1–2.6)	<0.001
Rosen et al.[16]	2002	Observational	20 severe SDB	11.1 (3.5)	CHQ-PF50[g]	—	76.8 (6.2)	—	—
			25 moderate SDB				85.2 (6.1)		
			50 obstructive symptoms				80.7 (16.1)		
			203 control				88.3 (14.5)		
de Serres et al.[2]	2000	Prospective cohort	100	6.2 (2.1–12.9)	OSD-6	1	4.5 (median)	3.0 (2.7–3.4)	—
Franco et al.[4]	2000	Prospective cohort	61	4 (1–12)	OSA-18	—	3.9 (median)	—	—

[a]The items on the OSA-18 and OSD-6 are both scored on a 7-point ordinal scale: the OSA-18 from 1 to 7 assessing the frequency of the specific symptom while the OSD-6 is scored from 0 to 6 assessing the severity of the symptom.

[b]Change scores for the OSA-18 and OSD-6 are calculated by subtracting the postoperative mean survey score from the preoperative mean survey score. Change scores range from –7.0 to 7.0, with negative numbers indicating deterioration and positive numbers indicating improvement in quality of life. Change scores of <0.5 indicate trivial change, 0.5 to 0.9 indicate small change, 1.0 to 1.4 indicate moderate change, and ≥1.5 indicate large change.

[c]The Tonsil and Adenoid Health Status Instrument airway and breathing subscale.

[d]The Child Health Questionnaire-version PF28 (CHQ-PF28) physical functioning subscale.

[e]The PedsQL™ 4.0 total parent-reported score.

[f]The CHQ-PF28 Physical Summary Score.

[g]The Child Health Questionnaire (CHQ-PF50) global general health score.

for the OSA children as compared to the control children.

SCHOOL PERFORMANCE

Behavioral and neurocognitive difficulties have been found in 8.5–63% of children with SDB.[8,15–20] The mechanisms responsible for neurocognitive impairment are largely unknown, but intermittent hypoxia, sleep fragmentation, and alveoloar hypoventilation resulting in hypercarbia are considered integral to their development.[21] Children with primary snoring but otherwise normal sleep study indices (obstructive apnea index of <1/h, apnea/hypopnea index [AHI] of <5/h, and no gas exchange abnormalities) have also been shown to have lower scores on measures of behavior and cognition using a battery of neurobehavioral tests as compared to control children, although the mean scores for both groups were still in the normal range.[22] Six studies using standardized behavioral and neurocognitive assessments have documented significant improvements in test scores after T&A in children with SDB, suggesting that neurocognitive deficits are potentially reversible.[5,8,15,17,23,24]

Studies evaluating the school performance of children with SDB are presented in Table 4.2. Five studies have demonstrated impaired academic performance in children with SDB. Montgomery-Downs et al.[29] collected validated questionnaires evaluating sleep and school performance from parents of 1010 disadvantaged preschoolers. Based on responses to questions about habitual snoring, 22% of the children were deemed to be at increased risk for SDB. The children at risk were significantly more likely to be sleepy during the day and less likely to rank higher-than-average for school performance than those not at risk.

Urschitz et al.[30] performed another cross-sectional study of 1144 third grade children who were evaluated by nocturnal pulse oximetry and whose parents completed an SDB questionnaire. Poor academic performance was based on the last school report. Although parental reports of snoring were significantly associated with poor academic performance, intermittent hypoxia was not independently associated with poor academic performance. In a follow-up study of 995 primary school children using similar methodology, Urschitz et al.[26] found that the nadir oxygen saturation was the only pulse oximetry variable significantly related to impaired school performance with a significant relationship between the degree of desaturation and impaired performance.

Goodwin et al.[18] performed a prospective study of 239 elementary school children who underwent a home PSG and whose parents completed a sleep habits questionnaire. Parental report of learning problems was significantly associated with a respiratory disturbance index (RDI) ≥ 5, or an RDI ≥ 1 with an associated 3% oxygen desaturation. The same group prospectively evaluated 149 elementary school children with home PSG and a cognitive evaluation using a battery of standardized tests. The children with an AHI ≥ 5 had weaker learning and memory than the group with an AHI < 5. Sleep fragmentation was negatively related to learning and memory. There was a negative relationship between AHI and memory, IQ, and math achievement. Hypoxemia was associated with a lower performance IQ.[28]

In contrast to the above studies, Chervin et al.[27] performed a cross-sectional study of 145 children in the second and fifth grades. Parents completed the SDB subscale of the Pediatric Sleep Questionnaire and teachers rated school performance using a 5-point scale. In a multiple regression model, poor school performance was predicted by low socioeconomic scores but not by SDB risk. Using similar methodology, Carvalho et al.[25] evaluated 79 children aged 8 years with SDB, 468 children with nonrespiratory sleep disorders, and 633 normal children. There was no significant difference in cognition between groups although first grade children with SDB who studied in the morning

Table 4.2 Impact of sleep-disordered breathing (SDB) on school performance in children

Author	Year	Design	n	Mean age in years (SD or range)	Methods	Results
Carvalho et al.[25]	2005	Prospective cohort	79 SDB 468 non-respiratory 633 normal	8.46 (1.08) 8.40 (1.10) 8.40 (1.09)	SDB and non-respiratory sleep disorders defined by Sleep Disturbance Scale for Children, cognition assessed by Bender Visual Motor Gestalt Test	No significant difference in cognition between groups, but 1st grade children with SDB who studied in the morning had higher odds for cognitive dysfunction than normals. Increasing odds of cognitive dysfunction with age in children with SDB
Urschitz et al.[26]	2005	Cross-sectional	995 primary school children	9.6 (0.7)	Children underwent nocturnal home pulse oximetry. Impaired academic performance in mathematics based on last school report	Nadir SpO$_2$[a] values only variable significantly associated with impaired performance with a significant relationship between degree of desaturation and impaired performance
Chervin et al.[27]	2003	Cross-sectional	145 children in 2nd & 5th grades	8.1 (0.4) & 11.1 (0.4)	Parents completed SDB subscale of Pediatric Sleep Questionnaire, teachers rated performance using 5-point scale, & scores from Wayne RESA Benchmark reading and math assessment obtained	In multiple regression models, poor school performance predicted by low socioeconomic score but not by SDB risk

(continued)

Table 4.2 (Continued)

Author	Year	Design	n	Mean age in years (SD or range)	Methods	Results
Goodwin et al.[18]	2003	Prospective cohort	239 elementary school children	6–11	Parents completed sleep habits questionnaire & unattended home PSG performed	Parent report of learning problem was significantly associated with RDI[b] ≥5 or RDI ≥1 with a 3% oxygen desaturation
Kaemingk et al.[28]	2003	Prospective cohort	149 elementary school children	8.36 (1.69)	All children evaluated by Wechsler Abbreviated Scale of Intelligence (WASI), Woodcock–Johnson Psycho-Educational Battery (WJ-R), the Children's Auditory Verbal Learning Test-2, and unattended home PSG. Parents completed Conners' Parent Rating Scale	Group with AHI[c] ≥5 (n=77) had weaker learning and memory than group with AHI <5 (n=72). Sleep fragmentation negatively related to learning and memory. Negative relationship between AHI and memory, IQ, and maths achievement. Hypoxemia associated with lower performance IQ
Montgomery-Downs et al.[29]	2003	Cross-sectional	1010 disadvantaged preschoolers	4.2 (0.53)	Parents completed questionnaires evaluating sleep and school performance	22% of children found to be at risk for SDB. This group was significantly more likely to be sleepy during the day and less likely to rank higher than average for school performance than those not at risk
Urschitz et al.[30]	2003	Cross-sectional	1144 3rd grade children	9.6 (0.7)	All children underwent home nocturnal pulse oximetry. Parents completed SDB	Snoring always was significantly associated with poor academic performance in maths, science, and spelling while snoring

(continued)

Table 4.2 (Continued)

Author	Year	Design	n	Mean age in years (SD or range)	Methods	Results
					questionnaire. Poor academic performance based on last school report	frequently was associated with poor performance in maths and spelling. Intermittent hypoxia did not show an independent association with poor academic performance
Gozal & Pope[31]	2001	Prospective cohort	791 7th & 8th grade children in top 25% (HP) of class and 797 in bottom 25% (LP) of class matched to HP[d]	13 to 14	Parents completed SDB and school performance questionnaire	Snoring in early childhood significantly more common in LP group than HP group (12.9% vs. 5.1%, $p < 0.00001$) but no significant difference in current snoring. Significantly more LP children had history of T&A[e] for SDB than HP children
Gozal[32]	1998	Prospective cohort, control group refused T&A	297 1st grade children in lowest 10th percentile, 54 with SDB, 24 T&A, 30 controls	1st grade	Parents completed SDB questionnaire and children underwent overnight pulse oximetry and transcutaneous CO_2 measurement. Academic grades obtained for school year preceding and school year after enrollment	297 studied and 54 demonstrated sleep associated gas exchange abnormalities. Mean grades increased significantly in study patients but not controls

[a]SpO_2=oxygen saturation; [b]RDI=respiratory disturbance index; [c]AHI=apnea/hypopnea index; [d]HP=high performance; LP=low performance; [e]T&A=adenotonsillectomy.

had higher odds of cognitive dysfunction than normals.

Only one study has evaluated improvement in academic performance after T&A. Gozal[32] evaluated 297 first grade children in the lowest 10th percentile of their class by overnight pulse oximetry and transcutaneous CO_2 measurement. Fifty-four children demonstrated sleep-associated gas exchange abnormalities of whom 24 underwent T&A. The mean grades of the children who underwent surgery increased significantly during the following academic year as compared to the children whose parents refused surgery. There was no academic improvement in the children with primary snoring and the children without SDB. These findings suggest that neurocognitive difficulties found in children with SDB are reversible with treatment.

To further evaluate the long-term impact of SDB in early childhood, Gozal and Pope[31] mailed questionnaires to the parents of seventh and eighth graders whose school performance was in the top 25% of the class or bottom 25% of the class, and who were matched for age, gender, race, school, and street of residence. Responses were obtained from 791 high performance children and 797 low performance children. Snoring in early childhood was significantly more common in the low performance group than the high performance group, but there was no significant difference in current snoring. Significantly more low performance children had a history of T&A for SDB than high performance children. The findings suggest that the neurocognitive impairments of pediatric SDB may not be fully reversible, especially if they occur during a critical period of brain development.

CONCLUSIONS

There is mounting evidence that SDB in children significantly impairs health-related quality of life and school performance. A few, mostly uncontrolled, studies document improvements after treatment by T&A, although it is not known whether the neurocognitive deficits are completely reversible. Larger, controlled prospective studies are needed to fully evaluate the daytime morbidities associated with pediatric SDB, determine the outcomes after treatment, and develop strategies to allow for their early recognition.

REFERENCES

1. Ali NJ, Pitson DJ, Stradling JR. Snoring, sleep disturbance, and behavior in 4–5 year olds. Arch Dis Child 1993; 68: 360–6.
2. de Serres LM, Derkay C, Astley S et al. Measuring quality of life in children with obstructive sleep disorders. Arch Otolaryngol Head Neck Surg 2000; 126: 1423–9.
3. de Serres LM, Derkay C, Sie K et al. Impact of adenotonsillectomy on quality of life in children with obstructive sleep disorders. Arch Otolaryngol Head Neck Surg 2002; 128: 489–96.
4. Franco RA, Rosenfeld RM, Rao M. Quality of life for children with obstructive sleep apnea. Otolaryngol Head Neck Surg 2000; 123: 9–16.
5. Goldstein NA, Post JC, Rosenfeld RM, Campbell TF. Impact of tonsillectomy and adenoidectomy on child behavior. Arch Otolaryngol Head Neck Surg 2000; 126: 494–8.
6. Sohn H, Rosenfeld RM. Evaluation of sleep-disordered breathing in children. Otolaryngol Head Neck Surg 2003; 128: 344–52.
7. Stewart MG, Friedman EF, Sulek M et al. Validation of an outcomes instrument for tonsil and adenoid disease. Arch Otolaryngol Head Neck Surg 2001; 127: 29–35.
8. Tran KD, Nguyen CD, Weedon J, Goldstein NA, Child behavior and quality of life in pediatric obstructive sleep apnea. Arch Otolaryngol Head Neck Surg 2005; 131: 52–7.
9. Stewart MG, Glaze DG, Friedman EM, O'Brian Smith E, Bautista M, Quality of life and sleep study findings after adenotonsillectomy in children with obstructive sleep apnea. Arch Otolaryngol Head Neck Surg 2005; 131: 308–14.
10. McLaughlin Crabtree V, Varni JW, Gozal D. Health-related quality of life and depressive symptoms in children with suspected sleep-disordered breathing. Sleep 2004; 27: 1131–8.

11. Mitchell RB, Kelly J, Call E, Yao N. Long-term changes in quality of life after surgery for pediatric obstructive sleep apnea. Arch Otolaryngol Head Neck Surg 2004; 130: 409–12.

12. Mitchell RB, Kelly J, Call E, Yao N. Quality of life after adenotonsillectomy for obstructive sleep apnea in children. Arch Otolaryngol Head Neck Surg 2004; 130: 190–4.

13. Mitchell RB, Kelly J, Outcome of adenotonsillectomy for severe obstructive sleep apnea syndrome. Int J Pediatr Otorhinolaryngol 2004; 68: 1375–9.

14. Flanary VA. Long-term effect of adenotonsillectomy on quality of life in pediatric patients. Laryngoscope 2003; 113: 1639–44.

15. Goldstein NA, Fatima M, Campbell TF, Rosenfeld RM. Child behavior and quality of life before and after tonsillectomy. Arch Otolaryngol Head Neck Surg 2002; 128: 770–5.

16. Rosen CL, Palermo TM, Larkin EK, Redline S. Health-related quality of life and sleep-disordered breathing in children. Sleep 2002; 25: 657–66.

17. Avior G, Fishman G, Leor A, Sivan Y, Kaysar N, Derowe A. The effect of tonsillectomy and adenoidectomy on inattention and impulsivity as measured by the Test of Variables of Attention (TOVA) in children with obstructive sleep apnea syndrome. Otolaryngol Head Neck Surg 2004; 131: 367–71.

18. Goodwin JL, Kaemingk KL, Fregosi RF et al. Clinical outcomes associated with sleep-disordered breathing in Caucasian and Hispanic children – the Tucson children's assessment of sleep apnea study (TuCASA). Sleep 2003; 26: 587–91.

19. Owens J, Opipari L, Nobile C, Spirito A. Sleep and daytime behavior in children with obstructive sleep apnea and behavioral sleep disorders. Pediatrics 1998; 102: 1178–84.

20. Rosen CL, Storfer-Isser A, Taylor HG. et al. Increased behavioral morbidity in school-aged children with sleep-disordered breathing. Pediatrics 2004; 114: 1640–8.

21. O'Brien LM, Gozal D. Behavioural and neurocognitive implications of snoring and obstructive sleep apnoea in children: facts and theory. Paediatr Respir Rev 2002; 3: 3–9.

22. O'Brien LM, Mervis CB, Holbrook CR et al. Neurobehavioral implications of habitual snoring in children. Pediatrics 2004; 114: 44–9.

23. Ali NJ, Pitson D, Stradling JR. Sleep disordered breathing: effects of adenotonsillectomy on behaviour and psychological functioning. Eur J Pediatrics 1996; 155: 56–62.

24. Owens J, Spirito A, Marcotte A, McGuinn M, Berkelhammer L. Neuropsychological and behavioral correlates of obstructive sleep apnea syndrome in children: a preliminary study. Sleep and Breathing 2000; 4: 67–77.

25. Carvalho LBC, Prado LF Silva L et al. Cognitive dysfunction in children with sleep-disordered breathing. J Child Neurol 2005; 20: 400–4.

26. Urschitz MS, Wolff J, Sokollik C et al. Nocturnal arterial oxygen saturation and academic performance in a community sample of children. Pediatrics 2005; 115: e204–e9.

27. Chervin RD, Clarke DF, Huffman JL. School performance, race, and other correlates of sleep-disordered breathing in children. Sleep Medicine 2003; 4: 21–7.

28. Kaemingk KL, Pasvogel AE, Goodwin JL et al. Learning in children and sleep disordered breathing: Findings of the Tucson children's assessment of sleep apnea (TuCASA) prospective cohort study. J Invest Neurosci 2003; 9: 1016–26.

29. Montgomery-Downs HE, Jones VF, Molfese VJ, Gozal D. Snoring in preschoolers: associations with sleepiness, ethnicity, and learning. Clin Pediatr 2003; 42: 719–26.

30. Urschitz MS, Guenther A, Eggebrecht E et al. Snoring, intermittent hypoxia and academic performance in primary school children. Am J Respir Crit Care Med 2003; 168: 464–8.

31. Gozal D, Pope DW. Snoring during early childhood and academic performance at ages thirteen to fourteen years. Pediatrics 2001; 107: 1394–9.

32. Gozal D. Sleep-disordered breathing and school performance in children. Pediatrics 1998; 102: 616–20.

CHAPTER 5

Sleep in aging

Andrew A Monjan

Sleep is essential to our well-being and occupies about a third of our lives. Without enough of it, we are subject to fatigue, clouded thinking, and diminished quality of life. For older people, these symptoms can be more than a matter of discomfort; they can lead to more serious complications. Falls resulting from fatigue and confusion, for example, can result in debilitating, costly injuries in this vulnerable population. The importance of recognizing and treating age-associated health problems, such as sleep disorders, takes on a new dimension as the USA's elderly population grows to record numbers. In the next 50 years, the aged will make up a progressively greater proportion of the general population (Figure 5.1).

Many older people are very healthy and have normal sleep. Many people believe that poor sleep is a normal part of aging, but it is not. In fact, many healthy older adults report few or no sleep problems. Sleep patterns change as we age, but disturbed sleep and waking up tired everyday are not part of normal aging. However, many older adults have sleep problems, which are often linked to underlying medical conditions. Abnormal sleep can cause disease but diseases can cause abnormal sleep.

THE PROBLEM

Sleep problems are among the most common health-related complaints of the elderly (Table 5.1), yet remarkably, often go unrecognized or are treated inappropriately.[1]

Insomnia affects about a third of the older population in the USA.[2,3] Insomnia, in fact, is the most prevalent sleep problem reported not only among the older, but across all population age groups within the industrialized countries of the world.[4,5] This inability to have restful sleep at night also results in excessive daytime sleepiness, attention and memory problems, depressed mood, falls, and lowered quality of life.[6–12] In some cases, physicians are not trained to recognize sleep disorders in their older patients. In others, physicians assume that sleep disorders are an inevitable part of aging, an assumption increasingly questioned by researchers. The old dogma that poor sleep is an inevitable and natural part of aging has not been supported.

Data indicate that in the elderly, age by itself does not predict incident complaints of insomnia, even in the presence of lowered sleep efficiency and decreased proportion of slow-wave sleep.[13,14] These changes begin in midlife, as do many of the diseases and disorders associated with aging (Figure 5.2).

However, both the prevalence and incidence of insomnia are markedly reduced in the healthiest older population (Figure 5.3).[15] The prevalence of insomnia and other sleep disorders is high in the population due to the growing numbers of elderly and the associated comorbidities, disease, changes in environment,

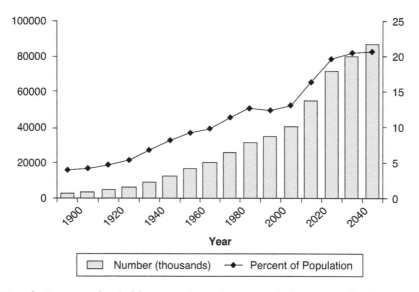

Figure 5.1 Population growth of older Americans (≥65 years). Source: Federal Interagency Forum on Aging related Statistics, 2004

Table 5.1 Prevalences of sleep problems in the elderly

Chronic sleep problem	Prevalence (%)
Any sleep complaint	57
Sleep apnea	24
PLMS[a]	45
Insomnia	29
Early morning awakening	19

Foley et al.[2]; Ancoli-Israel et al.[37]
[a]Periodic limb movements in sleep.

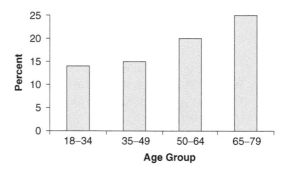

Figure 5.2 Prevalence of insomnia by age group. Source: Mellinger et al.[38]; Foley et al.[2]

or concurrent age-related processes common in late life that affect sleep.[16] Yet even physicians who correctly diagnose sleep disorders in their older patients might not be able to offer treatments because of a paucity of effective therapies for this prevalent condition. More precisely, there has been a paucity of research to discover the causes of sleep disorders and effective therapies to treat them.

THE SLEEP–WAKE CYCLE AND METABOLISM

At the cellular and molecular level, it has been shown that there are age-associated changes in afferent and efferent pathways of the suprachiasmatic nucleus (SCN), the biological clock that controls the circadian patterning of many neural, endocrine, and behavioral functions.

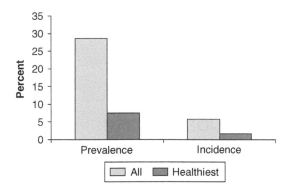

Figure 5.3 Percentage of prevalence and incidence of insomnia in the healthiest older population compared to the total older population. Source: Foley et al.[2,15]

It is quite possible that disruption in the integrative neural systems could have serious deleterious effects in the function of other organ systems. For example, shifts in biological clocks affect secretion and metabolism in a wide variety of neuroendocrine functions that influence not only the sleep–wake cycle but also metabolic functions and activities in organ systems.

A study using mice with a mutation that disrupts their circadian rhythms and produces fragmented sleep found a link between sleep disturbances and metabolic syndrome, a cluster of conditions shown to increase risk of heart attack, stroke, and diabetes, suggesting that the brain system controlling the sleep–wake cycle might play a role in regulating appetite and metabolism.[17] The mice with this mutation, when fed a regular diet, gained about as much weight as normal mice that were fed a high-fat diet, and showed even greater weight gain and changes in metabolism when fed a high-fat diet. This study in mice has brought to light the importance of the circadian clock on the regulation of processes regulating body weight and metabolism.

As has been found in human studies,[18] disruptions of the normal sleep–wake cycle alter the body's ability to regulate its energy balance, especially when there is an overloading of fat in the diet. Similar findings were found in a population-based longitudinal study of over a 1000 participants now between 45 and 75 years of age.[19] In those who slept less than 8 hours per night (about 75% of the sample), body mass index increased as sleep time decreased. Short sleep also was associated with reduced leptin and elevated ghrelin levels in the blood. Short sleep (<5 hours per night), as compared to 7 to 8 hours per night, also has been associated with: obesity during midlife (ages 32 to 49 years) but not later in life;[20] coronary heart disease in women (ages 45 to 65 years);[21] increased risk of incident diabetes;[22] and an increased risk of age-adjusted mortality.[21,23]

It now is evident that disturbance in sleep can also lead to changes in other body systems, especially the production of appropriate levels of hormones and the proper metabolic functioning.[18,24–27]

An interesting molecule discovered in the last decade is hypocretin (Hcrt), a hypothalamus-specific peptide that shares substantial nucleic acid sequences with the gut hormone secretin.[28] Hcrt protein is restricted to neuronal cell bodies in the dorsal and lateral hypothalamic areas. Two forms have been identified, Hcrt1 and Hcrt2, the latter being proposed as a peptide neurotransmitter. The brain cells that contain them make connections with many of the brain regions involved in regulating the sleep–wake cycle. The hypocretins may act as chemical signals involved in the mechanisms of homeostasis and alertness. Their functions have been proposed as being involved in co-ordination of autonomic functions and homeostasis, including feeding, blood pressure regulation, neuroendocrine regulation, thermoregulation, and the sleep–wake cycle. Their link to the aging nervous system remains to be established.

THE CIRCADIAN CLOCK

Shifts in the phase or amount of compounds released by such cycling systems may influence such activities as drug metabolism, nutrient absorption, and other basic physiologic functions essential to health. The relationship between sleep timing and the timing of the circadian rhythm of plasma melatonin secretion was investigated in a group of healthy young and older volunteers without sleep complaints.[29] The timing of sleep and the phase of the circadian melatonin rhythm were earlier in the older participants, although the duration of sleep was similar. Consequently, the older participants were waking at a time when they had higher melatonin levels, in contrast to younger participants, whose melatonin levels were relatively lower by wake time. These findings indicate that aging is associated not only with an advance of sleep timing and the timing of circadian rhythms, but also with a change in the internal phase relationship between the sleep–wake cycle and the output of the circadian pacemaker.

It now has been reported that the human circadian clock has a period of close to 24 hours (24 h 11 min), similar to other species, rather than about 25 hours as previously thought.[30] This study used a technique that controls for the confounding effects of entrainment (resetting) of the circadian clock by light and other non-photic synchronizers. This study found no difference in circadian period between healthy young and older individuals. This counters the belief that the circadian clock speeds up (shortens in duration) as we age. Furthermore, the stability of the circadian clock across adult ages indicates that precise circadian timing is vital to the health and well-being of humans. This study changes some fundamental assumptions about the causes of sleeplessness among the elderly. Again, poor sleep is not in itself a function of being old.

Other factors associated with aging, such as disease, changes in environment, or concurrent age-related processes, may contribute to problems of sleep in older persons. Studies on young adults have shown that entrainment of the circadian timing system can be achieved with much lower light intensities than was previously estimated. Light of indoor intensity can have a significant phase-shifting effect on the circadian pacemaker, and can suppress plasma melatonin secretion.[31] Older healthy adults show a shift in their sleep–wake cycle such that they awaken earlier relative to their melatonin rhythm than younger adults, which may be a cause for sleep disruption.[32]

THE MENOPAUSAL STATE

Recent studies are investigating the associations between peri- and postmenopause and sleep problems. Although sleep disruptions, insomnia, and the incidence of sleep-disordered breathing increase in midlife women, little is known about the relationship between menopause and sleep. The few data that now exist suggest that the sleep–menopause relationship is not merely one of age, but that a variety of relevant psychobiological factors contribute. Sleep in women during the menopausal transition is often reported to be disturbed. In one large epidemiological study utilizing polysomnography it was found that the likelihood of increased sleep-disordered breathing (SDB) over 6 months was significantly greater for women during peri- and postmenopause, compared with those of premenopausal status,[33] independent of age or body mass index. In addition, peri- and postmenopausal women using hormone therapy had lower but not statistically significant risks of SDB. A 10% increase in weight predicted a six-fold significant increase in the odds of developing moderate-to-severe SDB over a 4-year interval for 690 randomly selected participants in the study, excluding participants with weight change in excess of 20% of baseline weight. Women having > 10 nights with hot flashes per month had on average five more nights of restless sleep and four more nights of difficulty maintaining sleep and one more night of difficulty initiating sleep than did women reporting no night-time hot flashes; having < 10 night-time hot flashes was not strongly related to sleep complaints. The association between age and these complaints was slight, and menstrual status was not related to sleep complaints or depression.

EXCESSIVE DAYTIME SLEEPINESS AND COGNITION

A large epidemiological longitudinal study of older men (mean age of 76.6 years, range 71 to 93) investigated the association between sleep disturbances (insomnia and daytime sleepiness) and the incidence of dementia and cognitive decline.[34] It was found that there was a significant association between the self-report of excessive daytime sleepiness and the diagnosis of incident dementia three years later. The risk was twofold as compared to those not reporting daytime sleepiness, after adjusting for age and other factors. Incident cognitive decline also was significantly associated with excessive daytime sleepiness. In contrast, insomnia was not associated with either incident cognitive decline or dementia.

SOME THERAPEUTIC APPROACHES

Several therapeutic strategies, especially phototherapy and melatonin administration, are likely to become effective treatments for some of the insomnias associated with aging. The use of bright light therapy for phase disorders is now more commonplace. Behavioral modifications, such as stimulus control and sleep restriction, appear to be effective techniques for shortening the sleep latency and wake after sleep onset times.[35]

Melatonin treatment appears to be effective at physiologic levels in dealing with circadian dysynchrony. A double-blind placebo-controlled clinical trial of melatonin was conducted on a group of older individuals (age 50 years and older) with insomnia and a group without.[36] Self-reports of insomnia were confirmed by actigraphy as well as by polysomnography in the sleep laboratory. In addition to a placebo, each participant received different doses of melatonin (0.1, 0.3, and 3.0 mg) orally one-half an hour before the usual bedtime for 1 week in a random order, each followed by a 1-week washout period. The highest dose (3.0 mg), the dose commonly found in over-the-counter preparations, resulted in blood levels 10 to 20 times the normal physiologic levels which were produced by the lower doses. The most effective dose for improving the quality of sleep, measured as sleep efficiency or the proportion of time in bed actually sleeping, was 0.3 mg. The highest dose, like the lowest dose, also improved sleep efficiency, although to a lesser extent. However, the 3 mg dose also significantly reduced night-time body temperature and increased daytime melatonin levels. There was no relation found between a person's own endogenous melatonin levels and sleep efficiency. Individuals with normal sleep were unaffected by any dose of melatonin.

SOME NEW RESEARCH DIRECTIONS

Although there is a growing body of research on the aging circadian system, relatively little exists on the aging sleep homeostatic mechanisms. The brain mechanisms underlying age-dependent changes in the sleep homeostatic mechanisms are beginning to be understood. New studies are pursuing leads into the genetics of sleep. The relevance of the genetics of sleep to the problems of the older individual needs further stimulation. Similar to other recent findings that neuronal loss is not an inevitable consequence of aging, these data indicate that there is little evidence of an age-related loss of neurons that has been identified as playing a key role in the maintenance of sleep homeostasis. Thus, the age-related alterations in the control of sleep appear to not be due to loss of critical neurons, but to subtle changes within the cells and in their interactions with other brain cells involved in the control of sleep and alertness. The elucidation of these factors, such as the role played by adenosine in the induction of sleep, can lead to the development of more effective and targeted pharmacologic approaches to alleviate some of the problems of sleep that afflict over half of our older population.

Research also needs to be directed at the development of new and more effective therapeutic modalities that are targeted at correcting the underlying pathological mechanisms of sleep disorders rather than treating them symptomatically. However, until that time, clinical trials on the safety and efficacy of long-term use of hypnotic and somnolent agents are needed.

A large proportion of older nursing home residents have problems in night-time sleep and daytime wake. They often are treated for their sleep problems with hypnotic agents that may put them at risk for falls and confusion. Behavioral and environmental approaches may be more effective at dealing with these sleep problems, along with the identification of undiagnosed sleep apnea that could underlie some of them.

Research needs to further elucidate how the state of sleep debt is associated with decreased glucose tolerance and insulin sensitivity, elevated evening cortisol levels, and increased sympathetic activity. It appears that there are distinct changes in sleep quality that occur through the adult age span, and these changes also mark specific alterations in hormonal systems that are essential for metabolic regulation.

Sleep loss may increase the stress load, possibly facilitating the development of chronic conditions, such as obesity, diabetes, and hypertension, which have an increased prevalence in lower socioeconomic groups.

SUMMARY

Changes in daily sleep patterns are some of the most prominent behavioral and symptomatic changes that occur with aging. Understanding the age-related changes in the nervous system that underlie changes in sleep can lead to better means of primary and secondary prevention of these disorders and, thus, reduce the economic and social impacts of sleep disturbances in the older population.

REFERENCES

1. National Commission on Sleep Disorders Research. Wake up America: a national sleep alert. Vol 1: Executive summary and executive report. Bethesda MD: National Institutes of Health 1993.
2. Foley D, Monjan A, Brown SL et al. Sleep complaints among elderly persons: an epidemiologic study of three communities. Sleep 1995; 18: 425–32.
3. Ohayon MM. Sleep and the elderly. J Psychosom Res 2004; 56: 463–4.
4. Sateia MJ, Doghramji K, Hauri PJ, Morin CM. Evaluation of chronic insomnia. An American Academy of Sleep Medicine review. Sleep 2000; 23: 243–308.
5. Walsh JK, Benca RM, Bonnet M, et al. Insomnia: assessment and management in primary care. Am Family Physician 1999; 59: 3029–38.
6. Bixler EO, Vgontzas AN, Lin HM, Vela-Bueno A, Kales A. Insomnia in central Pennsylvania. J Psychosom Res 2002; 53: 589–92.
7. Brassington GS, King AC, Bliwise DL. Sleep problems as a risk factor for falls in a sample of community-dwelling adults aged 64–99 years. J Am Geriatr Soc 2000; 48: 1234–40.
8. Cricco M, Simonsick EM, Foley DJ. The impact of insomnia on cognitive functioning in older adults. J Am Geriatr Soc 2001; 49: 1185–9.
9. Foley D, Monjan A, Masaki K, et al. Daytime sleepiness is associated with 3-year incident dementia and cognitive decline in older Japanese-American men. J Am Geriatr Soc 2001; 49: 1628–32.
10. Jean-Louis G, Kripke DF, Ancoli-Israel S. Sleep and quality of well-being. Sleep 2000; 23: 1115–21.
11. Moore P, Bardwell WA, Ancoli-Israel S, Dimsdale JE. Association between polysomnographic sleep measures and health-related quality of life in obstructive sleep apnea. J Sleep Res 2001; 10: 303–8.
12. Stepnowsky C, Johnson S, Dimsdale J, Ancoli-Israel S. Sleep apnea and health-related quality of life in African-American elderly. Ann Behav Med 2000; 22: 116–20.
13. Ohayon MM, Carskadon MA, Guilleminault C, Vitiello MV. Meta-analysis of quantitative sleep parameters from childhood to old age in healthy individuals: developing normative sleep values across the human lifespan. Sleep 2004; 27: 1255–73.

14. Vitiello MV, Larsen LH, Moe KE. Age-related sleep change: gender and estrogen effects on the subjective–objective sleep quality relationships of healthy, noncomplaining older men and women. J Psychosom Res 2004; 56: 503–10.

15. Foley DJ, Monjan A, Simonsick EM, Wallace RB, Blazer DG. Incidence and remission of insomnia among elderly adults: an epidemiologic study of 6800 persons over three years. Sleep 1999; 22 (Suppl 2): S366–S72.

16. Ohayon MM, Zulley J, Guilleminault C, Smirne S, Priest RG. How age and daytime activities are related to insomnia in the general population: consequences for older people. J Am Geriatr Soc 2001; 49: 360–66.

17. Turek FW, Joshu C, Kohsaka A, et al. Obesity and metabolic syndrome in circadian clock mutant mice. Science 2005; 308: 1043–5.

18. Spiegel K, Leproult R, Van Cauter E. Impact of sleep debt on metabolic and endocrine function. Lancet 1999; 354: 1435–9.

19. Taheri S, Lin L, Austin D, Young T, Mignot E. Short sleep duration is associated with reduced leptin, elevated ghrelin, and increased body mass index. PLoS Med 2004; 1: e62.

20. Gangwisch JE, Malapsina D, Boden-Albala B, Heymsfeld SB. Inadequate sleep as a risk factor for density: analyses of the NHANES 1. Sleep 2005; 1289–96.

21. Ayas NT, White DP, Manson IE, et al. A prospective study of sleep duration and coronary heart disease in women. Arch Intern Med 2003; 163: 205–9.

22. Ayas NT, White DP, Al Delaimy WK, et al. A prospective study of self-reported sleep duration and incident diabetes in women. Diabetes Care 2003; 26: 380–4.

23. Kripke DF, Garfinkel L, Wingard DL, Klauber MR, Marler MR. Mortality associated with sleep duration and insomnia. Arch Gen Psychiatry 2002; 59: 131–6.

24. Spiegel K, Leproult R, L'Hermite-Baleriaux M, Copinschi G, Penev PD, Van Cauter E. Leptin levels are dependent on sleep duration: relationships with sympathovagal balance, carbohydrate regulation, cortisol, and thyrotropin. J Clin Endocrinol Metab 2004; 89: 5762–71.

25. Van Cauter E, Leproult R, Plat L. Age-related changes in slow wave sleep and REM sleep and relationship with growth hormone and cortisol levels in healthy men. J Am Med Assoc 2000; 284: 861–8.

26. Van Cauter E, Plat L, Copinschi G. Interrelations between sleep and the somatotropic axis. Sleep 1998; 21: 553–66.

27. Vgontzas AN, Papanicolaou DA, Bixler EO et al. Sleep apnea and daytime sleepiness and fatigue: relation to visceral obesity, insulin resistance, and hypercytokinemia [see comments]. J Clin Endocrinol Metab 2000; 85: 1151–8.

28. De Lecea L, Kilduff TS, Peyron C, et al. The hypocretins: hypothalamus-specific peptides with neuroexcitatory activity. Proc Natl Acad Sci USA 1998; 95: 322–7.

29. Duffy JF, Zeitzer JM, Rimmer DW, Klerman EB, Dijk DJ, Czeisler CA. Peak of circadian melatonin rhythm occurs later within the sleep of older subjects. Am J Physiol Endocrinol Metab 2002; 282: E297–E303.

30. Czeisler CA, Duffy JF, Shanahan TL, et al. Stability, precision, and near-24-hour period of the human circadian pacemaker. Science 1999; 284: 2177–81.

31. Duffy JF, Wright KP, Jr. Entrainment of the human circadian system by light. J Biol Rhythms 2005; 20: 326–38.

32. Duffy JF, Zeitzer JM, Rimmer DW, et al. Peak of circadian melatonin rhythm occurs later within the sleep of older subjects. Am J Physiol Endocrinol Metab 2002; 282: E297–E303.

33. Young T, Finn L, Austin D, Peterson A. Menopausal status and sleep-disordered breathing in the Wisconsin Sleep Cohort Study. Am J Respir Crit Care Med 2003; 167: 1181–5.

34. Foley DJ, Monjan AA, Masaki KH, Enright PL, Quan SF, White LR. Associations of symptoms of sleep apnea with cardiovascular disease, cognitive impairment, and mortality among older Japanese-American men. J Am Geriatr Soc 1999; 47: 524–28.

35. Morin CM, Hauri PJ, Espie CA, Spielman AJ, Buysse DJ, Bootzin RR. Nonpharmacologic treatment of chronic insomnia. Sleep 1999; 22: 1134–56.

36. Zhdanova IV, Wurtman RJ, Regan MM et al. Melatonin treatment for age-related insomnia. J Clin Endocrinol Metab 2001; 86: 4727–30.

37. Ancoli-Israel S, Kripke DF, Klaubes ME et al. Sleep-disordered breathing in community-dwelling elderly. Sleep 1991; 6: 486–95.

38. Mellinger QD, Balter M, Uhlenhuth EH. Insomnia and its treatment: prevelence and correlates. Arch Cien Psychiatry 1985; 42: 225–232.

CHAPTER 6

Sleeping environments

Alain Muzet

Sleep is a fundamental physiologic state and its normal achievement is essential for the living organism. However, sleep initiation and sleep maintenance are also influenced by environmental factors. These factors are generally not neutral for the sleeper and, depending on their nature, they can facilitate or disturb the sleep process. The sleeping environment can be quite non-stressful or extreme. Extreme sleeping environments can be encountered by mountain climbers or individuals engaged in single-sailor competitions. These exceptional situations, however, do not affect most of the population and thus do not figure prominently in public health impact assessments. Therefore, this chapter concentrates on those factors that are most often present in our sleeping environment and discusses their possible public health impact.

SLEEP AND THE AMBIENT TEMPERATURE

Ambient temperature is a fundamental physical characteristic of our living environment. However, large differences in ambient temperature exposure do exist depending on geographic location, climatic, and even cultural conditions. Despite these large variations, man tries, through the use of clothing and bedding, to maintain a much narrower range of temperatures in the immediate microclimate around the body, and thus across different cultures and environments

the average skin temperature shows relatively little variation. Within a certain range of ambient temperature, sleep structure appears to be moderately modified, while ambient temperatures that are too low or too high lead to important modifications in the sleep process. This is mainly due to the fact that the sleeping person does not benefit fully from the thermoregulatory system while being in this particular state. One of the new concerns, however, is the possible impact on human health of increasing exposure to higher temperatures over the next century due to predictions of global warming. This phenomenon could obviously affect our way of living and particularly of sleeping.

Thermo neutrality during sleep and the thermal comfort zone

During sleep, thermo neutrality can be defined as the ambient temperature range in which activation of neither cooling nor heating thermoregulatory mechanisms is needed to maintain endothermy. For uncovered and semi-nude persons thermo neutrality is around 32°C during sleep.[1] However, this temperature should be considered an average because of the existence of large differences between individuals. In fact, thermo neutrality during sleep is apparently sleep-stage dependent and thus fluctuates during the night.[2] With the use of sweat collection capsules stuck on the body skin one may record small changes in local sweating rates. With such a technique it has been possible to detect sweating occurring in slow-wave sleep (SWS: stages 3 and 4) for lower ambient temperatures than those necessary to stimulate sweating in stage 2 or in waking.[3] From a thermoregulatory point of view, sleep should therefore be regarded as a dynamic activity and certainly not as a uniform state.

Thermo neutrality is included within a larger thermal comfort zone where there should be no major sleep disturbance caused by the activation of thermoregulatory mechanisms. This means that, within this range of ambient temperature, maintenance of normal sleep patterns could be compatible with moderate changes in peripheral vasomotor and/or sweating responses. Of course, clothing and bed covering conditions of sleeping persons affect this thermal comfort zone. In a study where subjects slept wearing pyjamas under one cotton sheet and a wool blanket, Candas et al.[4] found that the microclimate temperature inside the bed varied from 28.6°C to 30.9°C, while the ambient temperature (air and wall temperatures being equal) varied from 16°C to 25°C.

Between these two ambient temperatures, which are usually encountered in everyday life, the quantitative measures of sleep, such as sleep stage latencies, time spent in each sleep stage, number and duration of nocturnal awakenings, and occurrence of phasic events such as transitory activation phases or arousals, were only slightly modified.[5,6] Candas et al.,[4] however, found that the mean amplitude of the rectal temperature variation during the night was strongly and inversely correlated with the ambient temperature recorded inside the bed. The investigators hypothesized that during sleep a person is able to build a microclimate by heat dissipation from his or her own body, and that this occurs in the very first part of the night. The warming of this 'climatic nest' is due to the heat transfer from the skin of the sleeper to the local environment by vasomotor changes. This heat loss is preferentially performed in the initial SWS,[7] where the thermoregulatory mechanisms are quite active and facilitate the lowering of core body temperature.[3] Similarly, the internal heat storage occurring prior to sleep, due to either a passive heating through a hot bath or an active heating through intensive physical exercise, induces an increased amount of SWS during the consequent sleep period.[8,9]

Therefore, a thermal equilibrium might appear between the body heat loss and the ambient temperature inside the bed. This explanation was confirmed by the fact that subjects showing large decreases in their rectal temperature during the night slept in hotter bed microclimates than those showing smaller rectal temperature decreases. These results were insufficient to determine exactly the limits of the thermal comfort zone during sleep. However, they indicate that this zone corresponds certainly to a broad range because the sleeping person can build, regulate, and keep almost constant a microclimate around his or her body by heat exchange processes that do not disturb sleep.

Thermoregulation and the stages of sleep

Being a homeothermic organism, man must regulate his temperature during sleep. This regulation depends on his or her thermal sensitivity and thermoregulatory responses to the variations of the environmental temperature.[10] The thermal sensitivity is still maintained in rapid eye movement (REM) sleep, and this sleep state is even more disturbed by thermal transients than SWS. Moreover, similarly to what has been already described during wakefulness, sensitivity to cooling during sleep appears to be greater than sensitivity to warming.[11]

In contrast to what has been described in animals,[12] the thermoregulatory responses of humans to elevated temperatures are not abolished during REM sleep.[13] The fact that the thermoregulatory system is less active, and the sweating response is less precisely regulated in REM sleep than in any other sleep stage, explains why the maintenance of homeothermic status during this sleep state becomes more difficult.[14] This can lead to a conflict between the necessity of temperature regulation of the body and the continuity of a sleep state that is less efficient for thermoregulation than other sleep stages.

Inside the thermal comfort zone, an inverse relationship has been found between the ambient temperature and the rhythmicity of occurrence of the successive REM phases. Thus, for ambient temperatures ranging from 13 to 25°C, the average REM sleep rhythmicity varies between 85 and 108 minutes.[15]

The effects of large variations in ambient temperature on sleep characteristics

The few studies that have considered the impact of large variations in ambient temperature on sleep have shown that exposure to heat or to cold leads to disturbed sleep structure, with an increased number of arousals and awakenings, together with a reduction in the amount of SWS and REM sleep fragmentation.[16–18] A reduction in the amount of SWS and REM sleep can be observed even for small increases above 32°C, the ambient temperature required for maintaining bodily thermo neutrality.[16,17] The effect of variation in ambient temperature during sleep can also be seen on the autonomic variables and especially on body temperature. Thus ambient temperature has an effect not only on the level, but also on the shape of the curve of the rectal temperature during sleep. Under cold conditions the body temperature decreases earlier and is sustained longer at a low level than under warm conditions.[19–21] The increase in heart rate in hot ambient conditions compared to the neutral environment has also been described during sleep in humans.[16] This increase in heart rate is often associated with a greater variation due to the increased number of body movements. The increase in body motility under high ambient temperature contributes to a more fragmented sleep, since body movements are often accompanied by awakenings or sleep stage changes.

In the short term, it appears that there is no adaptation to hot ambient temperatures during sleep, in spite of active thermoregulatory mechanisms.[22] In case of exposure to moderate cold, the time spent in SWS tends to increase but no noticeable changes in REM sleep have been found.[23]

Conclusion

The evidence indicates that environmental temperature plays an important role in the organization of human sleep. The reduced reactivity of the thermoregulatory system within sleep is compatible with the maintenance of this state as long as the ambient temperature is kept within the thermal comfort zone. Deviations from this zone, however, might induce important sleep disturbance, mainly due to increase in arousals and wakefulness periods. More research and a better understanding of these limits are certainly needed since there exist large differences between individuals.

SLEEP AND AMBIENT NOISE

Sleep disturbance is one of the major complaints from people exposed to ambient noise. The noise events, often defined as 'unwanted sounds', are perceived as environmental stressors, intruding into personal privacy and causing annoyance and a reduction in the individual's quality of life. They induce involuntary and, most of the time, unexpected reactions from the sleeper and their frequent occurrence may lead to a chronically stressful sleeping environment. It is sometimes suggested that individuals chronically exposed to noise might be more vulnerable to aggression from other factors, whether physical, chemical, or biological. If this is true, it would partially explain the close association between chronic noise exposure and the need for increased medical consultations.[24]

Transportation noise is the most common source of noise in our everyday environment. Traffic and railway noises, as well as noises from aircraft, are frequently encountered in large cities and surrounding areas. In developed countries, tens of millions of people are exposed to noise levels, during the daytime as well as at night, which could be considered deleterious to health. It is difficult to quantify these effects in a linear fashion. The impact of noise on human health is variable and depends on both its unitary and interactive characteristics including its intensity, frequency, complexity, duration (whether intermittent or continuous), and its particular meaning.

To some degree, sleep disturbance may be quantified by the number and duration of nocturnal awakenings, number of sleep stage changes, and modifications in amount and proper rhythms of particular sleep stages such as slow-wave sleep (SWS: stages 3 and 4) and rapid eye movement (REM) sleep, together with modifications in the autonomic functions (heart rate, blood pressure, vasoconstriction, and respiratory rate).

Shortening of the sleep period

Total sleep time can be reduced by longer time to fall asleep, premature final awakening, or increased number of nocturnal awakenings. It has been reported that intermittent noises with peak noise levels of 45 dB(A) and above can increase the time to fall asleep by a few minutes to 20 minutes.[25] On the other hand, sleep pressure is significantly reduced after the first 5–6 hours. Therefore, in the morning hours, noise events can more easily awake and prevent the sleeper from getting back to sleep. To the best of our knowledge no studies have been carried out on the long-term effects of chronic reductions in sleep time resulting from noise exposure.

Sleep awakenings

It seems obvious that noise occurring during sleep may provoke awakenings. The noise threshold for such a major disturbance depends on several factors. One of these factors is the sleeper's current stage of sleep: the threshold is particularly high in deep slow-wave sleep, while it is much lower in shallower sleep stages (stages 1 and 2). The awakening threshold also depends on physical characteristics of the noisy environment (intermittent, sharp rising noise occurring above a low background noise will be particularly disturbing) as well as noise signification.[26] Thus whispering the sleeper's name can awaken the person more easily than a much louder but neutral acoustic stimulus. Similarly, with an equivalent intensity, an alarm noise will awaken the sleeper more easily than a noise without any particular meaning.

Sleep stage modifications

Both SWS and REM sleep are considered as important stages of sleep which should be well protected. SWS appears to be an energy restoration state of the sleeping body, while REM sleep seems to be more related to mental and memory processes. Carter reported that SWS could be reduced in young sleepers exposed to intermittent noises.[27] We previously reported that REM sleep rhythmicity could also be affected by environmental noise exposure.[28] It is a common observation in all disturbed sleep studies (due to noise or extremes in ambient temperature) to see an increase in sleep stage changes such that the amount of time spent in shallow sleep increases at the expense of SWS and REM sleep. This instability of the sleep process might be detrimental if it becomes chronic. Its picture is close to that observed in chronic insomniacs and it would be important to explore the long-term evolution of such a sleep disturbance.

Autonomic responses

Awakenings and sleep stage modifications are not the only possible acute effects of noise on the sleep process itself. If in a similar population nocturnal awakenings can be provoked with peak noise levels of 55 dB(A) and above, disturbance of normal sleep sequence can be observed for peak noise levels between 45 and 55 dB(A). Thus, in order to protect noise-sensitive people, the World Health Organization recommended the following noise limits inside the bedroom: mean level ($L_{Aeq,8h}$) of 30 dB and maximal level (L_{Amax}) of 45 dB.[29] However, this does not mean that for lower noise levels there are no further effects on the sleeper. Autonomic responses such as increases in blood pressure and heart rate can also be found at much lower peak noise levels, indicating that the sleeping body still perceives the external stimuli, even if there is no consciousness or memory about the occurrence of these events.

These effects can be considered as minimal. However, they have not been found to habituate over long exposure times, in contrast to clear subjective habituation occurring in a few days.[30,31] The autonomic responses represent also reflex responses of the sleeping body to the external stimuli, which can be already observed at quite low intensity. The health effects of long-term repetition of such responses should be considered, especially in the case of multiple source noise exposure due to, for example, air traffic and surface traffic. The deleterious impact of this type of combined source noise pollution, which could possibly amount to thousands of discrete stimuli per night, would obviously be considerable for cardiovascular responses and other vital functions.

Physiologic sensitivity to noise

Physiologic sensitivity to noise depends also on the age of the sleeper. Thus, while electro-encephalographic modifications and awakening thresholds are, on the average, 10dB(A) higher in children than in adults, their cardiovascular sensitivity to noise is comparatively similar, if not greater.[32] Elderly individuals complain much more than younger adults about environmental noise. However, their spontaneous or other cause-related awakenings during the night sleep are also much more numerous. A confounding variable is the fact that melatonin secretion decreases in adults after the age of 55 years, the effect of which is to produce a greater amount of sleep fragmentation, and it is thus difficult in this group to evaluate the separate impact of environmental noise. This endogenously produced fragmentation of their night sleep tends also to lengthen their return to the sleeping state, and this certainly accounts for a significant part of their subjective complaints.

The main question about possible sensitive groups remains almost entirely unanswered. Most of the studies, in laboratories as well as in the home, have been done on groups of 'normal' people or, at least, populations where some specific pathologies have been systematically excluded.

Secondary effects of noise exposure during sleep

Not only may noise affect sleep but it may have some secondary effects during the following day. In a community study of exposure to road traffic noise, perceived sleep quality, mood and performance in terms of reaction time were all decreased following sleep which had been disturbed by road traffic noise.[33] Similarly, cognitive performance was decreased[34] and nocturnally secreted stress hormones were increased as a result of noise-disturbed sleep.[35] Subjective evaluation of reduced sleep quality is often the only way to evaluate the impact of noise at night. Sleep recordings are too costly and difficult to run on large samples of the population, while sleep questionnaires remain an easier way of collecting data in this case. However, subjective complaints are not always equivalent to objective (instrumental) measures. If the number of the noise events increases, the number of sleep modifications or awakenings also increases, although not proportionally. As indicated by Porter et al.,[36] noise heard at night will be more intrusive and noticeable than during the day. This is due to the reduced outside and inside background noises at night. The night-time period may thus be a time of greater noise sensitivity, especially in the case of intermittent events such as aircraft noise.

However, if the number of noise events is important and that noise level is high, a nocturnal awakening can be excessively prolonged and even constitute a premature final awakening of the night. Sleep disturbance occurring during the early part of the night and during the time just preceding usual awakening appears to be the most annoying.[25,37] In this case, sleep disturbances will lead to excessive daytime fatigue, often accompanied by daytime sleepiness with its specific effects in terms of low work capacity and increased accident rate.

Laboratory versus field studies: is there any systematic difference?

There is still a debate about existing differences between results obtained in the field compared to those obtained in laboratory studies. Indeed, field studies and laboratory experiments on noise-induced sleep disturbance show different results. Thus, Persons et al.[38] found large discrepancies between laboratory experiments and field settings regarding the variables analysed: arousals or awakenings and change to a lighter stage of sleep; the results showed a greater extent of sleep disturbance in the former than in the latter settings. In a recent study, however, Skanberg[39] found that results obtained by questionnaires and wrist actigraphy indicated that laboratory experiments do not exaggerate effects of noise on sleep when compared to field settings. In fact, it appears that the conflicting results depend, at least to some extent, on the type of sleep disturbance criteria. Comparison of the results based on the same methods in laboratory and field studies showed fairly good agreement for difficulties in falling asleep and reported sleep quality, whereas awakening reactions were much less frequently reported in the field studies.[40]

Long-term habituation to noise

A certain amount of habituation to noise does exist. If the noise load is not in excess, subjective habituation will occur in a few days or weeks. However, this habituation is not complete and the measured modifications of cardiovascular functions still remain unchanged over long periods of exposure. As suggested earlier, impairment to the cardiovascular system could be one of the long-term outcomes of this type of exposure.[27,41] However, in the absence of evidence this suggestion remains speculative.

What are the possible effects of noise-disturbed sleep on general health?

Of course, these effects depend on the magnitude and the repetition of sleep disturbance over long periods. To be awakened from a sound sleep can provoke anger or at least irritation in all but a few. However, it is through the reduction of quality of life during the waking hours that the greatest impacts of sleep disturbance are manifested. Excessive daytime fatigue accompanied by sleepiness, deterioration of normal behavior, expression of anger, lack of concentration and reduced work ability are often associated with chronic sleep deprivation. Often in these circumstances it is not possible to satisfy the need for an additional period of daytime rest. In fact, the subtle equilibrium between waking and sleeping states deteriorates to the detriment of both states' quality.

More generally, some health effects such as the increased use of prescription drugs around major airports[24] or increased rate of mental hospital admission[42] could also be related to night-time noise exposure. However, many confounding factors cannot be eliminated in these epidemiological studies, and therefore it remains difficult to generalize such results. Based on complaints received by the public relations departments of airports, it is apparent that the linkage between poor sleep quality and aircraft noise is well understood by the public. Most of the complaints refer to sleep disturbance, general fatigue, and anxiety. Noise is then clearly identified as a factor of stress and may be considered as the possible mechanism through which mental and physical health can be affected by noise.[43]

Of course, sleep disorders are based on a multiplicity of factors, but it is not unreasonable to infer that at least some of these may be related to environmental noise. In Europe, tens of millions of people complain chronically about poor sleep quality, with difficulty falling asleep and maintaining sleep being almost universally cited. Among this group, about 15% are using hypnotic drugs. For most of these people, and even to a greater extent for the hypnotic drug users, the main consequence of poor sleep quality is the subsequent impairment in the quality of life. Increase of fatigue and sleepiness, together with decrease in performance and productivity, have a major impact on both public health and the large-scale economy.

Conclusion

The permanent exposure to noise sources such as traffic, railways and aircraft constitutes a major annoyance for the concerned population. Although there is no real danger about the specific noise effect (deafness) for people living around airports or surface transport infrastructures, the non-specific effects, and particularly sleep disturbance, are major problems which lead to a substantial reduction in quality of life. Continuous high-level exposure can lead to detrimental effects in a hostile, angry, helpless population facing a major environmental aggression.

ELECTRIC AND MAGNETIC FIELDS

Although quite limited in terms of the people directly concerned, research over the last decade has identified several possible biological effects associated with exposure to electric and magnetic fields (for a review, see Ref. 44). Concerning the effects of these exposures in the occupational-intensity range on sleep polysomnography, results suggest that field exposure may disrupt human electroencephalographic activity during the night.[45,46] Similar findings were obtained more recently in older people, especially in women, with reductions in total sleep time, sleep efficiency, and in the duration of REM sleep.[47] It is worthy of note, however, that none of those exposed was able to detect when he or she was exposed to the fields, nor did they report any subjective symptoms. There is a need for further research in this area.

REFERENCES

1. MacPherson RK. Thermal stress and thermal comfort. Ergonomics 1973; 16: 611–23.
2. Libert JP, Candas V, Muzet A, Ehrhart J, Vogt JJ. Thermoregulatory adjustments to thermal transients during slow wave sleep and REM sleep in man. J Physiol (Paris) 1982; 78: 251–7.
3. Sagot JC, Amoros C, Candas V, Libert JP. Sweating responses and body temperature during nocturnal sleep in humans. Am J Physiol 1987; 252: R462–R70.
4. Candas V, Libert JP, Vogt JJ, Ehrhart J, Muzet A. Body temperature during sleep under different thermal conditions. In: Fanger PO, Valbjorn O, eds. Indoor Climate: Effect on Human Comfort, Performance and Health. Copenhagen: Danish Building Research Institute; 1979: 763–75.
5. Muzet A, Ehrhart J, Libert JP, Candas V. The effect of thermal environment on sleep stages. In: Fanger PO, Valbjorn O, eds. Indoor Climate: Effect on Human Comfort, Performance and Health. Copenhagen: Danish Building Research Institute; 1979: 753–61.
6. Ehrhart J, Muzet A, Candas V, Libert JP, Vogt JJ. Activation phases during human sleep in

different conditions of ambient temperature. In: Popoviciu L, Asgian B, Badiu G, eds. Sleep. Basel: Karger, 1980: 335–9.

7. Libert JP, Candas V, Muzet A, Ehrhart J, Vogt JJ. Thermoregulatory adjustments during SWS and REM sleep in man. In: Koella WP, ed. Sleep 1978. Basel: Karger, 1980: 305–7.

8. Bunnel DE, Agnew JA, Horvath SM, Jopson L, Wills M. Passive body heating and sleep: influence of proximity to sleep. Sleep 1988; 11: 210–19.

9. Horne JA, Reid AJ. Night time sleep EEG changes following body heating in a warm bath. Electroencephal Clin Neurophysiol 1985; 60: 154–7.

10. Kenshalo DR, Nafe JP, Brooks B. Variations in thermal sensitivity. Science 1961; 134: 104–5.

11. Haskell EH, Palca JW, Walker JM, Berger RJ, Heller HC. The effects of high and low ambient temperatures on human sleep stages. Electroencephal Clin Neurophysiol 1981; 51: 494–501.

12. Parmeggiani PL, Rabini C. Sleep and environmental temperature. Arch Ital Biol 1970; 108: 369–87.

13. Candas V, Libert JP, Muzet A. Heating and cooling stimulations during SWS and REM sleep in man. J Therm Biol 1982; 7: 155–8.

14. Glotzbach SF, Heller HC. Central nervous regulation of body temperature during sleep. Science 1976; 194: 537–9.

15. Muzet A, Ehrhart J, Candas V, Libert JP, Vogt JJ. REM sleep and ambient temperature in man. Intern J Neurosci 1983; 18: 117–26.

16. Karacan I, Thornby JI, Anch AM, Williams RL, Perkins HM. Effects of high ambient temperature on sleep in young men. Aviat Space Envir Med 1978; 49: 855–60.

17. Kendel K, Schmidt-Kessen W. The influence of room temperature on night sleep in man (polygraphic night-sleep recordings in the climatic chamber). In: Levin P, Koella WP, eds. Sleep 1973. Basel: S Karger, 1974; 423–5.

18. Muzet A, Libert JP, Candas V. Ambient temperature and human sleep. Experientia 1984; 40: 425–9.

19. Buguet A, Livingstone SD, Reed LD, Limmer RE. EEG patterns and body temperatures in man during sleep in arctic winter nights. Int J Biomet 1976; 20: 61–9.

20. Palca JW, Walker JM, Berger RJ. Thermoregulation, metabolism, and stages of sleep in cold-exposed men. J Appl Physiol 1986; 61: 940–7.

21. Buguet A, Rivolier J, Jouvet M. Human sleep patterns in Antarctica. Sleep 1987; 10: 374–82.

22. Libert JP, Di Nisi J, Fukuda H, et al. Effect of continuous heat exposure on sleep stages in humans. Sleep 1988; 11: 195–209.

23. Sewitch DE, Kittrell EMW, Kupfer DJ, Reynolds CF. Body temperature and sleep architecture in response to a mild cold stress in women. Physiol Behav 1986; 36: 951–7.

24. Knipschild P, Oudshoorn N. Medical effects of aircraft noise: drug survey. Int Arch Occup Environ Health 1977; 40: 197–200.

25. Öhrström E. Research on noise since 1988: present state. In: Vallet M, ed. Noise and Man, vol 3. Nice: INRETS, 1993: 331–8.

26. Muzet A, Réactivité de l'homme endormi. In: Benoit O, Foret J, eds. Le Sommeil Humain. Paris: Masson, 1992: 77–83.

27. Carter NL. Transportation noise, sleep, and possible after-effects. Environ Internat 1996; 22: 105–16.

28. Naitoh P, Muzet A, Lienhard JP. Effects of noise and elevated temperature on sleep cycle. Sleep Res 1975; 4: 174.

29. WHO. Noise and Health. Geneva: World Health Organization, 2000. WHO Local authorities, health and environment, No 36.

30. Muzet A, Ehrhart J. Habituation of heart rate and finger pulse responses to noise during sleep. In: Tobias JV, ed. Noise as a Public Health Problem. Rockville, MD: ASHA Report No 10, 1980: 401–4.

31. Vallet M, Gagneux JM, Clairet JM, Laurens JF, Letisserand D. Heart rate reactivity to aircraft noise after a long term exposure. In: Rossi G, ed. Noise as a Public Health Problem. Milan: Centro Ricerche E Studi Amplifon, 1983: 965–71.

32. Muzet A, Ehrhart J, Eschenlauer R, Lienhard JP. Habituation and age differences of cardiovascular responses to noise during sleep. In: Sleep 1980. Basel: Karger, 1981: 212–15.

33. Öhrström E, Rylander R, Bjorkman N. Effects of night time road traffic noise – an overview of laboratory and field studies on noise dose and subjective noise sensitivity. J Sound Vib 1988; 127: 441–8.

34. Wilkinson RT, Campbell KB. Effects of traffic noise on quality of sleep: assessment by EEG, subjective report, or performance the next day. J Acoust Soc Am 1984; 75: 468–75.

35. Maschke C, Breinl S, Grimm R, Ising H. The influence of nocturnal aircraft noise on sleep and on catecholamine secretion. In: Ising H,

Kruppa B, eds. Noise and Disease. Stuttgart: Gustav Fischer, 1993: 402–7.

36. Porter ND, Kershaw AD, Ollerhead JB. Adverse Effects of Night-time Aircraft Noise. London: National Air Traffic Services, report No 9964, 2000.

37. Fields JM. The Relative Effect of Noise at Different Times of the Day. NASA Langley Research Center, report No CR-3965, 1986.

38. Pearsons K, Barber D, Tabachnick B, Fidell S. Predicting noise-induced sleep disturbance. J Acoust Soc Am 1995; 97: 331–8.

39. Skanberg A. Road traffic noise-induced sleep disturbances: a comparison between laboratory and field settings. J Sound Vib 2004; 277: 465–7.

40. Öhrström E. Sleep disturbances caused by road traffic noise – studies in laboratories and field. Noise Health 2000; 18: 71–8.

41. Carter NL. Cardiovascular response to environmental noise during sleep. 7th International Congress on Noise as a Public Health Problem, Vol. 2. Sydney, Australia, 1998: 439–44.

42. Tarnopolsky A, Watkins G, Hand DJ. Aircraft noise and mental health: I. Prevalence of individual symptoms. Psychol Med 1980; 10: 683–98.

43. Kryter KD. The Effects of Noise on Man. Orlando, FL: Academic Press, 1985.

44. Olden K. NIEHS Report on Health Effects from Exposure to Power-line Frequency Electric and Magnetic Fields. Washington, DC: National Institutes of Health, 1999.

45. Åkerstedt T, Arnetz B, Ficca G, Paulsson LE. A 50-Hz electromagnetic field impairs sleep. J Sleep Res 1998; 8: 77–81.

46. Graham C, Cook MR. Human sleep in 60 Hz magnetic fields. Bioelectromagnet 1999; 20: 277–83.

47. Graham C, Sastre A, Cook MR, Gerkovich MM. Nocturnal magnetic field exposure: gender specific effects on heart rate variability and sleep. Clin Neurophysiol 2000; 111: 1936–41.

CHAPTER 7

Impact of sleeping environment on sleep quality

Gaby Bader

Whereas animals have rest–activity cycles driven by changes in light and temperature, humans are influenced by a variety of cues such as alarm clocks, alterations in the outdoor light (sunsets), rapid changes in temperature, and social activities. However, like other animals we also follow an internal rhythm. This endogenous rhythm, which follows a period of nearly 24 hours, drives sleep–wake cycles, modifications in body temperature and other physiologic parameters; but many decades ago, time-isolation experiments showed that humans have a natural tendency to sleep at a slightly different frequency from the most adaptive 24-hour rhythm. This circadian rhythm is closer to 25 hours and has to be reset each day – by *zeitgebers* or external cues. The circadian rhythm links sleep behavior to body temperature: body temperature decreases, not only as a function of circadian rhythm phase, but also as a function of sleep. When a person is asleep, central control of body temperature is decreased, and at certain sleep stages when this control is suspended the body relies on an equilibrium with its environment.

The autonomic nervous system (ANS) activity during sleep is a function of time and sleep stage. Hence external interventions can affect the ANS differently, depending on the sleep stage and the time of the night. With the onset of sleep, the autonomic balance shifts from sympathetic to parasympathetic dominance, with parasympathetic activity increasing and remaining at high level throughout non-rapid eye movement (NREM) sleep. During REM sleep it returns towards wakefulness values, remaining slightly higher. Sympathetic drive falls during NREM sleep and increases above wakefulness level during REM sleep. Hence there is a relative sympathetic dominance during wakefulness and REM sleep and relative parasympathetic dominance during NREM sleep.

Sleep-modulating sympathetic and parasympathetic activities control the variations of blood pressure and heart rate activity,[1] which are reduced during the nyctohemeral phase. Heart rate decreases at sleep onset and continues to fall through NREM sleep, under a combined circadian and sleep influence.[2] The fall in blood pressure under NREM sleep is entirely influenced by sleep.[3] During REM sleep, heart rate and blood pressure return either to waking level or above NREM sleep levels.

Human sleep patterns have changed dramatically over the last 100 years, beginning with industrialization, electric lighting and shift work, but more radically during the last 30 years with the development of electronic gadgetry, entertainment pressure and other massive intrusions in the night. Biological rhythms have become disturbed by the need to be always reachable and connected, diversions, extensive working hours, and social gatherings. The boundary between day and night activities is becoming blurred and the '24/7 society' will soon be a reality. In order to cope with all this pressure, sleep has been sacrificed. Sleep, a biological necessity, is now widely undervalued.

Bad sleep and disturbed circadian rhythms cause problems, which are at the root of many accidents, and when they become chronic they have long-term adverse effects on health, on the cardiovascular and endocrinologic systems, and on cognitive functioning.

Reduction in the amount of sleep makes it even more essential to have a sleep of optimal quality. All conditions having a possible impact on sleep have to be taken into consideration in order to promote 'good sleep'. Of prime importance are environmental factors including: ergonomics (quality and comfort of the bed system, bedlinen and sleepwear, pillows, etc.), and ambient conditions and microclimate changes (disturbing noises or variations of light in the bedroom, changes in external temperature or bad ventilation). Other external factors such as the position of the bed, high tension wires or electromagnetic fields have been reported to impede sleep.

These environmental factors may coexist, or interact, with maladaptive sleep and wake behaviors or physiologic dysfunctions, including allergies, age-related autonomic or hormonal disregulation, which further erode sleep quality. Solutions other than medical have to be found to address these disturbing causes (e.g., in the case of a snoring person, raising his or her head).[4] In this chapter the various environmental factors which may interfere with sleep are reviewed.

SOUND

Hearing is among the first senses to develop in humans. The fetus is sensitive very early on to surrounding sounds from both the physiologic milieu of the mother's body and the outside world. An unborn child learns early on to recognize the mother's voice. Most likely he or she learns to be appeased by these physiologic sounds while the outside noise, if aggressive, although filtered and dampened by the amniotic fluid, can have a negative impact.

We are, from birth to death, constantly surrounded by all sorts of sounds, generated by humans, traffic, nature, etc., or even endogenous sounds from breathing and the heartbeat. While some of these sounds are pleasant, many others are uncomfortable and stressful.

Noise

Noise is one of the most common physical agents of stress to which urban societies are exposed. Average levels of sounds have increased during the last 30 years – passing heavy traffic can yield a noise level of up to 90 dB – as well as the numbers and types of sources generating noise: alarm systems, telephone, traffic, background music in most public places, and so on.

Individuals surrounded by loud background occupational noise often complain of worsening nocturnal sleep quality. Industrial workers exposed to loud noise during the day have their night sleep efficiency decreased to less than 80%,[5] with an increase in sleep stage shifts, and a decrease in the total time spent in REM as well as slow-wave sleep. Furthermore, the inhibition of the nocturnal reduction in heart rate and elevated morning cortisol levels following noise exposure are indicative of a stress response.

The deleterious effect of night-time exposure to noise on sleep quality is well documented. The threshold of the noise effect is about 40 dB (corresponding to a low-level conversation), and a linear dose–response relationship exists between the peak noise level and changes in sleep architecture.[6] This is characterized by an increased number of awakenings, sleep stage changes and amount of light sleep[7] and a modification in sleep spindles (transient decrease during noise, with an increase during periods of silence). In daytime, impairment of mood and performance is observed.

The extents of these reactions depend on the information content of the noise and its acoustical parameters. They are also modified by situational conditions and by the individual's ability to get used to noise. Adaptation to 'habitual' or regularly occurring noise that is not too loud can be observed in people living on a busy street or along a railway, who learn to develop a rather good night's sleep. Paradoxically, some people who have adapted to chronically noisy sleep environments have difficulties in falling asleep in novel, quiet environments.

The central nervous system is preferentially sensitive to changes in the sensory environment and hence intermittent noise and sound with sudden variations in intensities or pitches – such as those produced at night by road traffic or air traffic near airports.

Among the conditions required to insure a good night's sleep, silence has been stressed in some early studies as being a primordial element[8] in inducing sleep, and a common thinking persists that a silent room is the best aural environment for sleep. However, total silence may be worrying and may even have adverse effects on sleep. Craig[9] reported as early as 1937 that individuals fell asleep sooner when subjected to disturbing sounds than in a perfectly quiet atmosphere. Some endogenous sounds, for example tinnitus, can be annoying and even unbearable if heard in a quiet atmosphere. So, long sensory deprivation, which was reported very early on[10] to induce sleep, can have a negative impact.

For good sleep it is essential not to avoid noises completely but to 'escape' from disrupting ones. Although much more is known about the negative impact of noise on sleep, sounds can also encourage sleep, by providing a distracting focus from thoughts at bedtime.

In the presence of continuous high-intensity sound, it becomes possible to endure a much higher level of noise. This is why background noise is frequently used to mask irregular sounds and patients suffering from tinnitus often use white noise to mask its disturbing impact.

On the other hand, if the ambient sound signals become monotonous, 'habituation' develops and relaxation can occur. Monotony of stimulation can hence induce sleep, and monotonous sounds have long been used as soporific agents. Infrasound (sounds below the hearing frequency limit, $< 20\,Hz$) can yield to drowsiness. Such sound is produced by vehicles in motion due to rolling, heavy duty tyres.

Music

Music, a combination of sound and rhythm, has always been known to have an appeasing effect on the mind. The general public as well as scientists have, since ancient times, recommended music as a therapeutic agent. Although music is universal, its perception can be nurtured. Humans of all ages have the capacity to process pitch materials. While sensory dissonance, a roughness produced by specific components of sound and universally rejected, seems to have a biological basis, harmony dissonance (the rejection of the roughness produced by the violation of the tonal principle) is culture based.[11]

Preferences for well-formed music can begin as early as toddlerhood.[12] Infants less than 1 year old are already very sensitive to many characteristics of music – the melody contour, the rhythm, the tempo, the intervallic dissonance. They prefer consonances over dissonances,[13] and fast, loud music over slow, quiet music.

However, harmony and tonality are the most difficult elements for young children to perceive.[14] Children below the age of 8 years do not generally seem to have the cognitive capacity to be attentive to harmony when simultaneously processing melodic and rhythmic information. (The processus of tonal relationships involves the right frontal lobe – inferior frontal cortex and insula.) This can stem from attention behavior, young children focusing their attention on the concrete form of the melody such as rhythm, pitch, and contour rather than abstract elements such as harmony and key. Noteworthy is the overlap between cognitive components of music processing and related components of non-musical tasks such as language.

Lullaby and babies

Mothers who maintain high levels of rhythmic/physical exercise during pregnancy, such as continuing to dance to music, influence their offspring.[15] Children of such women more often needed to be rocked to fall asleep during their first year compared with the control group. The women who danced also had more children who played musical instruments. This increased need to be rocked and the aptitude to play instruments may be related to the prenatal maternal rhythmic movements.

If a mother sings regularly while pregnant, her child is often soothed when hearing these songs. In premature infants, music appears to reduce stress. The lullaby is appreciated in most cultures as an effective tool in helping babies to fall asleep. For example, in Europe, Brahms-type lullabies are common and in Southern India the raga is said to improve falling asleep.[16] Nearly everyone can remember a time when our mother lulled us to dreamland by singing a melody. Softly singing or humming a tune stimulates the senses by way of a smooth massage leading easily to slumberland. Mothers habituate the babies to these sleepy-time tunes. Today, however, in westernized countries mothers unfortunately have less time to sing; they use instead mechanical or electronic devices to help induce sleep.

Music in children and adolescents

Children and adolescents are spending more time listening to music, and often go to bed with earphones plugged in, falling asleep with the music playing. What is the impact of background music on their quality of sleep?

This effect was recently studied in a randomized controlled trial of 86, primary school children in Taiwan.[17] Children in an experimental group were subjected to background music lasting 45 minutes at naptime and bedtime each day for 3 consecutive weeks. Sleep quality was measured using the Pittsburgh Sleep Quality Index prior to the test period and at its completion. Children who had listened to the music showed significant improvement in their global sleep quality over the test period, specially in sleep duration and sleep efficiency.

Impact of music on older adults

Few studies have focussed on the effects of music as a non-pharmacologic method of improving the quality of sleep. In the last decade a few reports were published on the effects of music on sleep quality in the elderly, leading to recommendations for using soothing music as a non-pharmacologic intervention for sleep, particularly for those in community dwelling situations.

In a study performed in 1995, 25 community-based elderly people complaining of sleep disturbances listened to classical music and New Age music before bedtime. According to sleep diaries 96% of them reported improvement in their sleep following this self-administered intervention.[18]

In another study, the use of music to promote sleep onset and increase sleep maintenance was tested among 52 women over the age of 70 years using individualized music protocol.[19] Music listening was shown to decrease time to sleep latency and awakenings during night-time. These women reported that they also derived more satisfaction from their sleep.

More recently,[20] in a controlled trial in Taiwan, 62 volunteers, both men and women, aged 60–83 years with difficulty in sleeping were randomly divided into equal numbers of a music group and a control group. The subjects were not using sleep medication or relaxation techniques, nor caffeine, and did not have psychologic or health impairment that could interfere with sleep. The music group was asked to listen to sedative music for 45 minutes at bedtime for 3 weeks. The subjects were able to select from both Chinese folk music and soft, slow, Western music known to reduce postoperative pain. Sleep quality was measured with the Pittsburgh Sleep Quality Index before and at the end of the study. The music group reported significantly better scores in overall sleep quality as early as the first week (35% improvement). Individuals in this group had shorter sleep latencies, longer night-time sleep, improved sleep efficiency and perceived sleep quality. The subjects also had lower heart and respiratory rates when listening to music, indicating increased relaxation aiding a restful sleep. They also functioned better during the daytime. Since the subjects continued to improve after the first week – mastering the technique of relaxation to the sedative music – the authors suggested a cumulative dose effect. In conclusion, listening to soft music at bedtime can be recommended to older adults with insomnia, helping them to sleep better and longer.

Ill patients and music

Music therapy to promote sleep is increasingly used in conditions of illness. The efficacy of music, alone or together with other complementary and alternative therapies, for sleep induction in critically ill patients has recently been reviewed.[21] Studies have shown that music therapy as well as massage promote relaxation and comfort leading to improved sleep in patients with insomnia. Reduction of noise or the playing of natural sounds (like those from the sea) can also yield improved sleep.

Music therapy and physiologic correlates of its effects

Music therapy has been used in many psychologic conditions with positive results. Gentle melodies and relaxing music are common non-pharmacologic methods to promote sleep,

as immersion in music helps the mind to defocus. In those who are not sleep deprived music can also help maintain arousal: increased sleep latencies were observed in both the Multiple Sleep Latency and the Maintenance Wakefulness tests.[22]

In a recent study, the effects of music therapy combined with progressive muscle relaxation were tested on the anxiety level and sleep patterns of 28 abused women residing in shelters.[23] During five consecutive days they listened to 20-minute music sessions together with a progressive muscle relaxation script. Therapy was found to improve sleep quality, as measured by the Pittsburgh Sleep Quality Index, and reduce anxiety.

But does music have intrinsic sleep promoting qualities or does its effect reflect only a conditioned response? What is the real impact of music on the ability to fall asleep? In one study of the psychophysiological effects of music on the human brain, the electroencephalograms (EEGs), electrocardiograms (ECGs), and electrooculograms were recorded from eight volunteers under three sound conditions.[24] The procedure started with 5 minutes of silence, followed by 11 minutes of listening to two types of music or two types of simulated music/noise (produced by a sound modulator, simulating by white noise the sound pressure variations of a given piece of music), and ended with another 5 minutes of silence. A total of 10 music and 10 simulated music conditions were used. While the subjects reported feeling pleasantly relaxed when listening to music, they felt uncomfortable and sleepy when listening to the simulated music. However, higher delta-EEG power densities were recorded at drowsiness and stage 1 sleep when a person listened to simulated music compared to when listening to pure music. The author concluded that, even during drowsiness and light sleep, physiologic consciousness was higher when listening to pure music and the differences in the EEG slow components during light sleep showed that the differences in consciousness had a physiological aspect and were indicative of differences in mental activity.

In another study, the EEG activity during relaxation technique (RT) and music listening was compared in 36 volunteers listening to either music tapes or RT audiotapes during a 6-week period.[25] The power spectral analysis of the EEG showed increase in the low frequency domain in many cortical regions, with a more pronounced theta activity for the RT condition. These findings are suggestive of widespread reductions in cortical arousals.

'Brain music' is one among the many attempts to treat insomnia with non-pharmacologic methods. The method is based on the transformation of EEG into music, whereby EEG segments corresponding to the different sleep states are selected from the polysomnogram (PSG) of the individual. The data are fed into a computer program to create the same brain wave patterns as when the individual is trying to sleep, then transformed into a soundtrack to generate unique and user-tailored 'meditative' music whose rhythmic and tonal sound patterns create a condition supposed to be conducive to sleep.[26]

Fifty-eight patients with insomnia were selected for a study and divided into a placebo ($n=14$) and an experimental ($n=44$) group. They were instructed to listen to 'brain music' at bedtime during 15 consecutive days. Sleep quality was evaluated with questionnaires, PSGs and EEGs performed before and after the treatment period. The results showed significant improvement in 80% of the patients as estimated by both the neuropsychologic and neurophysiologic methods as well as their subjective feelings. No side effects were reported.

Another group of investigators studied the ability of 'brain music' to assist in relaxation and improvement in the overall quality of sleep.[27] Ten volunteers listened to individually tailored brain music; eight more listened to music which had not been specially designed for them. Both groups experienced less anxiety after listening to the music over a 4-week period, but the effect was more pronounced in the group that listened to the personalized music.

Brain music reduced anxiety and improved sleep in those who had been suffering from insomnia for at least 2 years.

Hence, if effective, brain music therapy may represent a possible alternative for therapeutic management of insomnia and anxiety. Critics argue that anything relaxing and that pushes other noises, like traffic, out of the mind is going to help sleep.

Rhythms and ethnomusic

Is it only the melody, as in the lullabies, which has an impact? What is the role of the rhythm in music therapy?

The first rhythm that a fetus experiences is the heart beat of the mother. Hearing the regular beats of the heart may enhance the fetus's feeling for rhythms. It is very likely that this first rhythm will leave traces and unconsciously be associated with the security of the womb.

A mother has a tendency to put her crying baby more often on the left side of her breast rather than on the right side, whatever her handedness. It is suggested that the baby is appeased when hearing the mother's heart beat. Infants fall asleep listening to the 'music of the heart'.

In an interesting study, Betterman et al.[28] investigated musical rhythms in the dynamics of the heart period. They analyzed 24 ECGs of 96 healthy volunteers, transforming the heart period tachograms into binary symbol sequences, resembling the percussive rhythm found in African music. Using an analysis technique derived from jazz theory they established a hierarchical rhythm pattern scheme and classified the different rhythm patterns obtained. They observed that, during sleep, certain classes of rhythms developed in a cyclically recurrent manner, specific to individuals, while other classes disappeared. Most interestingly, the most frequent classes developed from phase-locking processes in autonomic regulation, such as between respiratory and cardiac cycles.

Heart period patterns can be interpreted as musical rhythms, particularly during night sleep. This method may have potential use in music therapy applications, especially considering that many insomniacs, while lying awake during the night, can often hear the sound of their heart rhythm.

While the cardiac rhythm can be transformed in appeasing sonic rhythm, has a musical rhythm any effect on the heart rhythm, and is it possible to modulate the heart rhythm with a musical rhythm? Attempts to use synchronization of heart rhythm and music therapy in relaxation therapy, intended to improve falling asleep, were randomly made in 28 cancer patients with chronic pain.[29] During 14 days the patients were trained in relaxation therapy, including listening to a 30-minute lullaby-like rhythmic music with gradually decreasing speed. The investigators analyzed the degree of synchronization between heart rate and the musical beat (co-ordination of systole and musical central time point) on the first and the last day. Time of falling asleep, patient's subjective evaluation, pain intensity and use of analgesics were recorded. The results were compared to a control group not submitted to this training. The experimental trained group showed, together with an improvement in falling asleep and decreased consumption of medication, an increased co-ordination of heart rate and musical beat; also the group showed a very stable 2:3 synchronization, especially at a musical tempo between 42 and 48 beats/min. Hence, lullaby-like music, at least within a special range of tempi and rhythms, can induce a trainable synchronization of heart rate, associated with a relaxation reaction and improved sleep.

Mechanical devices

There are many different types of music and sound-making devices on the market that can assist in the relaxation process. They are said to help falling asleep faster, sleeping more deeply, and waking refreshed! They can be grouped in two classes.

Musical devices These may be variously described as classical music, electronic music eschewing the pulsating beat of techno, soothing melodies, syncopated rhythms and gentle sound effects, or primitive and tribal music featuring more organic sounds, as well as diverse non-electronic instruments such as the sitar, flutes, harpsichords, chimes and bells, with often rhythmic drumming (similar to the beats found in a tribal drum circle), chanting or throat sounds.

Non-musical devices These are sound effects with various soothing natural, relaxation-oriented sounds such as waterfalls, ocean waves, wind, rain, whale songs, and water drops. One can also find recordings of other types of sounds such as those of busy city streets, fire engines, and airplanes, which are designed for city dwellers who become anxious when it is just too quiet!

The effectiveness of music as a therapeutic tool in dealing with insomnia varies from individual to individual. Depending on the patient and type of insomnia, what works for one person will not necessarily work for another. Some people will have better results with rhythm and gentle percussion, while others will respond more positively to melody or nonlinear compositions. Some will react to constant repetition, while others will benefit from randomness.

LIGHT

Light profoundly impacts humans through the stimulation of the visual system, eliciting physiologic and alerting responses and powerfully regulating the circadian system.

Seasonal affective disorder (SAD) is a well-known circadian rhythm pathology, affecting particularly those who live at the extremities of the hemispheres. These, mostly healthy people experience depressive mood in the darker period of the year, particularly at the beginning of the autumn and the spring. Light has been proved to be an effective treatment, although many sufferers exposed to bright light experience side effects such as nausea, headaches, visual discomfort, and eye strain. Light can either advance or delay the body clock depending on its timing in relation to a person's circadian rhythms. Hence, not only the intensity but also the timing of light is important when considering light therapy for treating circadian disorders.

Light intensity is the *zeitgeber* controlling the biological clock and the secretion of melatonin. Light, even at low intensity, inhibits melatonin release. Hence efficient drapes and shades should be used in the bedroom to avoid external light entering, especially in the early hours of the morning in summer. Light also influences sleep indirectly depending on the habits acquired; for example, while some people need total darkness to sleep, others like a dim light in their bedroom in order to achieve relaxation.

Like sound, light vibrations at particular frequencies, i.e. colors, might have impact on a human's physiology (certain individuals can perceive sounds as colors and vice versa. The famous composers Rimsky-Korsakoff and Scriabin were reported to have this kind of synesthesia.)

It is commonly accepted that colors can affect the mood, and emphasis is now being put on selecting the right surrounding colors in the bedroom, some colors being more relaxing than others, generally blues and greens. Reds and yellows have been found to be less soothing. The recommendation is to use neutral (pale) color in the background, adding colorful tones through the furniture and, even better, through the lighting.

While full-spectrum bright white illumination is generally used in light therapy, recent advances have shown that the wavelength of the light has a major impact. A recent study has shown that dim red light (1 lux at 652 nm) increased the circadian period in mice [30] and, in humans, exposure to 2 hours of monochromatic

light at 460 nm (blue) in the late evening induced a greater melatonin suppression than light at 550 nm, with a greater alerting response and increased body temperature and heart rate.[31]

The rod and cone cells of the retina, responding best to white full-spectrum light, have long been considered to be responsible for mediating light and thus its effect. Recently, a small population of photosensitive retinal ganglion cells has been found to play a key role in the regulation of the non-visual photic responses (behavioral responses to light, pineal melatonin synthesis, and papillary light reflex). These cells, which project to the suprachiasmatic nucleus, synthesize melanopsin, a photopigment opsin, which mediates these non-visual photic responses and contributes to circadian entrainment.[32] Melanopsin cells respond to a specific bandwidth in the range of 446–477 nm, which corresponds to the blue portion of the light spectrum, and is fundamentally different from the rod and cone photoreceptor peaks. These cells might also be responsible for detecting changes in the intensity of the light. It has been suggested that patients with circadian rhythm disorders might have a deficiency of melanopsin cells, and hence cannot distinguish daylight signals to adjust their rhythms.

Different levels of light illumination intensity influence the behavioral and autonomic regulation of body temperature in humans. When healthy women were exposed to high (700 lux) or low (70 lux) light intensities at different room temperatures (26 or 20°C for 30 min), their peripheral skin blood flow was decreased and they felt cooler following exposure to the cooler environment and the low illumination.[33] It was suggested that vasoconstriction seems to occur strongly in dim light.

Strong evening light can disturb nocturnal sleep. Individuals exposed to dim light (150 lux) or bright light (3000 lux) from 7 p.m. to 9.30 p.m. for 5 days had, after exposure to the bright light, a shift of their rhythm as expressed by the delay of the nadir of their core temperature.[34] Sleep quality and ease of falling sleep were also worsened. So, in order to prepare for sleep, it is recommended to avoid strong illumination prior to bedtime.

Sensing temperature changes at bedtime can influence the choice of night clothing. Evening exposure to bright light, which suppresses the nocturnal rise of melatonin, inhibits or reduces the evening decline of core temperature. The thermal sensibility to cold becomes sharper compared with evening dim light exposure, affecting dressing behavior.[35]

Daytime levels of light intensity can influence the circadian rhythm of the body temperature and have an impact on the subjective feeling of temperature at night, on nocturnal body temperature and likely on sleep. Exposure to low light intensity (200 lux) for only 2 days is enough to induce a phase delay of the core temperature rhythm,[36] and in sleep-deprived individuals exposure to bright light during daytime reduces the impact of sleep loss on sleepiness levels as compared to dim light.[37]

Exposure to bright light (4000 lux) during daytime for several hours increases the evening melatonin secretion and lowers core temperature during nocturnal sleep as compared to a dim light exposure (100 lux);[38] the peripheral skin temperature gets higher in the evening and during sleep. This makes the thermal sensibility to cold slower in the evening, as compared to exposure to dim light in daytime, with also an impact on night dressing behavior: when exposed during daytime to illumination of low intensity (10 lux), subjects dressed more quickly and preferred to wear thicker clothing than after exposure to the bright light condition.[39]

Even the color of the clothes selected is influenced by light intensity during daytime, and people prefer warmer colors when exposed to dim light in daytime.[40]

ODOR

Aromas produced by essential oils or herbs (decoctions or infusions applied as compresses) have been used for centuries for their assumed properties as hypnotics, analgesics, antiseptics, soporifics, or aphrodisiacs and for inducing sweating as well as urination.

Olfaction has different properties compared to the other senses. Its effect is immediate but not constant, it fades very quickly and eventually disappears. Air movement is necessary for continuous olfaction, the odoriferous molecules having to be replaced by fresh ones. The fading effect can be countered by the smelling of different odors; however, even so there is an effect of habituation and tiredness and after a while olfaction becomes less and less acute. There is also a sex-based difference in odor preference and it was recently reported that the olfactory response to and preference for aromas are modulated, in women, by the menstrual cycle, and those taking contraceptive pills are, for example, more receptive to food odors than to sexual related odors.

Furthermore, this sense is unique in that it has the property to retrieve immediately old memories. Marcel Proust reported this experience in his masterwork *A la recherche du temps perdu*, where the sudden smelling of small cakes, called madeleines, flashed back all his childhood memories.

It is therefore likely that smells which unfold memories can have a psychological impact. They can help or hinder relaxation, depending on the positive or negative content of the memory they raise.

In the past decades there has been an increase in research examining the connection between olfaction and mood, behavior, and performance; aromatherapy is becoming very popular as a complementary alternative treatment in many conditions. Its use, alone or combined with massage, is reported to help relaxation and to improve both sleep onset and sleep quality. Lavender, sandalwood, ylang-ylang, camomile, marjoram, camphor, basil, rose, neroli and jasmine are are recommended against insomnia. The skin seems to be responsive somehow to essential oils and, according to proponents of aromatherapy, can be sensitive to odors; hence massaging the body with aromatic oils could combine the beneficial effect of massage itself with the properties of the essences. While massage has an obvious effect on relaxation, the question remains whether there is any direct impact of olfaction on sleep. Inhalation of essential oils can induce side effects such as headaches, nausea, and allergy. Hence, if intended to be used at night, aromas should be recommended cautiously.

The physiology of odor perception is still partially unknown. The rod-like olfactory neural cell has one end emerging directly from the olfactory bulb in the brain and terminates in the roof of the nasal passage as a dozen or so tiny hairs embedded in a thin layer of mucus. Hence the hairs are unprotected extensions of the cells providing a direct interaction between the source of stimulation and the neurons. The olfactory system is unique since, with its short pathway, it has an immediate and direct effect on the nervous system. Therefore, we cannot exclude the fact that most odors have some effect on the body, even in the absence of awareness.

While asleep, people can be exposed to various unwanted smells developed by the surroundings in the bedroom, the bed system, or even their own breath and perspiration. However, it is still unclear whether the human body responds to odors presented during sleep.

Olfactory stimulation (peppermint) during stage 2 sleep was reported to produce autonomic (heart rate, respiration), behavioral (awakening) and central (EEG) responses[41] and subjects exposed to jasmine odor were found to have a better sleep quality and enhanced cognitive task performance but less vigor when awakening in the morning.[42] However, in a more recent investigation the results were negative. The arousal thresholds of an auditory tone were compared to two odorants, peppermint and pyridine, tested at various concentrations.[43] While the rate of awakening efficiency of the auditory tones was more than 75% of all the trials, 92% of the subjects responded to both odors only in stage 1 sleep, while pyridine alone produced a response in 45% of the subjects in stage 2 sleep, but not in the other sleep stages. Thus, in this study odors seemed ineffective to interrupt sleep.

Although the odo-alarm remains fictional, waking up in surroundings with agreeable and discrete fragrances could have some positive impact. The market is thus offering gadgets that release refreshing fragrances 10 to 30 minutes prior to the activation of an alarm clock.

TEMPERATURE, HUMIDITY, VENTILATION, ALLERGY

A thermoregulatory function has been suggested for sleep (i.e., sleep functions to preserve energy,[44] or REM sleep acts to warm the brain[45]). Temperature influences sleep architecture, and conversely, sleep has a strong influence on homeostatic regulation of body temperature.

Temperature is mainly regulated by water evaporation through breathing and by the release of human body heat through the skin. Temperature in the sleeping environment, within the bedroom or/and in the bed, can have a deep impact on the quality of sleep. Too low heat insulation or extreme cold (i.e., <16°C) will cool off the body, causing shivering and muscle stiffness, thus disturbing sleep. A high heat insulation or a too warm environment (i.e., 24°C) can cause restlessness and transpiration, resulting in an increase of relative humidity, both conditions leading to sleep disturbances, reductions in both REM and NREM sleep, and increased wakefulness. Furthermore, moist skin is more sensitive to shear forces.

Sleeping body temperature depends on room temperature, the sleeping system, the fabrics of the bed clothing and garments. The insulation capabilities of a mattress depend on its core (for instance, latex or polyurethane having higher insulation than springs) and on its top layers (wool having a good ability to retain air[46] and so on). The subject's health status, age and gender, and medication also play an important role in thermoregulation.

The ability to sweat decreases with age;[47] in women subjected to passive heating, sweating onset regulating core temperature has been reported to be delayed compared with men,[48] and those taking contraceptives have higher nocturnal temperature than men.[49] On the other hand, when the ambient temperature decreases, women feel cooler during the luteal period of the menstrual cycle than during the follicular phase and have a higher metabolic rate.[50]

Although low temperatures are more bearable to most people, the ability to maintain a sleep state has been observed to be impaired in a mildly cold sleeping environment.[51] In an early study, an ambient temperature (21°C) was found to be more disruptive to sleep than warmer ones, with individual sensitivity to cold.[52] Generally, a person tends to remain immobile in a cold bedding, avoiding unnecessary shifts of position.

Temperature influences sleep architecture even within thermoneutrality, while non-neutral thermal environments accentuate NREM sleep and wakefulness. Continuous heat exposure (35°C) was reported to reduce total sleep time and increase the amount of wakefulness.[53] However, in rats, chronic exposure to warm temperatures increased the amount of sleep, specially that of paradoxical sleep, whereas cold increased wakefulness.[54]

REM sleep is more sensitive than NREM sleep to changes of ambient temperature even within thermoneutrality. This is more of a problem late in the night, when REM sleep predominates.

During REM sleep thermal regulation of the body is decreased or suppressed, resulting in the body temperature varying with the temperature of the environment, the human body becoming poikilothermic. Body temperature variation during this sleep stage can result in awakenings. The inability to thermoregulate in REM sleep affects the response to temperature changes: sweating and shivering occurring in response to extreme temperatures in NREM sleep cease during REM sleep.

Extreme low (<-5°C) and high ($>+25$°C) temperature can affect REM sleep duration. The length of the REM cycle decreases when the ambient temperature increases from 13 to 25°C[55] or more,[53] and also if the body is exposed to a nocturnal cold atmosphere (slow-wave sleep is not affected).[56]

In small infants, a mild increase in body temperature secondary to changes in ambient temperature (20–30°C) resulted, especially during REM, in an increased occurrence of central apneas associated with oxygen saturation drops. The parasympathetic activity was observed to be lower and the basal heart rate higher with shorter RR intervals.[57]

A drop in temperature is thought to be a 'soporific' signal for the body. A close association has been found between decreased body temperature by distal vasodilatation (and increased distal temperature) and initiation of sleep.[58] A gently declining body temperature is thought to trigger the onset of sleep. Paradoxically, however, in insomniacs, heat loss from the distal skin regions appears to be greater than normal.

Body temperature follows a circadian rhythm. It is a solid marker of the biological clock. The warmest point (acrophase) is reached in the late afternoon/early evening, while the coolest point (nadir) occurs after midnight between 2.00 and 4.00 a.m. and rises by the time REM is occurring in abundance, during the second half of the night. Ideally the temperature of the sleeping environment should follow the circadian rhythm, decreasing during the evening and increasing in the early morning. In some species, specially in heterothermic but even in some mammals, cyclic changes in ambient temperature can entrain this rhythm.[59]

Exposure to passive heat in the afternoon and evening has no significant effect on the sleep pattern that night if the person sleeps in thermoneutrality (30°C). However, sleep is disturbed, restless and less efficient, with reduction of REM sleep, if the night ambient temperature is high (35°C).[60] On the other hand, subjects exposed during their night sleep to a slightly cold environment showed, on a following daytime recovery sleep, an increase in REM sleep duration.[61]

Sleep deprivation can also influence the temperature effect and may modify the thermoregulatory response, especially in a cold environment, where higher sensations of cold and shivering have been reported.[62] However, a recent study did not show significant differences in rectal temperature or heat production when the subjects were exposed for 180 minutes to cold air following 33 hours of sleep deprivation.[63]

Bed clothing and sleep garments

The composition of the constituent materials affects the exchange of heat and moisture between the body, the clothing and the layers of the bedding. Hence the top layers of the bed, the bed clothes and night garments should preferably be made of natural materials such as cotton, wool, linen, or silk. Sheets and blankets can easily be adjusted to the ambient temperature. Quilts are popular since they sit snugly around the body.

If used, sleepwear has to be adequate, loose and comfortable in order not to disturb sleep. For good sleep comfort, thin, loose-fitting nightwear, pyjamas, night-shirt or negligé should be recommended. Tight clothing may cause the person to feel restricted and result in awakenings. On the other hand, too loose a garment can twist tightly around the body if a person moves about too much during sleep, causing restriction and hindering posture changes.

There are also specific requirements to be considered. People with perspiration and allergy problems should choose adequate bedding materials. Women feel cooler in the luteal phase if the ambient temperature is low, and they have a tendency to wear thicker clothing.

Air, humidity and ventilation

Air composition in the bedroom and the amount of moisture in the sleeping environment are important factors contributing to sleep quality.

The human body releases hundreds of millilitres of moisture during the night, in certain conditions up to 1 litre. One-third of this moisture evaporates in breathing, two-thirds are emitted through the body surface. This release of moisture through the skin should not be confused with perspiration, and is in fact greater in volume than perspiration.

Ideally, the relative humidity between the skin and the sheet/mattress should stabilize within half an hour and should remain under 75%. In order to prevent mildew formation on the bottom of the mattress, or a clingy feeling to the sheets or the mattress surface, moisture has to be transported and absorbed by the environment, that is, the nightwear, bed clothing, mattress, and head pillow.

Overly dry air can irritate the upper airway and bronchial passages, resulting in coughing and awakenings. Electrical humidifiers or a bowl of water in the room address this problem. Opening a window improves the room ventilation. Excessive humidity can raise body temperature and result in uncomfortable perspiration, leading to arousals; this can be enhanced by the fact that, in humid conditions, sweat is slow to evaporate.

Exposure to humid heat increases sweating, which disrupts sleep and increases wakefulness more during the initial segment of the sleep period than during the later part.[64] Hence air conditioning should preferably be used in the initial hours of sleep.

Sleeping naked, without covers in a humid environment, will allow the body to remain damp, and this can result in a chill. Soft, moisture absorbing nightwear and sheets of cotton or linen are recommended. Head cooling during sleep may help decrease sweating,[65] while increasing air circulation, for example, with a fan, will help decrease humidity.

Body movements during sleep can improve ventilation, although this is not enough. Mattresses should also allow for adequate heat and humidity flow. Those made of latex, for instance, have very poor ventilation properties compared with spring mattresses. To decrease the risk of creating breeding grounds for house dust mites, mattresses should be ventilated regularly and turned around.

The effect of air ions on humans has been the subject of much debate. While an excess of positive ions may cause discomfort, including headaches, nausea, and nasal congestion, negative ions have been reported to bestow beneficial effects. Men exposed for at least six hours to negative ions felt more relaxed and less tired.[66] The mode of action seems to be through the respiratory system. Negative ions are more concentrated in fresh air, and they are produced by lightning, waterfalls and other natural processes. Air ionizers are electrical devices producing negative air ions. They have been used for the treatment of seasonal winter depression.[67]

In a study, pyjamas with negative air ions were worn during night sleep. The rectal temperature was observed to be more reduced and the elevation of salivary IgA more marked than when not wearing this clothing.[68]

House dust mite allergy

The house dust mite is a microscopic scavenger (< 0.5 mm) which eats what is available. It has no eyes nor organized respiratory systems. With its eight legs, each with a sucker and hooks, it moves easily on carpets, curtains, clothing, blankets, soft toys, and old furniture. The mite colonizes nest sites whenever it finds suitable conditions, that is warmth, darkness, and moisture, which explains why, even though it never drinks, its body weight consists of 80% water. Its lifespan is about 3 months.

In the bedroom, mattresses and head pillows are important seedbeds; the mites breed on organic debris, mainly flakes of human skin. The mite's digestive system creates up to 20 dung droppings a day. This desiccated excrement can remain suspended in still air (e.g., an unventilated room) for almost half an hour, enough time to be easily inhaled by unsuspecting people, causing allergic reactions (coughing,

asthma, irritation in the eyes, dermatitis), which manifests specially during the night.[69] Genetically predisposed individuals (atopic family or history of allergy) are more vulnerable to the mite. The allergy is not originated by dust or the mite itself but by very invasive allergens (dermatophagoides) produced in the intestinal canal during degradation of organic dirt.

Mites develop best in a temperature of 20–25°C and relative air moisture of 70–75%. Bedrooms with high temperature, high humidity, and lack of ventilation are ideal breeding grounds. In the bedding dust, besides the mites, other micro-organisms and fungi living on the mite excrement can be found in abundance, some of them also pathogenic.

Mattresses tend to accumulate allergen rather rapidly. In a study, 51 mattresses used during 8–25 months had a median concentration of total major allergens of 0.5 µg/g. The allergen concentration was found to be above the risk level (2 µg/g) in 56% of the mattresses.[70]

Neither spring, foam nor heated water mattresses are immune from producing mite allergy. Attempts have been made to reduce mite allergen in the bedroom by treating carpets and bedding with chemicals, encasing the mattresses or developing new fabrics. Treatment of pillows, mattresses, and duvets with acaricide (benzyl benzoate) seemed to be ineffective.[71]

The efficiency of encasing mattresses with anti-allergic covers is controversial. In some studies allergen-impermeable bed covers did not show a decrease in the mite antigen level,[72] while in others, the use of anti-allergic mattress covers has been shown to be effective in patients who are asthmatic and allergic to the house dust mite.[73] In an investigation comparing a control group using only regular cotton bed sheets with an experimental group using partial encasement of the mattress with an impermeable membrane (a nylon sheet underneath the regular cotton bed sheet), it was found that the nylon sheet reduced the migration of mite antigens from the mattress to the surface of the cotton bed sheet during the study period of 6 months.[74] The use of washable blanket covers of synthetic fibres or cotton also significantly reduced the allergen exposure.[70]

A novel way to fight dust mites has been to impregnate mattresses with permethrin (450 mg/m² permethrin in polyester netting weighing 35 g/m²). In a 27-month field test, the permethrin-impregnated bedding significantly reduced allergen concentrations of dust mite without side effects.[75]

In conclusion, it is practically impossible to get rid of the mites. Allergic symptoms can be lessened by keeping air humidity lower than 55% and limiting the exposure to the dung pellets by correct hygiene, good ventilation, and aeration of the bed. Synthetic top layers that can be washed above 60°C can be recommended.

THE SLEEPING SYSTEM

The sleeping system, that is the mattress and its supporting structure, is one of the most important ergonomic factors that influence sleep. An adequate sleeping system should fulfill different needs, depending on individual requirements, and has to be appropriate for the different sleeping postures. Muscles have to relax, decreasing the load of the intervertebral disks. A good resting place is the one that allows the entire musculoskeletal system to recuperate. An incorrect sleeping position or a sleeping system which is ergonomically insufficiently adapted and which does not support the vertebral column appropriately can result in unsatisfactory sleep with daytime tiredness – and most likely back pain on waking.

Sleeping position and posture shifts during sleep

To remain still conserves energy and helps falling asleep. Most people develop a specific body position to sleep – the best for relaxation and energy conservation. However, body position at sleep onset changes during sleep.

Posture changes are necessary to avoid muscle stiffness and pressure overloading of soft tissue. Too long periods of immobility may be harmful to the soft tissues and the musculoskeletal system, resulting in stiffness. In fragile people, such as children or elderly, long periods of immobilization may also have an impact on their respiration.[76]

Movements occur often before a shift in sleep stage. During deep sleep there is a minimal amount of movement, and generally during REM only brief twitches in the small muscles of the arms and legs can occur.

The number of movements during sleep is 10–20 per hour. Adults shift positions between 15 and 40 times per night, with about 2–4 major position shifts per hour.[77,78] Increase of body movement reflects fragmented sleep of bad quality: poor sleepers change position more frequently; they also sleep more often in the supine position than good sleepers.[77]

Spine support

While bed manufacturers used to have little, if any, interest in considering the physiological aspects of sleeping, attention has been focussed on ergonomic features, mainly the relationship between the bed and its impact on the spine. An interesting review has recently been published.[79]

Almost everybody experiences back pain at some time during their life. Most complaints arise from the lumbar area: pain is often caused by overloading of the spinal column, for instance, when adopting a damaging posture or performing sudden movements. Even soft tissues can be damaged by this overload. In these cases intervertebral discs function as absorbers of the shock.[80]

These discs consist mostly of water. Following a loading of the spine for a few hours, part of the fluid is lost (up to 10%). When the body is resting in a horizontal position, the intervertebral discs are unloaded and rehydrate. Recuperation of the lost water helps them regain their elasticity.[81] (This effect also causes the body to elongate approximately 1–2 cm (2%) during sleep.[82]) Hence it is essential that the vertebral column remains unloaded as much as possible during sleep. But a prolonged incorrect rest posture during sleep can result in loading. A good support of the vertebral column should optimally distribute the load, restoring the physiologic shape of the spine, thus relieving daily stress and reducing low back pain.

The question remains as to what is the optimal spinal curvature one should have during sleep? Should the lumbar lordosis be flattened? Classically, a good sleeping position is thought to be achieved when the spine adopts its natural, upright position, preserving the lumbar lordosis. For a lateral sleeping posture, it is generally assumed that an optimal support should allow the spine to be in a straight line in order to distribute the loading of the vertebral column symmetrically.[83]

Both body weight distribution and body dimension influence the position of the spine in any resting position and on any support. Since the human body will strive for minimal loading while sleeping, healthy people will automatically try to adjust their sleeping posture to their sleeping system. Bending the knees and hip joints to an angle of 45 degrees, a position naturally adopted by most people sleeping in a lateral position, relaxes the iliopsoas muscle and smoothes the lumbar lordosis.

The bed

There are different types of bed on the market, using horizontal or vertical coil springs and other materials. Manufacturers advertise the 'sleep-improving' qualities of their products showing, for example, how the contour of the bed conforms to that of the body.

Very few controlled studies[78] have been made that address the impact of sleep surfaces on sleep quality, and the few published reports have failed to demonstrate significant differences in sleep quality of healthy adults.[84,85] Young people sleep well regardless of the sleeping conditions, while adults can be affected by the sleeping surface. For instance, Suckling et al.[86] found that mobility increased when sleeping on a firm surface, and the depth and subjective estimates of sleep decreased.

Sleeping surfaces and mattresses

The core of most of the mattresses consists of either latex, spring, foam (such as polyurethane), or fluids. Some manufacturers combine these materials; for example, a core of springs with a cover of foam or latex.

Latex mattresses are composed of particles of foam rubber. Depending on the type of moulding, various elastic behaviors can be obtained with different stiffness zones, each zone being able to deform independently. Latex has a very good heat insulation but low air permeability, and the firmness is directly dependent on the density of the latex.

The advantage of the **spring mattress** is that stiffness can be adjusted. The wire thickness of the spring is mainly responsible for the elasticity. Spring mattresses support the body well: the greater the number of springs used, the better the support. Spring mattresses have good ventilation, but also low thermal insulation. Springs can have different shapes. Pocket springs are springs individually wrapped into 'sockets' and mounted in rows; they offer better support since they can deform independently of each other.

Foam mattresses are light, and easy to handle; they have a good thermal insulation and permeability as well as elasticity, with a small hysteresis. The characteristics of foam mattresses allow a wide variety of stiffness for a given density.

Water beds distribute weight evenly and can provide the right support, but they can provoke oscillations which disturb stability. They can limit motility and if not well designed can alter the microclimate, with bad ventilation and humidity.

The cover of the mattress functions as a protective top layer; it distributes contact pressure, and regularizes humidity and temperature. It should be adequately treated against dust mites and bacteria, and should not be allergenic. Thus the material of the cover should preferably be synthetic or natural.

- *Wool* has very good absorption and good thermal properties.
- *Silk* has poor thermal qualities but can absorb a lot of moisture and is suitable for people who sweat profusely. It has also good antiallergic properties.
- *Cotton* has poor thermal insulation so is suitable for warm climates. Although able to absorb large quantities of moisture it feels sticky at low moisture levels. It has good antibacterial properties.

Futon beds, traditionally used in Japan, are becoming more popular in Europe. The mattresses are made only with natural material. A thick cotton quilt is stuffed with layers of cotton wadding, sometimes combined with wool, and placed on a slatted support of rice straw or wood (in Europe). The sleeping surface moulds well to the body and the natural fibres allow good air circulation.

The material can absorb large quantities of moisture; therefore these mattresses need to be shaken regularly and aired.

Mechanical characteristics of mattresses

- *Hysteresis* measures the energy dissipated in the mattress. It should be minimized to avoid too much energy consumed in moving and changing posture. Latex mattresses have a better hysteresis than those with visco-elastic foams.
- *Density* of the mattress is representative of its fatigue resistance. The higher the density, the better the resistance, but also the greater the surface stiffness.
- *Stability* is an important feature of mattresses. If not stable enough (e.g., water beds) a sleeping surface can react to body movements by oscillating. Proprioceptive mechanisms to stabilize the sleeping posture

will stimulate continuous muscle activity, keeping some muscle groups under constant stress.
- *Elasticity* represents the force needed to dent the mattress and is reflected in its firmness. Elasticity is the feature of the sleeping surface that provides correct body support. With visco-elastic materials such as polyurethane, elasticity is dependent on the velocity of deformation, while elasticity of pure elastic material is constant.

People with back problems should take particular notice of the mechanical features of the bed, especially with regard to back support. Among other properties, pressure-relieving qualities are important. Ideally, the material properties of the mattress should be adjusted to each individual.

Mattress support: firm or soft?

Soft mattresses If a sleeping system is too soft, the contact areas between the body and the bed will be more widespread. The body will sink deeply into the mattress, especially the heavy parts. Although this position will prevent blood circulation problems and help some muscles to relax, it is certainly not the best relaxing position for the spine. In a lateral posture, the spine will be loaded asymmetrically, while in a supine sleeping position the pelvis will sink backward, yielding an excessive smoothing of the lumbar lordosis.

Sinking into the mattress will also limit body mobility. With a soft sleeping surface and large contact area, the body sinks into the mattress which may press against the skin, causing the local temperature to increase along with a tendency to compensatory sweating that may lead to arousals. The feeling of a moist surface will further disturb sleep.

Hence, an overweight person sleeping on a soft mattress will sag into it, the pelvic girdle sinking into the mattress. Small movements which normally should be enough to adjust position and avoid stiffness will be inefficient to change posture: the body will fall back into the hollow space. More energy will be needed for every change in position, which can result in arousals. On the other hand, if the heat dispersion of the supporting material is not good, a heat pocket surrounding the body can easily develop, resulting in disturbed sleep. Overly soft beds can also numb sensations.

Firm mattresses   If the sleeping system is too firm, the vertebral column can be incorrectly supported. When lying in a supine position the pelvis can first protrude forward due to the tension of the iliopsoas muscle, and when the muscle relaxes the pelvis will bend backward, flattening the lumbar lordosis.

In a lateral posture, only the large and heavy parts of the body, such as the pelvis and the shoulders, will be supported while the lumbar region will bend downward. By flexing the spine laterally, a firm mattress can induce locally increased pressure peaks.

So when sleeping on too firm surfaces, body weight will not be distributed evenly. Reducing areas of body contact with the sleeping surfaces increases pressure and shear forces on the skin and soft structures, compressing the vascular bed and resulting in a shortage of blood and oxygen supply to the tissues. If pronounced and persistent this can result in ischemia. Hence in order to limit the duration and level of contact pressure, body movements will increase.

Heavy persons could benefit from a firm mattress in order to avoid the pelvic girdle sinking deeply into the bed. A lean person sleeping on a firm surface will have increased risks of compression of some peripheral nerves, for example, at the elbows or blood vessels, especially at places where there are no fatty tissues or muscles to distribute contact forces, with the skin being squashed between the bones and the sleep surface. In supine position, the risk areas include the elbow, the scapula, and the heel; in the lateral posture the risk areas include the ankle, the knee, and the shoulder. This results in paresthesia, increased movements and posture adjustments, resulting in restlessness and arousals. Sleep becomes fragmented. Muscles will not relax adequately and this may slow down the rehydration of the intervertebral discs, with risks for back pain and stiffness when waking up, as well as the feeling of non-refreshed night sleep.

It is noteworthy that for subjects with pronounced back pain or injury, a firm mattress can yield temporary stress relief at the level of pain or injury and hence be preferred by the suffering subjects.[87]

Specific surfaces   Pressure-relieving mattresses do not always yield the expected results. For instance, some heavy parts of the body, such as the pelvic girdle, might sink into the mattress, causing it to sag, whereas other parts will rise up, resulting in an asymmetrically loaded spine.

Some manufacturers offer mattresses with different localized elastic properties, for example, firmer at the pelvic zone and softer at the shoulder, by placing pocket springs with different properties in a matrix, which deform independently. If well designed, these mattresses can provide a good support of the spine.

Bed size

A bed should be wide enough to allow for easy movements and posture changes, and should be at least 15–20 cm longer than the height of the sleeping person. The bed should preferably not be flat on the floor but elevated to enable good air circulation and convenient access getting in and out of bed.

Habituation and adaptation to changing sleeping system

People get used to the supporting pressure exerted on different parts of their body. Adapting to a new underlying sleeping surface can take many days.[78,88] Due to this adaptation, a temporary worsening of the back support can develop, even when one changes to a better sleeping system.

In a recent study,[88] 16 healthy and active adult men with regular working hours and without sleep disorders or allergy were investigated in a double-blind, cross-over study. The participants were studied at home, first sleeping in their habitual bed for 3 days. The next 6 weeks they slept in three different beds, changing bed after a 2-week period. The beds were outwardly similar in appearance but had different firmness. Sleep was estimated using both subjective estimates of sleep quality and objective measurements (actigraphy, sensor pads, and standard polysomnography). Significant changes in sleep quality were observed related to bed firmness. The effect of the beds was observed to change with time, often with a decreased impact at the end of the test period as compared to the initial days, suggesting a period of adaptation to the new sleeping surface.

This effect can be psychophysiological in nature which can take effect either at the beginning or end of the test. Initially there may be a 'placebo-like' effect related to the novelty and excitement of experiencing a new bed, which fades out after a few days. Toward the end of the test an 'anxious' expectancy develops when the individual awaits another bed. The effect can also be secondary to some changes in the bed's physical features: after a few nights of use and pressure, there may be a mechanical settling changing the characteristics of the bed. However, since the same beds were used for all the participants, this mechanical adaptation would have acted for the first user but not for the others.

Pillows

A pillow should be designed to support the head and the neck optimally in order to release the tension of the muscles supporting the head. While a soft pillow might feel comfortable and supportive, it can also hinder head movements during sleep, requiring more energy with risks of awakenings.

During sleep there is a tendency for the upper airways to become narrower, worsening breathing, especially in people who are overweight or over 40 years old. It is therefore important that the pillow does not further disturb breathing by wrongly positioning the head in relation to the cervical spine and thus narrowing the airways further. Ideally, when lying in a supine position the entire vertebral column should be in a straight line. If the pillow is too soft, breathing can also be worsened by allowing the head to sink into it.

Temperature under the head can increase during the night, especially if the material in the pillow is of poor quality. This can result in local sweating and awakenings. Pillows should hence have good thermal properties to allow rapid dissipation of heat below the head.

The type of filling of the pillow should be carefully considered, since it can produce allergic reactions such as rhinitis resulting in mucus secretion which obstructs the upper airway and disturbs sleep. Soft pillows are recommended for people sleeping on their stomach. Firm pillows should be used if sleep is mainly in the supine or lateral positions. Anatomically shaped pillows filled with water or with flexible thermosensitive materials adjusting 'automatically' to the shape of the head are reported to be very supportive. Feather filled pillows that mould very well to the shape of the head can cause allergies. Those made with synthetic material are less allergenic and can easily be washed.

Some pillows on the market contain material with magnetic properties supposed to promote sleep by increasing 'blood flow' in the head or 'optimizing the electrical activity of the brain'. There are many anecdotal reports about the positive influence of magnetic fields on health and sleep quality. It remains a very controversial issue and to our knowledge there are no major controlled studies yet supporting such claims.

It has become fashionable to place herbal sachets underneath the pillow to benefit from the sleep-inducing properties of these herbs.

Conclusions

The choice of a firm or soft mattress is not a matter of likes and dislikes: it should be done in consideration of individual needs.

The anthropometric features of a person should be weighed when choosing between a soft or a firm sleeping surface. Obese or lean, tall or short people do not have the same needs for sleep surfaces. Men and women probably have different requirements related to their different body contours. Furthermore, the health status of an individual should influence the choice of sleeping surface.

Back support qualities are very important. By combining different materials correctly (springs, latex, polyurethane) optimal correct support quality can be achieved. Support properties can be optimized by combining different stiffness zones – however, an incorrect assignment can do more harm than good.

An ideal sleeping system should also offer optimal spine support, with minimal deformities allowing freedom and easiness of movements as well as the possibility of posture changes, thus posing the least possible resistance and demanding minimal energy. It should be soft enough to avoid compression and therefore increased body movements and sleep disruption, but it should not be so soft as to hinder natural movements and posture changes.

Most of the properties of a sleeping system do not stand the test of time; all mattresses, even the most fatigue-resistant ones, lose some elasticity after a few years. Hence a mattress is not a piece of furniture that can be kept indefinitely; it has to be changed when needs be.

Bed and room disposition

Some people believe that the room disposition and bed placement can influence sleep, positively or negatively. In recent years the Asian concept of *Feng Shui* has become a popular approach to furniture arrangement in the home and workplace. *Feng Shui*, originally used to find the most appropriate burial site for the dead, is a belief that well-being can be enhanced by harmonizing the energy emanating from the Earth that flows throughout the environment.

Feng Shui is supposed to balance the two opposite but complementary forces which harmonize this energy: the *yin* and the *yang*. Used in the bedroom, it is expected to make surroundings both relaxing through the *yin*, promoting sleep, and energizing through the *yang*, optimizing alertness upon waking. The concept is to have a geometrically regular, minimalist and simply decorated bedroom, free from clutter. Visually stimulating items such as mirrors or hanging clothes are avoided as well as anything not associated with sleep, such as a TV or computer. The bed is placed in certain energy fields, avoiding interrupting the flow of energy, hence is placed between a door and a window and its position allows the lying person to see people entering the room. The bed is raised off the floor to let the energy flow around the bed and the head of the bed is directed toward a position particular to the sleeping person, in relation to the signs of the zodiac!

CONCLUSIONS

Stress, long days and sleepless nights wear on the body, leading to tiredness, fatigue, dulled reflexes and worsening of cognitive functions, as well as a decreased resistance of the defense systems. The few hours devoted to rest should foster a sleep of optimal quality.

Sleep is controlled by many factors, and environmental sleeping conditions can promote or prevent sleep. Other points which should also be addressed concern the invasion of entertainment equipment in everyday life and in the bedroom, such as TV and computers. Watching late TV programs is emotionally disturbing and/or visually stimulating, resulting in increased awakenings and difficulty to unwind, thus delaying sleep. This is becoming an acute problem particularly for teenagers, who often have already a biological tendency for phase delay in their circadian rhythms.

It is essential to increase public awareness about these issues. Many manufacturers of bedroom fixtures and bed systems are becoming conscious of the importance of these points and are trying to develop more adequate furnishings. A closer collaboration should evolve between these manufacturers, sleep researchers, and specialists in the domain of surroundings, light, sounds, and air.

To be successful when confronted with the many disturbing factors associated with a modern lifestyle, the art and conditions of sleep will need to become more dynamic, adjusting to the specific situations of the sleeping person and his or her environment.

REFERENCES

1. Trinder J, Kleiman J, Carrington M, et al. Autonomic activity during human sleep as a function of time and sleep stage. J Sleep Res 2001; 10: 253–64.

2. Burgess HJ, Trinder J, Kim Y, Luke D. Sleep and circadian influences on cardiac autonomic nervous system activity. Am J Physiol 1997; 273: H1761–H8.

3. Kerkhof GA, Van Dongen HPA, Bobbert AC. Absence of endogenous circadian rhythmicity in blood pressure? Am J Hypertens 1998; 11: 373–7.

4. Bader G, Eder DN. Elevating the head of the bed during sleep reduces snoring. [abstract]. World Association of Sleep Medicine, Berlin 2005.

5. Gitanjali B, Ananth R. Effect of acute exposure to loud occupational noise during daytime on the nocturnal sleep architecture, heart rate, and cortisol secretion in healthy volunteers. J Occup Health 2003; 45: 146–52.

6. Kawada T. Effects of traffic noise on sleep: a review. Nippon Eiseigaku Zasshi 1995; 50: 932–8.

7. Libert JP, Bach V, Johnson LC, et al. Relative and combined effects of heat and noise exposure on sleep in humans. Sleep 1991; 14: 24–31.

8. Vorwahl, Radiogefahren. Z Psychol Hyg 1929; 2: 71–4.

9. Craig DR. An investigation of basic skin resistance levels during sleep under differing conditions. Psychol Bull 1937; 34: 559.

10. Struempell A. Ein Beitrag zur Theorie des Schlafes. Pfluegers Arch 1878; 15: 573–4.

11. Tramo MJ, Cariani PA, Delgute B, Braida LD, Neurobiological foundations for the theory of harmony in Western tonal music. Ann NY Acad Sci 2001; 930: 992–1015.

12. Lamont A. Toddler's musical preferences. Ann NY Acad Sci 2003; 999: 518–19.

13. Trainor LJ, Tsang CD, Cheung VHW. Preference for sensory consonance in 2- and 4-month-old infants. Mus Percept 2002; 20: 187–94.

14. Costa-Giomi E. Young children's harmonic perception. Ann NY Acad Sci 2003; 999: 477–84.

15. Bellieni CV, Cordelli DM, Bagnoli F, Buonocore G. 11- to 15-year-old children of women who danced during their pregnancy. Biol Neonate 2004; 86: 63–65.

16. Gitanjali B. Effect of the Karnatic music raga 'Neelambari' on sleep architecture. Indian J Physiol Pharmacol 1998; 42: 119–22.

17. Tan LP. The effects of background music on quality of sleep in elementary school children. J Music Ther 2004; 41: 128–50.

18. Mornhinweg GC, Voignier RR. Music for sleep disturbance in the elderly. J Holist Nurs 1995; 13: 248–54.

19. Johnson JE. The use of music to promote sleep in older women. J Community Health Nurs 2003; 20: 27–35.

20. Lai HL, Good M. Music improves sleep quality in older adults. J Adv Nurs 2005; 49: 234–44.

21. Richards K, Nagel C, Markie M, Elwell J, Barone C. Use of complementary and alternative therapies to promote sleep in critically ill patients. Crit Care Nurs Clin North Am 2003; 15: 329–340.

22. Bonnet MH, Arand DL. The impact of music upon sleep tendency as measured by the multiple sleep latency test and maintenance of wakefulness test. Physiol Behav 2000; 71: 485–92.

23. Hernandez-Ruiz E. Effect of music therapy on the anxiety levels and sleep patterns of abused women in shelters. J Music Ther 2005; 42: 140–58.

24. Ogata S. Human EEG responses to classical music and simulated white noise: effects of a musical loudness component on consciousness. Percept Mot Skills 1995; 80: 779–90.

25. Jacobs GD, Friedman R. EEG spectral analysis of relaxation techniques. Appl Psychophysiol Biofeedback 2004; 29: 245–54.

26. Levin Yal. 'Brain music' in the treatment of patients with insomnia. Neurosci Behav Physiol 1998; 28: 330–5.

27. Kayumov L, Soare K, Serbine O, et al. Brain music therapy for treatment of insomnia and anxiety. Sleep 2002; 25 (Suppl): A241.

28. Bettermann H, Amponsah D, Cysarz D, van Leeuwen P. Musical rhythms in heart period dynamics: a cross-cultural and inter-disciplinary approach to cardiac rhythms. Am J Physiol 1999; 277: H1762–H70.

29. Reinhardt U. Investigations into synchroni-sation of heart rate and musical rhythm in a relaxation therapy in patients with cancer pain. Forsch Komplementarmed 1999; 6: 135–41.

30. Hofstetter JR, Hofstetter AR, Hughes AM, Mayeda AR. Intermittent long-wavelength red light increases the period of daily locomotor activity in mice. J Circadian Rhythms 2005; 3: 8.

31. Cajochen C, Munch M, Kobialka S, et al. High sensitivity of human melatonin, alertness, thermoregulation, and heart rate to short wave-length light. J Clin Endocrinol Metab 2005; 90(3): 1311–16.

32. Gooley JJ, Lu J, Fischer D, Saper CB. A broad role for melanopsin in nonvisual photore-ception. J Neurosci 2003; 23(18): 7093–106.

33. Kim SH, Jeong WS. Influence of illumination on autonomic thermoregulation and choice of clothing. Int J Biometeorol 2002; 46(3): 141–44.

34. Kubota T, Uchiyama M, Hirokawa G, et al. Effects of evening light on body temperature. Psychiatry Clin Neurosci 1998; 52(2): 248–9.

35. Tokura H, Kim HE. How does light intensity influence evening dressing behavior in the cold? J Physiol Anthropol Appl Human Sci 2005; 24(1): 37–40.

36. Park SJ, Tokura H. Effects of different light intensities during the daytime on circadian rhythm of core temperature in humans. Appl Human Sci 1998; 17(6): 253–7.

37. Phipps-Nelson J, Redman JR, Dijk DJ, Rajaratnam SM. Daytime exposure to bright light, as compared to dim light, decreases sleepiness and improves psychomotor vigilance performance. Sleep 2003; 26(6): 695–700.

38. Aizawa S, Tokura H. Exposure to bright light for several hours during the daytime lowers tympanic temperature. Int J Biometeorol 1997; 41(2): 90–3.

39. Kim HE, Tokura H. Influence of different light intensities during the daytime on evening dressing behavior in the cold. Physiol Behav 1995; 58(4): 779–83.

40. Kim SH, Tokura H. Visual alliesthesia–cloth color preference in the evening under the influ-ence of different light intensities during the day-time. Physiol Behav 1998; 65(2): 367–70.

41. Badia P, Wesensten N, Lammers W, Culpepper J, Harsh J. Responsiveness to olfactory stimuli pre-sented in sleep. Physiol Behav 1990; 48(1): 87–90.

42. Raudenbush B, Koon J, Smith J, Zoladz P. Effects of odorant administration on objective and subjective measures of sleep quality, post-sleep mood and alertness, and cognitive performance. North Am J Psychol 2003; 5(2): 181–92.

43. Carskadon MA, Herz RS. Minimal olfactory perception during sleep: why odor alarms will not work for humans. Sleep 2004; 27(3): 402–5.

44. Berger RJ. Bioenergetic functions of sleep and activity rhythms and their possible relevance to aging. Fed Proc 1975; 34: 97–102.

45. Wehr TA. A brain-warming function for REM sleep. Neurosci Biobehav Rev 1992; 16: 379–97.

46. Dickson PR. Effect of a fleecy woolen underlay on sleep. Med J Aust 1984; 140(2): 87–9.

47. Inoue Y, Shibasaki M, Ueda H, Ishizashi H. Mechanisms underlying the age-related decre-ment in the human sweating response. Eur J Appl Physiol Occup Physiol 1999; 79(2): 121–6.

48. Grucza R, Lecroart JL, Hauser JJ, Houdas Y. Dynamics of sweating in men and women dur-ing passive heating. Eur J Appl Physiol Occup Physiol 1985; 54(3): 309–14.

49. Baker FC, Selsick H, Driver HS, Taylor SR, Mitchell D. Different nocturnal body tempera-tures and sleep with forced-air warming in men and in women taking hormonal contraceptives. J Sleep Res 1998; 7(3): 175–81.

50. Kim HE, Tokura H. Effects of the menstrual cycle on dressing behavior in the cold. Physiol Behav 1995; 58(4): 699–703.

51. Sewitch DE, Kittrell EM, Kupfer DJ, Reynolds CF 3rd. Body temperature and sleep architec-ture in response to a mild cold stress in women. Physiol Behav 1986; 36(5): 951–7.

52. Haskell EH, Palca JW, Walker JM, Berger RJ, Heller HC. The effects of high and low ambient temperatures on human sleep stages. Elec-troencephalogr Clin Neurophysiol 1981; 51(5): 494–501.

53. Libert JP, Di Nisi J, Fukuda H, et al. Effect of continuous heat exposure on sleep stages in humans. Sleep 1988; 11(2): 195–209.

54. Mahapatra AP, Mallick HN, Kumar VM. Changes in sleep on chronic exposure to warm and cold ambient temperatures. Physiol Behav 2005; 84(2): 287–94.

55. Muzet A, Ehrhart J, Candas V, Libert JP, Vogt JJ. REM sleep and ambient temperature in man. Int J Neurosci 1983; 18(1–2): 117–26.

56. Ozaki H, Nagai Y, Tochihara Y. Physiological responses and manual performance in humans following repeated exposure to severe cold at night. Eur J Appl Physiol 2001; 84(4): 343–9.

57. Franco P, Szliwowski H, Dramaix M, Kahn A. Influence of ambient temperature on sleep characteristics and autonomic nervous control in healthy infants. Sleep 2000; 23(3): 401–7.

58. Van den Heuvel CJ. Anderson R, Ferguson SA. No link between distal vasodilatation and sleep onset latency in insomniacs. Sleep 2005; 28 (Suppl): A241.

59. Francis A, Coleman G. Ambient temperature cycles entrain the free-running circadian rhythms of the stripe-faced dunnart. J Comp Physiol [A] 1990; 167: 357–62.

60. Di Nisi J, Ehrhart J, Galeou M, Libert JP. Influence of repeated passive body heating on subsequent night sleep in humans. Eur J Appl Physiol Occup Physiol 1989; 59(1–2): 138–45.

61. Dewasmes G, Loos N, Candas V, Muzet A. Effects of a moderate nocturnal cold stress on daytime sleep in humans. Eur J Appl Physiol 2003; 89(5): 483–8.

62. Savourey G, Bittel J. Cold thermoregulatory changes induced by sleep deprivation in men. Eur J Appl Physiol Occup Physiol 1994; 69(3): 216–20.

63. Caine-Bish NL, Potkanowicz ES, Otterstetter R, Glickman EL. Thermal and metabolic responses of sleep deprivation of humans during acute cold exposure. Aviat Space Environ Med 2004; 75(11): 964–8.

64. Okamoto-Mizuno K, Tsuzuki K, Mizuno K, Iwaki T. Effects of partial humid heat exposure during different segments of sleep on human sleep stages and body temperature. Physiol Behav 2005; 83(5): 759–65.

65. Okamoto-Mizuno K, Tsuzuki K, Mizuno K. Effects of head cooling on human sleep stages and body temperature. Int J Biometeorol 2003; 48(2): 98–102.

66. Buckalew LW, Rizzuto A. Subjective response to negative air ion exposure. Aviat Space Environ Med 1982; 53(8): 822–3.

67. Terman M, Terman JS, Ross DC. A controlled trial of timed bright light and negative air ionization for treatment of winter depression. Arch Gen Psych 1998; 55: 875–82.

68. Wakamura T, Sato M, Sato A, et al. Preliminary study on influence of negative air ions generated from pajamas on core body temperature and salivary IgA during night sleep. Int J Occup Med Environ Health 2004; 17(2): 295–8.

69. Owen S, Morganstern M, Hepworth J, Woodcock A. Control of house dust mite antigen in bedding. Lancet 1990; 335(8686): 396–7.

70. Mosbech H, Jensen A, Heinig JH, Schou C. House dust mite allergens on different types of mattresses. Clin Exp Allergy 1991; 21(3): 351–5.

71. Weeks J, Oliver J, Birmingham K, Crewes A, Carswell F. A combined approach to reduce mite allergen in the bedroom. Clin Exp Allergy 1995; 25(12): 1179–83.

72. Luczynska C, Tredwell E, Smeeton N, Burney P. A randomized controlled trial of mite allergenimpermeable bed covers in adult mite-sensitized asthmatics. Clin Exp Allergy 2003; 33(12): 1648–53.

73. Rijssenbeek-Nouwens LH, Oosting AJ, De Monchy JG, et al. The effect of anti-allergic mattress encasings on house dust mite-induced early- and late-airway reactions in asthmatic patients. A double-blind, placebo-controlled study. Clin Exp Allergy 2002; 32(1): 117–25.

74. Jirapongsananuruk O, Malainual N, Sangsupawanich P, Aungathiputt V, Vichyanond P. Partial mattress encasing significantly reduces house dust mite antigen on bed sheet surface: a controlled trial. Ann Allergy Asthma Immunol 2000; 84(3): 305–10.

75. Cameron MM, Hill N. Permethrin-impregnated mattress liners: a novel and effective intervention against house dust mites (Acari: Pyroglyphididae). J Med Entomol 2002; 39(5): 755–62.

76. Chapell MS. Respiratory problems during sleep in infants and the elderly and possible relation to mattress compression. Sleep 1993; 16(4): 391.

77. De Koninck JM, Lorrain D, Gagnon P. Sleep positions and position shifts in five age groups: an ontogenic picture. Sleep 1992; 15(2): 143–9.

78. Bader G, Engdal S. The influence of bed firmness on sleep quality. Appl Ergonom 2000; 31: 487–97.

79. Haex B. Back and Bed: Ergonomic Aspects of Sleeping. London: CRC Press/M Dekker; 2005.

80. Nachemson A, Elfstrom G. Intravital dynamic pressure measurements in lumbar discs. Scand J Rehabil Med 1970; 1 (Suppl): 1–40.

81. Adams MA, Hutton WC. The effect of posture on the fluid content of lumbar inter-vertebral discs. Spine 1983; 8(6): 665–71.

82. Krag MA, Cohen MC, Haugh LD, Pope MH. Body height change during upright and recumbent posture. Spine 1990; 15(3): 202–7.

83. Gracovetsky SA, Farfan A. The optimum spine. Spine 1986; 11(6): 543–73.

84. Kleitman N. Sleep and Wakefulness. Chicago, IL: University of Chicago Press, revised 1963.

85. Buysse DJ, Reynolds III, CF. Insomnia. In: Thopry MJ, ed, Handbook of Sleep Disorders. New York: Dekker Inc, 1999: 375–433.

86. Suckling EE, Koening EH, Hoffman BF, Brooks C. The physiological effects of sleeping on hard and soft beds. Human Biol 1957; 29: 274–88.

87. Garfin SR, Pye SA. Bed design and its effect on chronic low back pain – a limited controlled trial. Pain 1981; 10(1): 87–91.

88. Bader G, Blomqvist C. The impact of bed firmness on sleep. Sleep 2002; 25 (Suppl): A392–393.

CHAPTER 8

Interaction between sleep and stress in shift workers

Torbjörn Åkerstedt

A close relationship exists between quality of sleep and the demands of the workplace. Sleep has a number of effects on the speed and efficiency of work performance. Conversely, work takes up most of our waking time and can have a significant influence on both the duration and quality of sleep. Perhaps the two most important effects of aspects of work on sleep experience are the number of hours worked and the amount of stress produced by the job tasks. Additionally, factors such as physical workload may contribute to the overall stress of the job. The effects of these work characteristics on sleep are profound and will be the focus of this chapter.

STRESS AND SLEEP

The core problem of stress with regard to sleep is that stress produces significant physiologic activation, which is in conflict with the inherent requirement of physiologic deactivation during sleep. The sections below review the basic concept of stress, and various studies that have examined its influence on sleep quality and daytime alertness.

The concept of stress

From a general perspective, psychosocial stress refers to 'the rate of wear and tear in the organism', and the biological definition of stress refers to the non-specific response to any demand[1] to increase the chances of survival of an individual who is facing a life-threatening situation. More specifically, stress is determined by 'the balance between the perceived demands from the environment and the individual's resources to meet those demands'.[2,3]

Contemporary physiologic stress models derive from Cannon's[4] and Selye's pioneering work.[1] Selye[5] proposed a model of stress, the general adaptation syndrome (GAS), composed of three stages: alarm, resistance, and exhaustion. These reflected the physiologic non-specific response to a challenge. The resistance stage of GAS has profound energy requirements, which, if persistent over time, deplete the person's capacity and lead to exhaustion.

Cannon[4] developed the concept of the 'fight–flight' response, which linked the emotional perception of a 'threat' to physiologic changes in the periphery. Markers of the fight–flight response are the catecholamines, epinephrine and norepinephrine, and other physiologic indicators associated with the autonomic nervous system.[6,7] Thus, the sympathetic adrenal medullary (SAM) system is activated when the individual feels threatened, irrespective of whether the requirement is to battle or to escape the emergency.

The hypothalamo-pituitary-adrenocortical (HPA) axis is also fundamental in the stress reaction. When the SAM system is activated and neuropeptides like corticosteroid-releasing hormone and vasopressin are released, they in turn stimulate adrenocorticotropic hormone release into the general blood circulation within the pituitary.[6,8] An increase or decrease in the HPA axis and SAM system produces abnormal levels of mainly cortisol and catecholamines into the blood.[9–11] These stress systems interact with the major endocrine and gastrointestinal and immune systems through complex stimulatory and inhibitory feedback pathways.[12]

Long-term effects of stress are described as 'allostasis', being the ability of the body to increase or decrease the activation level of vital functions to new steady states that are dependent on the characteristics of the challenge and the person's emotions and appraisal of events.[13] The resulting 'allostatic load' represents the cumulative cost to the body when the systems start to malfunction after a stressful event.[14] It is suggested that serious pathophysiology can occur if overload is not relieved in some way.[13] Clearly, one of the outcomes may be insomnia.

One of the leading psychosocial measures in work stress research is the demand/control model of Karasek[15] and Theorell.[16] Thus, high demands and low decision latitude have been found predictive of cardiovascular and other types of disease.[17–20] A somewhat different approach is that of Siegrist and his contrast between effort and resources.[21] In this model 'immersion' has an important role, representing major commitment and effort. Another important work-related factor may be the amount of social support received at work. Several studies have indicated the impact of lack of such support on cardiovascular disease, depression, and other outcomes.[16]

Connection between sleep and stress

Considering the physiologic activation involved in the stress response it seems logical to expect a connection with sleep. The evidence is, however, surprisingly modest, at least in terms of studies of causal connections. Nevertheless a number of cross-sectional epidemiologic studies point to a strong link between stress and sleep.[22–24] In fact, stress is considered the primary cause of persistent psychophysiologic insomnia.[25] In one study of life events, Cernovsky[26] demonstrated a clear increase in negative life events before an outbreak of insomnia.

Partinen et al.[27] investigated several occupational groups and found disturbed sleep to be most common among manual workers and much less so among physicians or managing directors. Geroldi et al.[28] found in a retrospective study of older individuals (above the age of 75 years) that former white collar workers reported better sleep than blue collar workers. Kupperman et al.[29] reported fewer sleep problems in individuals who were satisfied with their work.

In one of the more detailed epidemiological studies, Ribet et al.[30] studied more than 21 000 subjects in France, using a sleep disturbance index and logistic regression analysis. It was found that shift work, a long working week, exposure to vibrations, and 'having to hurry' appeared to be the main risk factors, controlling for age and gender. Disturbed sleep was more frequent in women and in older age groups.[24,31,32]

The work stressor most closely linked to disturbed sleep may be 'work under high demands'.[23,24,30,33] Åkerstedt et al.[33] found that the strongest item of the demand index was 'having to exert a lot of effort at work' – not simply 'having too much to do', for example. It was also found that when 'not being able to stop thinking about work in the evening' was added to the regression this variable took over part of the role of work demands as a predictor. This suggests that it may not be work demands *per se* that are important, but rather their non-remitting character. Lack of social support at work is also a risk indicator for disturbed sleep.[33] Poor (general) social support has been associated, for instance, with sleep complaints in Vietnam war veterans,[34] even if the amount of work available is rather limited.

In addition, epidemiologic studies have shown a connection between disturbed sleep and later occurrence of stress-related disorders such as cardiovascular disease[35–37] and diabetes type II.[38] The mechanism has not been identified but both lipid as well as glucose metabolism are impaired in relation to experimentally reduced sleep.[39]

Burnout is another result of long-term stress and is a growing health problem in many Western countries.[40] In Sweden, burnout is estimated to account for most of the doubling of long-term sickness absence since the mid-nineties.[41] The characteristic clinical symptoms of the condition are excessive and persistent fatigue, emotional distress, and cognitive dysfunction.[42,43] Self-reports of disturbed sleep are pronounced in patients scoring high on burnout.[44,45]

Stress and polysomnography

A number of laboratory studies of stress and sleep have been carried out, but the stressors have been rather artificial (e.g., an unpleasant movie) and the results unclear.[22] It is probably the case that the stressor needs to be of real significance to the individual in order to have any effect.

The number of physiologic investigations of the effects of common life stress on sleep is surprisingly low. In addition, the stress levels that are used in such studies are fairly modest. Thus, there have been studies looking at students' sleep the night before a big exam, sleep before a day of skydiving, sleep when on call, or sleep before an early awakening.[46–49] The results indicate a slightly negative effect on sleep efficiency and the amount of deep sleep.

Other results suggest that it is the worrying and the tension before the following sleep or before the next day that are most important.[50–52] Sleep appears to contain less slow-wave sleep (SWS) under such circumstances and this supports the notion that the anticipation of difficulties is important in the stress reaction.

It has also been shown that sleep is disturbed under threats to national security, for example, after the nuclear accident at Three Mile Island, USA, and during the scud missile attacks on Israel during the Gulf War.[53,54] The effect of losing a life partner has in one study been shown to have surprisingly modest effects – mainly an increase in rapid eye movement (REM) intensity.[55]

Post-traumatic stress disorder (PTSD) is another well-established cause of disturbed sleep, even if many of the more common indicators of sleep quality (sleep latency, efficiency of sleep, total length of sleep, and amount of stages 3 and 4) are only moderately affected.[56–59] Instead it appears that its major effect is to disturb REM sleep, in particular by either increasing or reducing its duration, and by increasing its intensity. The disorder also increases the number of awakenings. The unpleasant dreams associated with traumatic memories also tend to produce conditioned avoidance responses in affected individuals, resulting in postponements on a daily basis of retiring or of even entering the sleeping area.

Clinical aspects

In patients with primary insomnia there is an increased incidence of stress markers, including elevated cortisol levels, increased heart rate, and above-average body temperature[60–63]. In anxiety–associated insomnia, repeated stress that occurs frequently interferes with the normal sleep process.[64] This, in turn, gives rise to worrying about the next time one has to go to bed, which in turn disrupts sleep, and so on. This vicious circle leads to an adjustment of the stress-regulating system and the establishment of a higher base level for physiologic activation.

Recently, reports from several countries have suggested that the phenomenon of burnout is increasing.[40] Burnout is defined as extreme fatigue due to long-term exposure to stress[65] and is the main cause of the doubling of sickness absence in Sweden since the mid-nineties.[41] Questionnaire studies usually show pronounced increases of reports of disturbed sleep[44] and recently it has been demonstrated that sleep polysomnography is characterized by a high degree of disturbed sleep,[66,67] as well as reduced SWS, long sleep and REM latencies, and other indicators of abnormal sleep.

SHIFT WORK AND SLEEP/ WAKEFULNESS

The key problem with shift work in relation to sleep and wakefulness is that the night shift component requires work when the circadian clock drives the physiology towards deactivation and that sleep is displaced to a time of day when the circadian clock drives the physiology towards activation. This results in a conflict with consequences for disturbed sleep and alertness. The concept of shift work is introduced below and then its links to sleep and alertness are discussed.

Shift work

'Shift work' is an imprecise concept, although it usually refers to a work-hour system in which a relay of employees extends the period of production beyond the conventional 8-hour day. There are four major types of shift work: day work, permanently displaced work hours, rotating shift work, and roster work.

Day work involves work periods somewhere between approximately 7 a.m. and 7 p.m. *Permanently displaced work hours* requires the individual to work either a morning shift (approximately 6 a.m. to 2 p.m.), an afternoon shift (approximately 2 p.m. to 10 p.m.), or a night shift (approximately 10 p.m. to 6 a.m.). *Rotating shift work* involves alternation between two or three shifts. Two-shift work usually involves morning and afternoon shifts, while three-shift work also includes the night shift. Three-shift work is often subdivided according to the number of teams that are used to cover the 24 hours of a work cycle; this is usually three to six teams, depending on the speed of rotation (number of consecutive shifts of the same type).

Roster work is similar to rotating shift work but may be less regular, more flexible, and less geared to specific teams. It is used in service-oriented occupations, such as transport, health care, and law enforcement. In most industrialized countries, approximately one-third of the population has some form of 'non-day work' (shift work).[68] About 5 to 10% of them have shift work that includes night work.

In Europe, approximately 20% of the population in the European Union have work shifts that include night hours.[69] Among the member states, the UK, Austria, Finland, Ireland and France report more than 20% of males working nights, at least occasionally. Those with the lowest proportions of night shift workers are Portugal and Spain (< 15%). Among women the prevalence of night work is 10%, with Finland (15%), Ireland (15%), and the UK (14%) being the highest and Portugal (7%) and Spain (7%) the lowest.

The US Bureau of Labor Statistics Current Population Survey in May 1997 indicated that 82.9% of full-time wage and salary earners work regular daytime hours. Alternate schedules worked included evening shifts (4.6%), employer-arranged irregular schedules (3.9%), night shifts (3.5%), and rotating shifts (2.9%). A rough estimate of the amount of night work in the USA would be 6.4–11%, depending on the proportion of night work involved among the group 'employer-arranged irregular schedules'.

In most parts of Asia, Africa, and South America the figures vary between 1% and 10%, depending on the degree of industrial development.

Sleep in shift work

Early[70–74] as well as more recent studies[30] indicate that the dominant health problem reported by shift workers is disturbed sleep and wakefulness. At least three-fourths of the shift workers are affected[75] and insufficient sleep is often given as the reason for leaving shift work.

The night sleep *before* the first night shift is usually rather long,[76] starts rather early, and lasts to around 8 o'clock in the morning, or somewhat beyond. It is frequently (30–50% prevalence) associated with napping in the afternoon before the first night shift, especially if the preceding main sleep has been short.

Sleep after a night shift is usually initiated 1 hour after the termination of the shift,[76–78] with very little variation (30–60 min standard deviation) between individuals. The study by Pilcher et al.[78] also showed that most sleep reduction occurred after rotating night shifts – permanent night work seemed to allow slightly longer sleep.

About a third of the shift workers add a late afternoon nap between subsequent night shifts.[76,77,79] The nap duration often exceeds 1 hour and the prevalence of napping increases with decreasing length of the prior main sleep.[80,81] The nap thus seems to be a compensation for insufficient prior sleep.

The long-term effects of shift work on sleep are rather poorly understood. However, Dumont[82] found that the amount of sleep/wake and related disturbances in present-day workers were positively related to their previous experience of night work. Guilleminault[83] found an over-representation of former shift

workers with different clinical sleep/wake disturbances appearing at a sleep clinic. Recently, we have shown that in pairs of twins discordant on night work exposure, the exposed twin reported somewhat deteriorated sleep quality and health after retirement.[84]

Polysomnography and night work

Electroencephalographic (EEG) studies of rotating shift workers and similar groups have shown that duration of sleep during the day sleep is 1–4 hours shorter than sleep at night.[85–90] The shortening is due to the fact that sleep is terminated after only 4–6 hours, without the individual being able to return to sleep. The sleep loss is primarily accounted for by reductions in stage 2 sleep and REM sleep (dream sleep). Stages 3 and 4 ('deep' sleep) do not seem to be affected. Furthermore, the time taken to fall asleep (sleep latency) is usually shorter. Also, night sleep before a morning shift is reduced but is terminated artificially and the awakening is usually difficult and unpleasant.[79,91–93]

Interestingly, day sleep does not seem to improve much across series of night shifts.[94,95] It appears, however, that night workers sleep slightly better (longer) than rotating workers on the night shift.[96–98]

Subjective alertness

With respect to the prevalence of perceived sleepiness, a wealth of questionnaire studies suggest that the overwhelming majority of shift workers experience sleepiness in connection with night shift work, whereas daywork is associated with only marginal or no sleepiness.[72,74,99–106] The studies by Verhaegen's[103] and Paley's[106] groups are somewhat unusual in that they had an experimental design and showed that reported fatigue increased on entering and decreased on leaving shift work.

In many studies a majority of shift workers admitted to having experienced involuntary sleep on the night shift, whereas this was rare on day-oriented shifts.[107–110] Between 10% and 20% reported falling asleep during night work.

Ambulatory EEG recordings verify that incidents of actual sleep occur during night work in, for example, process operators.[89] Other groups, such as train drivers or truck drivers, showed clear signs of falling-asleep incidents when driving at night.[111–113] This occurs toward the second half of the night and appears as repeated bursts of alpha and theta EEG activity, together with closed eyes and slow undulating eye movements. As a rule the bursts are short (1–15 seconds) but frequent, and seem to reflect letdowns in the effort to fend off sleep. Approximately one-fourth of the subjects recorded show the EEG and electrooculographic patterns of fighting with sleep. This is clearly a larger proportion than that found in subjective reports of falling-asleep episodes.

As may be expected, sleepiness on the night shift is reflected in performance. One of the classic studies in this area was carried out by Bjerner et al.[114] who showed that errors in meter readings over a period of 20 years in a gas works had a pronounced peak on the night shift. There was also a secondary peak during the afternoon. Similarly, Brown[115] demonstrated that compared to daytime performance the speed with which telephone operators connected calls was considerably slower at night. Hildebrandt et al.[116] found that train drivers failed to operate their alerting safety devices more often at night than during the day. Most other studies of performance have used laboratory type tests and demonstrated, for example, reduced reaction time or poorer mental arithmetic performance on the night shift.[92,98] Flight simulation studies have, furthermore, shown that the ability to 'fly' a simulator,[117] or to carry out a performance test[118] at night may decrease to a level corresponding to that after moderate alcohol consumption (>0.05% blood alcohol).

The sleepiness induced by irregular work hours also causes increased accident risks. This is particularly obvious in connection with road transport. Thus Harris[119] and Hamelin[120] and others[121–123] convincingly demonstrated that single vehicle truck accidents have, by far, the greatest probability of occurring at night (early morning). Similar results have been presented for other car accidents.[124] Apparently, fatal accidents are particularly common in connection with early morning driving.

Furthermore, the (US) National Transportation Safety Board (NTSB) found that 30–40% of all US truck accidents are fatigue-related (and grossly underestimated in conventional reports). Recently, the latter investigation was extended to search for the immediate causes of fatigue-induced accidents.[125] It was found that the most important factor was the amount of sleep obtained during the preceding 24 hours and split-sleep patterns, whereas the length of time driving seemed to play a minor role. The NTSB also found that the Exxon Valdez accident in 1989 was due to fatigue, caused by reduced sleep and extended work hours.[126] In a new report published by NTSB, the current situation is summarized by the US Department of Transport's investigations into fatigue in the 1990s.[127] The extent of fatal, fatigue-related accidents is considered to be around 30%. This is approximately equivalent to the level of incidence in the air-traffic sector, while similar accidents at sea have an estimated occurrence of slightly less than 20%.

For conventional industrial operations fewer data are available[128,129] but indicate that overall accidents tend to occur, not surprisingly, when activity is at its peak. These values, however, do not take account of the prevalence of work hours at different times of day. The most carefully executed study, from car manufacturing, seems to indicate a moderate increase (30–50%) in accident risk on night shift work.[130] Most other studies also show an increase in accident rates on the night shift,[131–135] but not all.

It is also believed that the (night-time) nuclear plant meltdown at Chernobyl, in the Former Soviet Union, was due to human error related to work scheduling.[68] Similar observations have been made for the Three Mile Island reactor accident and the near-miss incidents at the David Beese reactor in Ohio and at the Rancho Seco reactor in California. Several studies have tried to evaluate the costs to society of alertness-related accidents and loss of performance (which does not necessarily reflect only the costs of shift work). One estimate is that the cost of these accidents and performance reductions exceeds $40 billion per year in the USA.[136] Others have claimed this to be a gross overestimation,[137] but the costs are still considerable. Still, it should be emphasized that it is not clear to what extent night shift fatigue may have been the main causal factor.

The mechanism behind disturbed sleep and wakefulness

Whereas living conditions may play a role in the negative effects on sleep, the main reason for the fact that daytime sleep is usually shorter than that at night has to do with the influence of circadian rhythms. The more sleep is postponed from the evening towards noon next day, the more truncated it becomes and when noon is reached the trend reverts.[85,138] Thus, sleep during the morning hours is strongly interfered with, despite the sizable sleep loss that, logically, should enhance the ability to maintain sleep.[139]

Also homeostatic influences control sleep. For example, the expected 4–5 hours of daytime sleep, after a night spent awake, will be reduced to 2 hours if a normal night's sleep precedes it and to 3.5 hours if a 2-hour nap is allowed.[140] Thus, the time of sleep termination depends on the balance between the circadian and homeostatic influences. The circadian homeostatic regulation of sleep has also been demonstrated in great detail in studies of forced or spontaneous desynchronization under conditions of temporal isolation and ad lib sleep hours.[139,141]

As with sleep, the two main factors behind sleepiness and performance impairment are circadian and homeostatic factors. Their effects may be difficult to separate in field studies but

are clearly discernible in laboratory sleep deprivation studies[142] as well as in studies of forced desynchronization.[143] Alertness falls rapidly after awakening but gradually levels out as wakefulness is extended. The circadian influence appears as a sine-shaped superimposition upon this exponential fall in alertness.[144]

Individual differences and shift work sleep disorder

It has often been observed that some shift workers have more difficulties than others. Among the cited factors that are thought to inhibit adjustment to night work are the diurnal 'type' of person one is (being an evening or morning person), age, and having an excessive need for sleep.[145] The limited findings regarding these influences, however, are limited and prevent firm conclusions. Whatever the causes, the symptoms resulting from an inability to adjust to shift work are inevitably excessive fatigue/sleepiness and non-restorative sleep.[146]

At present it is thought that the sleep/wake problems in shift work fulfill the criteria for disease, which has received a diagnostic classification: 'Shift work sleep disorder' (SWSD). *The Diagnostic and Statistical Manual of Mental Disorders (DSM IV)*[147] defines shift work sleep disorder (SWSD) as 'report of difficulty falling asleep, staying asleep, or non-restorative sleep for at least 1 month' and it must be associated with 'a work period that occurs during the habitual sleep phase'. The recent version of the *International Classification of Sleep Disorders* (ICSD)[148] lists excessive daytime sleepiness as an additional criterion for the syndrome. Note that normal night sleep and normal daytime alertness should be present when the individual is not working nights. See also Reid and Zee[149] for a recent review of SWSD as a circadian rhythm sleep disorder (CRSD).[149]

In one recent attempt to estimate the prevalence of SWSD the authors arrived at 10% of a population of shift workers.[150] Insomnia was defined according to DSM IV[147] as 'difficulties falling asleep, staying asleep or experiencing non-restorative sleep for at least 1 month'. The definition of SWSD[151] included the symptoms listed above (including excessive sleepiness) but occurring 'sometimes' or 'often' and with a severity of at least 6 on a 1–10 scale. The Epworth sleepiness scale level for excessive sleepiness was 13 (usually 10). Excessive sleepiness in this study was 24.7% in night workers, 20.3% in rotating workers and 15.5% in day workers. Using the established cut-off at 10, the values were 44.8%, 35.8%, and 32.7%, respectively. Interestingly, those shift workers who suffered from insomnia or excessive sleepiness also showed a higher prevalence of ulcers, depression, sleepiness-related accidents, missed work days, missed family/social events, etc. than those without sleep/sleepiness problems. These differences were not seen in day workers. In another study of 400 shift workers it was found that among the 8% of the sample who had a very negative attitude to work hours there was a greater proportion of sleepiness and sleep complaints.[152]

The fact that SWSD is now recognized as a classifiable disorder will increase the likelihood that it will be seen as a candidate condition for pharmacologic treatment. Perhaps indicative of a new trend in viewing the disorder is a recent study by Czeisler et al.,[153] who found that the alertness-enhancing drug modafinil decreased night shift sleepiness in terms of subjective, behavioral, and physiologic measures. Still, reduced sleep and alertness in connection with night shift work are extremely common, and further work is needed identify and test effective treatments for this important disorder.

CONCLUSIONS

The present chapter suggests that psychosocial stress and work hours are important causes of shortened or disturbed sleep as well as sleepiness, especially in the case of shift work. This raises the question of what might be the results of a combination of stress and shift work. There is also a certain similarity between the stress and night work effects. In both cases sleep appears to be interfered with by an increase in metabolic rate, which in turn is induced by stress and the biological clock. Strategies for addressing the physical and psychologic stresses associated with shift work could possibly include metabolism-reducing techniques, such as relaxation treatment or perhaps melatonin supplements in combination with light therapy. Some research has suggested that these may have beneficial effects on job stress and circadian rhythm disruption.

Other countermeasures with respect to shift work could include a provision for more free time for recuperation, napping to compensate for sleep loss, or revised scheduling, so that there are fewer night shifts in a row (in rotating systems).[154] None of these have, however, been shown to dramatically ameliorate sleep/wake problems in shift work. With respect to stress-induced insomnia recent developments in cognitive behavioral therapy are promising.[155]

REFERENCES

1. Selye H, ed. The Stress of Life. New York: McGraw Hill, 1956.
2. Frankenhaeuser M. A psychobiological framework for research on human stress and coping. In: Appley HH, Trumbull R, eds. Dynamics of Stress: Physiological, Psychological and Social Perspective. New York: Plenum Press, 1986: 101–16.
3. Lundberg U. Methods and applications of stress research. Technol Health Care 1995; 3: 3–9.
4. Cannon WB. The emergency function of the adrenal medulla in pain and the major emotions. Am J Physiol 1914; 33: 356–72.
5. Selye H. The general adaptation syndrome and the diseases of adaptation. J Clin Endocrinol 1946; 6: 117–231.
6. Dunn AJ, Berridge CW. Physiological and behavioral responses to corticotropin-releasing factor administration: is CRF a mediator of

anxiety or stress responses? Brain Res Rev 1990; 15: 71–100.

7. Brown MR. Neuropeptide-mediated regulation of the neuroendocrine and autonomic responses to stress. In: McCubbin J, Kaufman P, Nemeroff C, eds. Stress, Neuropeptides, and Systemic Disease San Diego: Academic Press 1991: 73–93.

8. Rock JP, Oldfield EH, Schulte HM, et al. Corticotropin releasing factor administered into the ventricular CSF stimulates the pituitary-adrenal axis. Brain Res 1984; 323: 365–8.

9. Sapolsky RM, Krey LC, McEwen BS. Stress down-regulates corticosterone receptors in a site-specific manner in the brain. Endocrinology 1984; 114: 287–92.

10. McEwen B, Albeck D, Cameron H, et al. Stress and the brain: a paradoxical role for adrenal steroids. In: Litwack G, ed. Vitamins and Hormones. New York: Academic Press Inc, 1995: 371–402.

11. Folkow B. Physiological aspects of the 'defence' and 'defeat' reactions. Acta Physiol Scand 1997; 640: 34–7.

12. Chrousos GP, Gold PW. The concepts of stress and stress system disorders. J Am Med Assoc 1992; 267: 1244–52.

13. McEwen BS, Wingfield JC. The concept of allostasis in biology and biomedicine. Horm Behav 2003; 43: 2–15.

14. McEwen BS. Protection and damage from acute and chronic stress: allostasis and allostatic overload and relevance to the pathophysiology of psychiatric disorders. Ann N Y Acad Sci 2004; 1032: 1–7.

15. Karasek RA. Job demands, job decision latitude and mental strain. Implications for job redesign. Adm Sci Q 1979; 24: 285–308.

16. Theorell T. The Demand-Control-Support Model for studying health in relation to the work environment: an interactive model. In: Orth-Gomér K, Schneiderman N, eds. Behavioral Medicine Approaches to Cardiovascular Disease Prevention. Lawrence Erlbaum Associates, Mahwah, NJ: 1996: 69–85.

17. Alfredsson L, Spetz C-L, Theorell T. Type of occupation and near-future hospitalization for myocardial infarction and some other diagnoses. Int J Epidemiol 1985; 14: 378–88.

18. Hammar N, Alfredsson L, Theorell T. Job characteristics and the incidence of myocardial infarction. Int J Epidemiol 1994; 23: 277–84.

19. Toomingas A, Theorell T, Michélsen H, Nordemar R. Associations between self-rated psychosocial work conditions and musculoskeletal symptoms and signs. Scand J Work Environ Health 1997; 23: 130–9.

20. Theorell T, Tsutsumi A, Hallquist J, et al. Decision latitude, job strain, and myocardial infarction: a study of working men in Stockholm. Am J Public Health 1998; 88: 382–88.

21. Siegrist J. A Theory of occupational stress. In: Dunham J, ed. Stress in the Workplace. Past, Present and Future. London: Whurt Publisher 2000: 52–65.

22. Åkerstedt T. Sleep and stress. In: Peter JH, Podszus T, von Wichert P, eds. Sleep Related Disorders and Internal Diseases. Heidelberg: Springer Verlag, 1987: 183–91.

23. Urponen H, Vuori I, Hasan J, Partinen M. Self-evaluations of factors promoting and disturbing sleep: an epidemiological survey in Finland. Social Sci Med 1988; 26: 443–50.

24. Ancoli-Israel S, Roth T. Characteristics of insomnia in the United States: results of the 1991 National Sleep Foundation survey. I. Sleep 1999; 22(Suppl 2): S347–S53.

25. Morin CM, Rodrigue S, Ivers H. Role of stress, arousal, and coping skills in primary insomnia. Psychosom Med 2003; 65: 259–67.

26. Cernovsky ZZ. Life stress measures and reported frequency of sleep disorders. Percept Mot Skills 1984; 58: 39–49.

27. Partinen M, Eskelinen L, Tuomi K. Complaints of insomnia in different occupations. Scand J Work Environ Health 1984; 10: 467–9.

28. Geroldi C, Frisoni GB, Rozzini R, De Leo D, Trabucchi M. Principal lifetime occupation and sleep quality in the elderly. Gerontology 1996; 42: 163–9.

29. Kuppermann M, Lubeck DP, Mazonson PD, et al. Sleep problems and their correlates in a working population. J Gen Internal Med 1995; 10: 25–32.

30. Ribet C, Derriennic F. Age, working conditions, and sleep disorders: a longitudinal analysis in the French cohort ESTEV. Sleep 1999; 22: 491–504.

31. Karacan I, Thornby JI, Anch M, et al. Prevalence of sleep disturbances in a primarily urban Florida county. Social Sci Med 1976; 10: 239–244.

32. Bixler EO, Kales A, Soldatos CR. Sleep disorders encountered in medical practice: a national survey of physicians. Behav Med 1979; 9: 1–6.

33. Åkerstedt T, Fredlund P, Gillberg M, Jansson B. Work load and work hours in relation to disturbed sleep and fatigue in a large representative sample. J Psychosom Res 2002; 53: 585–8.

34. Fabsitz RR, Sholinsky P, Goldberg J. Correlates of sleep problems among men: the Vietnam era twin registry. J Sleep Res 1997; 6: 50–60.

35. Parish JM, Shepard JW. Cardiovascular effects of sleep disroders. Chest 1990; 97: 1220–6.

36. Nilsson P, Nilsson J-Å, Hedblad B, Berglund G. Sleep disturbances in association with elevated pulse rate for the prediction of mortality – consequences of mental strain? J Int Med 2001; 250: 521–9.

37. Leineweber C, Kecklund G, Janszky I, Åkerstedt T, Orth-Gomér K. Poor sleep increases the prospective risk for recurrent events in middle-aged women with coronary disease. The Stockholm Female Coronary Risk Study. J Psychosom Res 2003; 54: 121–7.

38. Nilsson P, Rööst M, Engström G, et al. Incidence of diabetes in middle-aged men is related to resting heart rate and difficulties to fall asleep [abstract]. 7th International Congress of Behavioural Medcine, Helsinki, Finland, 2002.

39. Åkerstedt T, Nilsson PM. Sleep as restitution: an introduction. J Int Med 2003; 254: 6–12.

40. Weber A, Jaekel-Reinhard A. Burnout syndrome: a disease of modern societies? Occup Med 2000; 50: 512–17.

41. RFV. Långtidssjukskrivna – egenskaper vid 2003 års RFV-LS-undersökning. Stockholm. 2004: 4, Riksförsäkringsverket, 2003.

42. Kushnir T, Melamed S. The Gulf War and its impact on burnout and well-being of working civilians. Psychol Med 1992; 22: 987–95.

43. Melamed S, Kushnir T, Shirom A. Burnout and risk factors for cardiovascular diseases. Behav Med 1992; 18: 53–60.

44. Melamed S, Ugarten U, Shirom A, et al. Chronic burnout, somatic arousal and elevated salivary cortisol levels. J Psychosom Res 1999; 46: 591–8.

45. Grossi G, Perski A, Ekstedt M, et al. The morning salivary cortisol response in burnout. J Psychosom Res 2005; 59: 103–11.

46. Lester BK, Burch NR, Dossett RC. Nocturnal EEG-GSR profiles: the influence of presleep states. Psychophysiology 1967; 3: 238–48.

47. Holdstock TL, Verschoor GJ. Student sleep patterns before, during and after an examination period. J Psychol 1974; 4: 16–24.

48. Beaumaster EJ, Knowles JB, Maclean AW. The sleep of skydivers: a study of stress. Psychophysiology 1978; 15: 209–13.

49. Becker-Carus C, Heyden T. Stress-Wirkungen in Labor- und Realsituationen in Abhängigkeit von REM-Schlaf und psychophysiologischer Aktivation. Z Exp Angew Psychol 1979; XXVI: 37–52.

50. Torsvall L, Åkerstedt T. Disturbed sleep while being on call. An EEG study of apprehension in ships' engineers. Sleep 1988; 11: 35–8.

51. Kecklund G, Åkerstedt T. Objective components of individual differences in subjective sleep quality. J Sleep Res 1997; 6: 217–20.

52. Kecklund G, Åkerstedt T, Lowden A. Morning work: effects of early rising on sleep and alertness. Sleep 1997; 20: 215–23.

53. Davidson L, Fleming R, Baum A. Chronic stress, catecholamines, and sleep disturbance at Three Mile Island. Human Stress 1987; 13: 75–83.

54. Askenasy JJM, Lewin I. The impact of missile warfare on self-reported sleep quality. Part 1. Sleep 1996; 19: 47–51.

55. Reynolds III CF, Hoch CC, Buysse DJ, et al. Sleep after spousal bereavement: a study of recovery from stress. Biol Psychiatry 1993; 34: 791–7.

56. Ross RJ, Ball WA, Dinges DF, et al. Motor dysfunction during sleep in posttraumatic stress disorder. Sleep 1994; 17: 723–32.

57. Dow BM, Kelsoe JR, Gillin JC. Sleep and dreams in Vietnam PTSD and depression. Biol Psychiatry 1996; 39: 42–50.

58. Mellman TA, Nolan B, Hebding J, Kulick-Bell R, Dominguez RA. Polysomnographic comparison of veterans with combat-related PTSD, depressed men, and non-I11 controls. Sleep 1997; 20: 46–51.

59. Pillar G, Malhotra A, Lavie P. Post-traumatic stress disorder and sleep – what a nightmare! Sleep Med Rev 2000; 4: 183–200.

60. Monroe L. Psychological and physiological differences between good and poor sleepers. J Abnormal Psychol 1967; 72: 255–64.

61. Johns MW, Gay TJA, Masterton JP, Bruce DW. Relationship between sleep habits, adrenocortical activity and personality. Psychosom Med 1971; 33: 499–508.

62. Goodyear MDE. Stress, adrenocortical activity and sleep habits. Ergonomics 1973; 16: 679–81.

63. Bonnet MH, Arand DL. Metabolic rate and the restorative function of sleep. Physiol Behav 1996; 59: 777–82.

64. Bonnet MH, Arand DL. Hyperarousal and insomnia. Sleep Med Rev 1997; 1: 97–108.

65. Maslach C, Schaufeli WB, Leiter MP. Job burnout. Ann Rev Psychol 2001; 52: 397–422.

66. Söderström M, Ekstedt M, Åkerstedt T, Nilsson J, Axelsson J. Sleep and sleepiness in young individuals with high burnout scores. Sleep 2004; 17: 1369–77.

67. Ekstedt M, Söderström M, Åkerstedt T, Nilsson J, Perski A. Disturbed sleep and fatigue in occupational burnout. Scan J Work Environ Health 2006; 32: 121–31.

68. Mitler MM, Carskadon MA, Czeisler CA, et al. Catastrophes, sleep and public policy: consensus report. Sleep 1988; 11: 100–9.

69. Eurostat. Employment in Europe 1996. European Commission, Brussels 1996. Eurostat, Labour Force Survey, 1997.

70. Graf O, Pirtkien R, Rutenfranz J, Ulich E, eds. Nervose Belastung im Betrieb. I. Nachtarbeit und Nervose Belastung. Westdeutscher Verlag, 1958.

71. Thiis-Evensen E. Shift work and health. Ind Med Surg 1958; 27: 493–7.

72. Menzel W, ed. Menschliche Tag-Nacht-Rhythmik und Schichtarbeit. Basel: Schwabe, 1962.

73. Aanonsen A, ed. Shift Work and Health. Oslo: Universitetsforlaget, 1964.

74. Andersen JE. Three-Shift Work. Copenhagen: Socialforskningsinstitutet, 1970.

75. Åkerstedt T. Shift work and disturbed sleep/ wakefulness. Sleep Med Rev 1998; 2: 117–28.

76. Knauth P, Rutenfranz J. Duration of sleep related to the type of shift work. In: Reinberg A, Vieux N, Andlauer P, eds. Night and Shift Work: Biological and Social Aspects. Oxford: Pergamon Press, 1981.

77. Tepas DI. Shiftworker sleep strategies. J Hum Ergol 1982; 11: 325–36.

78. Pilcher JJ, Lambert BJ, Huffcutt AI. Differential effects of permanent and roating shifts on self-report sleep length: a meta-analytic review. Sleep 2000; 23: 155–63.

79. Åkerstedt T, Kecklund G, Knutsson A. Spectral analysis of sleep electroencephalography in rotating three-shift work. Scand J Work Environ Health 1991; 17: 330–6.

80. Åkerstedt T, Torsvall L. Napping in shift work. Sleep 1985; 8: 105–9.

81. Rosa R. Napping at home and alertness on the job in rotating shift workers. Sleep 1993; 16: 727–35.

82. Dumont M, Montplaisir J, Infante-Rivard C. Insomnia symptoms in nurses with former permanent nightwork experience. In: Koella WP, Obal F, Schulz H, Visser P, eds. Sleep '86. Stuttgart: Gustav Fischer Verlag, 1988: 405–6.

83. Guilleminault C, Czeisler S, Coleman R, Miles L. Circadian rhythm disturbances and sleep disorders in shift workers (EEG Suppl no. 36). In: Buser PA, Cobb WA, Okuma T, eds. Kyoto Symposia. Amsterdam: Elsevier, 1982: 709–14.

84. Ingre M, Åkerstedt T. Effect of accumulated night work during the working lifetime on subjective health and sleep in monozygotic twins. J Sleep Res 2004; 13: 45–8.

85. Foret J, Lantin G. The sleep of train drivers: an example of the effects of irregular work schedules on sleep. In: Colquhoun WP, ed. Aspects of Human Efficiency. Diurnal Rhythm and Loss of Sleep. London: The English Universities Press, 1972: 273–81.

86. Foret J, Benoit O. Structure du sommeil chez des travailleurs à horaires alternants. Electroencephalogr Clin Neurophysiol 1974; 37: 337–44.

87. Matsumoto K. Sleep patterns in hospital nurses due to shift work: an EEG study. Waking Sleeping 1978; 2: 169–73.

88. Tilley AJ, Wilkinson RT, Drud M. Night and day shifts compared in terms of the quality and quantity of sleep recorded in the home and performance measured at work: a pilot study. In: Reinberg A, Vieux N, Andlauer P, eds. Night and Shift Work. Biological and Social Aspects. Oxford: Pergamon Press, 1981: 187–96.

89. Torsvall L, Åkerstedt T, Gillander K, Knutsson A. Sleep on the night shift: 24-hour EEG monitoring of spontaneous sleep/wake behavior. Psychophysiology 1989; 26: 352–58.

90. Mitler MM, Miller JC, Lipsitz JJ, Walsh JK, Wylie CD. The sleep of long-haul truck drivers. New Engl J Med 1997; 337: 755–61.

91. Dahlgren K. Adjustment of circadian rhythms and EEG sleep functions to day and night sleep among permanent night workers and rotating shift workers. Psychophysiology 1981; 18: 381–91.

92. Tilley AJ, Wilkinson RT, Warren PSG, Watson WB, Drud M. The sleep and performance of shift workers. Hum Factors 1982; 24: 624–41.

93. Kecklund G. Sleep and Alertness: Effects of Shift Work, Early Rising, and the Sleep Environment [PhD thesis]. Stress Research Report 1996; 252: 1–94.

94. Foret J, Benoit O. Shiftwork: the level of adjustment to schedule reversal assessed by a sleep study. Waking Sleeping 1978; 2: 107–12.

95. Dahlgren K. Long-term adjustment of circadian rhythms to a rotating shiftwork schedule. Scand J Work Environ Health 1981; 7: 141–51.

96. Kripke DF, Cook B, Lewis OF. Sleep of night workers: EEG recordings. Psychophysiology 1971; 7: 377–84.

97. Bryden G, Holdstock TL. Effects of night duty on sleep patterns of nurses. Psychophysiology 1973; 10: 36–42.

98. Tepas DI, Walsh JK, Moss PD, Armstrong D. Polysomnographic correlates of shift worker performance in the laboratory. In: Reinberg A, Vieux N, Andlauer P, eds. Night and Shift Work: Biological and Social Aspects. Oxford: Pergamon Press, 1981: 179–86.

99. Wyatt S, Mariott R. Night work and shift changes. Br J Ind Med 1953; 10: 164–77.

100. Thiis-Evensen E. Shift work and health. Proceedings of the XII International Congress of Occupational Health (Helsinki), 1957: 97–105.

101. Mott PE, Mann FC, McLoughlin Q, Warwick DP, eds. Shift Work – the Social, Psychological and Physical Consequences. Ann Arbor, MI: University of Michigan Press, 1965.

102. Åkerstedt T, Torsvall L. Experimental changes in shift schedules – their effects on well-being. Ergonomics 1978; 21: 849–56.

103. Verhaegen P, Maasen A, Meers A. Health problems in shift workers. In: Johnson LC, Tepas DJ, Colquhoun WP, Colligan MJ, eds. Biological Rhythms and Shift Work. New York: Spectrum, 1981: 271–82.

104. Wagner JA, Garcia MM. Mine equipment operators' perceptions concerning alertness and shift rotation. Proceedings of the Human Factors Society 30th Annual Meeting 1986: 571–5.

105. Gold DR, Rogacz S, Bock N, et al. Rotating shift work, sleep, and accidents related to sleepiness in hospital nurses. Am J Public Health 1992; 82: 1011–14.

106. Paley MJ, Tepas DI. Fatigue and the shift-worker: firefighters working on a rotating shift schedule. Hum Factors 1994; 36: 269–84.

107. Prokop O, Prokop L. Ermüdung und Einschlafen am Steuer. Zbl Verkehrsmed 1955; 1: 19–30.

108. Kogi K, Ohta T. Incidence of near accidental drowsing in locomotive driving during a period of rotation. J Hum Ergol 1975; 4: 65–76.

109. Åkerstedt T, Torsvall L, Fröberg JE. A questionnaire study of sleep/wake disturbances and irregular work hours. Sleep Res 1983; 12: 358.

110. Coleman RM, Dement WC. Falling asleep at work: a problem for continuous operations. Sleep Res 1986; 15: 265.

111. Caille EJ, Bassano JL. Validation of a behavior analysis methodology: variation of vigilance in night driving as a function of the rate of carboxyhemoglobin. In: Mackie RR, ed. Vigilance. New York: Plenum Press, 1977: 59–72.

112. Torsvall L, Åkerstedt T. Sleepiness on the job: continuously measured EEG changes in train drivers. Electroencephalogr Clin Neurophysiol 1987; 66: 502–11.

113. Kecklund G, Åkerstedt T. Sleepiness in long distance truck driving: an ambulatory EEG study of night driving. Ergonomics 1993; 36: 1007–17.

114. Bjerner B, Holm Å, Swensson Å. Diurnal variation of mental perfomance. A study of three-shift workers. Br J Ind Med 1955; 12: 103–10.

115. Brown RC. The day and night performance of teleprinter switchboard operators. Occup Psychol 1949; 23: 121–6.

116. Hildebrandt G, Rohmert W, Rutenfranz J. 12 and 24 hour rhythms in error frequency of locomotive drivers and the influence of tiredness. Int J Chronobiol 1974; 2: 175–80.

117. Klein DE, Brüner H, Holtman H. Circadian rhythm of pilot's efficiency, and effects of multiple time zone travel. Aerospace Med 1970; 41: 125–32.

118. Dawson D, Reid K. Fatigue, alcohol and perfomance impairment. Nature 1997; 388: 235.

119. Harris W. Fatigue, circadian rhythm and truck accidents. In: Mackie RR, ed. Vigilance. New York: Plenum Press, 1977: 133–46.

120. Hamelin P. Lorry driver's time habits in work and their involvement in traffic accidents. Ergonomics 1987; 30: 1323–33.

121. Langlois PH, Smolensky MH, Hsi BP, Weir FW. Temporal patterns of reported single-vehicle car and truck accidents in Texas, USA during 1980–1983. Chronobiol Int 1985; 2: 131–46.

122. Lavie P, Wollman M, Pollack I. Frequency of sleep related traffic accidents and hour of the day. Sleep Res 1987; 16: 275.

123. Horne JA, Reyner LA. Sleep related vehicle accidents. Br Med J 1995; 310: 565–7.

124. Åkerstedt T, Kecklund G, Hörte L-G. Night driving, season, and the risk of highway accidents. Sleep 2001; 24: 401–6.

125. NTSB. Factors That Affect Fatigue in Heavy Truck Accidents. Washington, DC: National Transportation Safety Board. Safety Study 1995; NTSB/SS-95/01.

126. NTSB. Grounding of the US Tankship Exxon Valdez on Bligh Reef, Prince William Sound near Valdez, Alaska, March 24, 1989. Washington, DC: National Transportation Safety Board. Maritime Accident Report 1990; NTSB/MAR-90/04.

127. NTSB. Evaluation of US Department of Transportation: Efforts in the 1990s to Address Operation Fatigue. Washington, DC: National Transportation Safety Board, 1999. Safety Report NTSB/SR-99/01.

128. Ong CN, Phoon WO, Iskandar N, Chia KS. Shiftwork and work injuries in an iron and steel mill. Appl Ergonomics 1987; 18: 51–6.

129. Wojtczak-Jaroszowa J, Jarosz D. Time-related distribution of occupational accidents. J Safety Res 1987; 18: 33–41.

130. Smith L, Folkard S, Poole CJM. Increased injuries on night shift. Lancet 1994; 344: 1137–9.

131. Menzel W. Zur Physiologie und Pathologie des Nacht und Schichtarbeiters. Arbeitsphysiologie 1950; 14: 304–18.

132. Andlauer P. The Effect of Shift Working on the Workers' Health. European Productivity Agency, TU Information Bulletin 29, 1960.

133. Pradhan SM. Reaction of workers on night shift. Proceedings of the xvi International Congress of Occupational Health, Tokyo, 1969.

134. Quaas M, Tunsch R. Problems of disablement and accident frequency in shift and night work. Studia Laboris et Salutis 1972; 4: 52–65.

135. Smith P. A study of weekly and rapidly rotating shift workers. Int Arch Occup Environ Health 1979; 43: 211–20.

136. Leger D. The cost of sleep-related accidents: a report for the National Commission on Sleep Disorders Research. Sleep 1994; 17: 84–93.

137. Webb WB. The cost of sleep-related accidents: a reanalysis. Sleep 1995; 18: 276–80.

138. Åkerstedt T, Gillberg M. The circadian variation of experimentally displaced sleep. Sleep 1981; 4: 159–69.

139. Czeisler CA, Weitzman ED, Moore-Ede MC, Zimmerman JC, Knauer RS. Human sleep: its duration and organization depend on its circadian phase. Science 1980; 210: 1264–7.

140. Åkerstedt T, Gillberg M. A dose–response study of sleep loss and spontaneous sleep termination. Psychophysiology 1986; 23: 293–7.

141. Dijk D-J, Czeisler CA. Contribution of the circadian pacemaker and the sleep homeostat to sleep propensity, sleep structure, electroencephalographic slow waves, and sleep spindle activity in humans. J Neurosci 1995; 15: 3526–38.

142. Fröberg J, Karlsson CG, Levi L, Lidberg L. Circadian variations of catecholamine excretion, shooting range performance and self-ratings of fatigue during sleep deprivation. Biol Psychol 1975; 2: 175–88.

143. Dijk DJ, Duffy JF, Czeisler CA. Circadian and sleep–wake dependent aspects of subjective alertness and cognitive performance. J Sleep Res 1992; 1: 112–17.

144. Folkard S, Åkerstedt T. A three process model of the regulation of alertness and sleepiness. In: Ogilvie R, Broughton R, eds. Sleep, Arousal and Performance: Problems and Promises. Boston: Birkhäuser, 1991: 11–26.

145. Härmä M. Sleepiness and shiftwork: individual differences. J Sleep Res 1995; 4 (Suppl 2): 57–61.

146. Axelsson J, Åkerstedt T, Kecklund G, Lindqvist A, Attefors R. Hormonal changes in satisfied and dissatisfied shift workers across a shift cycle. J Appl Physiol 2003; 95: 2099–105.

147. Francis A, Pincus H, First M. Diagnostic and Statistical Manual of Mental Disorders. Washington, DC: American Psychiatric Association. 1994.

148. AASM. International Classification of Sleep Disorders – Diagnostic and Coding Manual. Chicago, IL: American Academy of Sleep Medicine. 2001.

149. Reid KJ, Zee PC. Circadian rhythm disorders. Semin Neurol 2004; 24: 315–25.

150. Drake CL, Roehrs T, Richardson G, Walsh J, Roth T. Shift work sleep disorder: prevalence and consequences beyond that of symptomatic day workers. Sleep 2004; 27: 1453–62.

151. AASM. International Classification of Sleep Disorders, Revised: Diagnostic and Coding Manual. Chicago, IL: American Academy of Sleep Medicine, 2001.

152. Axelsson J, Åkerstedt T, Kecklund G, Lowden A. Tolerance to shift work – how does it relate to sleep and wakefullness? Int Arch Occup Environ Health 2004; 77: 121–9.

153. Czeisler CA, Walsh JK, Rosh T. Modafinil for excessive sleepiness associated with shiftwork sleep disorders. N Engl J Med 2005; 353: 476–86.

154. Åkerstedt T, Landström U. Work place countermeasures of night shift fatigue. Int J Ind Ergonomics 1998; 21: 167–78.

155. Morin CM. Insomnia treatment: taking a broader perspective on efficacy and cost-effectiveness issues. Sleep Med Rev 2004; 8: 3–6.

CHAPTER 9

Sleepiness, sleep disorders, and accidents

Pierre Philip and Jaques Taillard

During the last 15 years several major epidemiological studies have drawn attention to the prevalence of sleepiness and sleep disorders among the general population.[1-3] Major industrial catastrophes have also been associated with sleepiness.[4] In 2002, industrial and traffic accidents were the ninth leading cause of death in the world and will become the third leading cause by 2020.[5] Sleepiness at the wheel[2,6] has been identified as one of the major reasons for fatal crashes and highway accidents caused by automobile and/or truck drivers. Young drivers are over-represented in these sleep-related accidents, although no clear differentiation has been made concerning the cause of sleepiness itself; that is, whether it was due to self-induced sleep deprivation or simply to a greater vulnerability to the effects of sleep loss.

In view of the huge cost of traffic accidents, the European Union has set a goal to reduce the number of highway deaths in 2010 by 50%, and consequently a vast program of road safety has been initiated. In order to achieve the challenging objective of preventing 20 000 traffic-related deaths per year, it is essential to have a clear understanding of their root causes. In view of the projected 50% increase in commercial traffic which is expected to occur over the next 10 years in Europe and in many other countries, there is now an urgent need to identify the causes of accidents and to develop new strategies to prevent them.

For many years fatigue has been associated with the risk of accidents but the causes of this problem have remained unclear. Night-time driving or driving for long periods were associated with accidents, but few reports differentiated fatigue from sleepiness. In the early 1990s, epidemiological data began to identify sleepiness as a cause of accidents.[7-9] Since then many articles have been published to try to discriminate behavioral from pathologic causes of sleepiness in drivers.

Another important point refers to the relationship between sleepiness, fatigue, and performance. Indeed, a vast majority of sleep-deprived workers or drivers curtail their sleep to increase their hourly workload. It is therefore critically important to discriminate the role of excessive work from sleep deprivation in the risk of accidents. We will review in this chapter the main references regarding behavioral, pathologic and iatrogenic causes of sleep-related accidents. We will also try to extrapolate from recent experimental results the possible strategies which might be used to decrease sleep-related accidents.

FATIGUE, SLEEPINESS, PERFORMANCE LOSS, AND INTER-INDIVIDUAL VULNERABILITY

As stated above, sleep loss apparently has different effects in separate age groups, and young drivers especially are over-represented in sleep-related accidents.

In the late 1990s we carried out a study[10] which supported the conclusion that driving for long and uninterrupted periods affected young and old drivers unequally. On trips of shorter duration young drivers (18–25 years) had significantly better performance records than older drivers (45–55 years), but the relationship between age and performance was reversed for long duration trips. These results have now been confirmed in a new sleep deprivation study[11] in which we showed that young subjects showed much greater losses in their reaction times than mature subjects after 24 hours of wakefulness. Interestingly we did not find any differences between young and mature subjects in terms of sleepiness and self-estimation of performance. This finding could be interpreted to mean that young people do not detect their own sleepiness and performance loss as easily as older people and therefore could be more prone to sleep-related accidents.

The relationships among fatigue, sleepiness and performance decrements may account for some of the age-related differences noted above. Using real driving in a long-distance experimental study,[12] we showed that fatigue perceived during the stops was a poor predictor of future driving impairment when sleepiness during the stops showed more accurately the future number of inappropriate line crossings. These findings imply that major revisions in public health messages about driving need to be undertaken. These issues will be discussed later in this chapter.

SLEEPINESS, BEHAVIOR AND ACCIDENTS

One of the best areas in society to look for the relation between sleep deprivation and accidents is shift work, in as much as night work is associated with sleepiness and sleep loss.[13] Relevant to this point is the argument that many of the most dramatic accidents in modern times have been 'fatigue accidents'. For example, the (night-time) nuclear plant meltdown at Chernobyl was due to human error related to work scheduling. Similar arguments have been made for the Three Mile Island reactor accident, the near-miss incidents at the David Beese reactor in Ohio and at the Rancho Seco reactor in California, the disaster in Bhopal, the Space Shuttle explosion as well as the grounding of the oil tanker Exxon Valdez.[14] However, these events[4] only constitute anecdotal evidence and merely serve as illustrations of possible links between sleep loss and accidents.

Traffic accidents are much more common and affect many more people in modern societies. Drivers are supposed to be healthy and responsible but lack of information on sleep hygiene and work or social pressure can explain a lot of sleep deprivation among this population. Until the mid-1990s, no study clearly demonstrated the main factors responsible for sleep-related accidents. We questioned, apart from organic sleep disorders, whether modifications of the sleep–wake schedules could be responsible for sleepiness at the wheel. Studying large populations of drivers,[15,16] we demonstrated that long-distance driving was very frequently associated with sleep curtailment. Our first study[16] was carried out on a freeway rest stop area in 1993, and showed that 50% of drivers ($n=567$) reduced their sleep duration in the 24 hours before departure for a long-distance journey. Ten per cent of drivers had had no sleep in the 24 hours before the interview. These stunning results could have been explained by a selected sample of exhausted drivers that we recruited at a rest area. Therefore, we decided to run a larger study in partnership with the highway patrol to confirm our results.[16] We randomly stopped 2196 automobile drivers at a freeway tollbooth. Fifty per cent of the drivers decreased their total sleep time in the 24 hours before the interview compared with their regular self-reported sleep time; 12.5% presented a sleep debt >180 minutes and 2.7% presented a sleep debt >300 minutes. Being young, commuting to work, driving long distances, starting the trip at night, being an 'evening' person, being a long sleeper during the week, and sleeping in at the weekend were risk factors significantly associated with sleep debt.

A posteriori, our sleep deprivation study on the effects of age on sleep deprivation and performance[11] combined with our epidemiological reports[10,16] tend to show that young drivers combine exposure and vulnerability to sleep loss.

Our previous epidemiological studies found clear associations among the personal characteristics of car drivers, work conditions, and sleep restriction. We therefore decided to study a population of truck drivers[17] on a week of work to confirm our results. A team of interviewers spent a week at a rest stop area and interviewed professional drivers. The drivers completed a questionnaire concerning sleep–wake habits and disorders experienced during the previous 3 months. In addition, they were asked to complete a sleep and travel log that included their usual work and rest periods during the previous 2 days. They answered questions concerning working conditions and reported their caffeine and nicotine intake during their trips. A total of 227 drivers, mean age 37.7 ± 8.4 years (96.2% acceptance rate), participated in the study. The drivers were found to have a fairly consistent total nocturnal sleep time during their working week, but on the last night at home prior to the new working week there was an abrupt earlier wake-up time associated with a decrease in nocturnal sleep

time. Of the drivers, 12.3% had slept less than 6 hours in the 24 hours prior to the interview and 17.1% had been awake more than 16 hours. Our study showed that shifting sleep schedules between work and rest periods could generate long episodes of enforced wakefulness. This type of sleep deprivation is rarely investigated, and is usually not taken into consideration when creating work schedules, but nevertheless has pronounced effects on driver performance. Unsuspected shifts occur at the onset of a new working week. Even if safety is a major concern for this population of drivers and their companies, sleep hygiene education for truck drivers is still far from perfect.

In a study of professional US truck drivers, Mitler et al.[18] recorded the electroencephalogram (EEG) of 20 drivers on four different work schedules. This study demonstrated a mean duration of sleep of 4.78 hours in a 5-day period. Fifty-six per cent of drivers presented at least six non-continuous minutes of EEG-recorded sleep during the driving sessions. The vast majority of these micro-sleep episodes occurred during the late night and early morning.

In 1995, a study by the National Transportation Safety Board on fatal accidents in professional truck drivers[8] showed that the mean duration of sleep among drivers was below 6 hours of sleep in the last 24 hours before the accident. Almost 10 years later, Connor et al.[2] showed that sleepiness at the wheel increased the risk of causing a traffic accident by 8.2-fold. Sleeping less than 5 hours in the 24 hours before the accident and driving between 2 a.m. and 5 a.m. were also significant risk factors for accidents (odds ratio [OR] = 2.7 and 5.6, respectively). Finally, other studies[2,19,20] have shown that shift work, multiple jobs, or extensive duration of work were associated with sleep-related accidents.

All these reports on sleep deprivation and driving have pointed to a link between traffic accidents and sleep–wake schedules.

SLEEP DISORDERS AND ACCIDENTS

Narcolepsy is a major pathology responsible for excessive daytime somnolence, and it has also been studied as a risk factor for traffic accidents. Aldrich[21] showed that narcolepsy patients presented a higher risk of sleep-related accidents than patients suffering from sleep apnea. Multiple sleep latency tests (MSLTs) did not correlate with the rate of accidents among sleepy patients. However, the number of patients in the study with MSLTs was quite limited (46 apneics, 22 narcoleptics, 17 patients with excessive daytime somnolence due to other causes), which could explain the lack of power of the study.

It is worth noting that in all sleep pathologies victims of accidents had sleep latencies lower than controls.

Teran-Santos et al.[22] published a case–control study on the risk of car accidents among apneic subjects. The case patients were 102 drivers who received emergency treatment at hospitals, after highway traffic accidents. The controls were 152 patients randomly selected from primary care centers and matched with case patients for age and sex. As compared with those without sleep apnea, patients with an apnea–hypopnea index (AHI) of 10 or higher had an OR of 6.3 (95% confidence interval, 2.4 to 16.2) for having a traffic accident. This relation remained significant after adjustment for potential confounders, such as alcohol consumption, visual-refraction disorders, body mass index, years of driving, age, history with respect to traffic accidents, use of medications causing drowsiness, and sleep schedule.

George and Smiley[23] published complementary data on the relationship between the AHI and the risk of accidents. In this study on 460 apneic patients, only the most severe patients (AHI > 30) presented an accident risk factor that was higher than that of controls.

Stoohs et al.[24] performed an integrated analysis of recordings of sleep-related breathing disorders, and self-reported automotive and company-recorded automotive accidents in 90 commercial long-haul truck drivers. Seventy-eight per cent of the drivers had an oxygen desaturation index (ODI) ≥ 5 per hour of sleep; 10% had an ODI ≥ 30 per hour of sleep. About 20% of drivers presented symptoms indicating very regular sleep disturbances. Truck drivers with sleep-disordered breathing had a twofold higher accident rate per mile than drivers without sleep-disordered breathing. Accident frequency was not dependent on the severity of the sleep-related breathing disorder.

Hakkanen and Summala[6] carried out a study of professional drivers. Two separate groups consisting of both long-haul ($n = 184$) and short-haul ($n = 133$) truck drivers were surveyed to examine the frequency of driver sleepiness-related problems at work during the previous 3 months and to assess the incidence of sleep apnea syndrome symptoms. Over 20% of the long-haul drivers also reported having dozed off at least twice while driving. Near-misses due to dozing off had occurred in 17% of these drivers. Factors indicating sleep apnea syndrome occurred in 4% of the long-haul drivers and in only two short-haul drivers.

All these studies, even if they report a great variability of prevalence of obstructive sleep apnea syndrome among occupational drivers (possibly explained by different diagnostic methods), confirm the risk of traffic accidents for apneic patients. Sleepiness at the wheel is obviously a main symptom to investigate in conjunction with the severity of the disease (AHI > 30).

Knowing this risk, a major question is how can accidents involving these patients be reduced? In 2001 George[25] studied the impact of continuous positive airway pressure (CPAP) treatment on risk of motor vehicle accidents in 210 non-professional drivers who were suffering from obstructive sleep apnea (OSA). The results indicated that CPAP therapy was definitely associated with a reduction in the risk of motor vehicle accidents due to OSA. These results strongly support the recommendation that drivers who have experienced sleepiness while on the road should take steps to find out the potential cause of the problem. In particular they should seek confirmation from a sleep clinic concerning whether they might have a disordered breathing problem such as OSA, and whether CPAP therapy might be indicated.

DRUGS AND TRAFFIC ACCIDENTS

Although many publications[26–30] associate drugs affecting the central nervous system, both prescription and non-prescription, with an increased risk of accidents, the inter-relationship of these drugs with sleep disorders and traffic accidents has been poorly studied. Many of the drivers questioned have been non-professionals or even retired and, in as much as the interviews were retrospective, little or no information has been made available on the level of alertness in the minutes before the accident.

Only one study evaluated the risk of drug-related accidents and sleep disorders among occupational drivers. Howard et al.[31] measured the prevalence of excessive sleepiness and sleep-disordered breathing and assessed accident risk factors in 2342 respondents to a questionnaire distributed to a random sample of 3268 Australian commercial vehicle drivers and another 161 drivers among 244 invited to undergo polysomnography. More than half (59.6%) of drivers had sleep-disordered breathing and 15.8% had OSA syndrome. Twenty-four per cent of drivers had excessive sleepiness. Sleepiness measured by the Epworth sleepiness scale was associated with an increased risk of accidents. Among these drivers, narcotic analgesic drugs and antihistamine use were also associated with an increasing risk of accidents.

ECONOMIC IMPACT OF SLEEPINESS AT THE WHEEL

In the early 1990s Léger[32] estimated the annual cost of sleep-related accidents in the USA at $43 billions per year. Almost 10 years later,

Sassani et al.[33] calculated the cost–benefit of OSA syndrome treatments regarding traffic accidents. More than 800 000 drivers were involved in OSA syndrome-related motor-vehicle collisions in the year 2000, which cost $15.9 billion and 1400 lives.[35] In the USA, treating all drivers suffering from OSA syndrome with CPAP would cost $3.18 billion, save $11.1 billion in collision costs, and save 980 lives annually.

CONCLUSION

Sleep hygiene and hours of work are very important factors to take into consideration for improving industrial and road safety. Due to these scientific findings, several governments and some truck companies have in recent years developed a greater interest in sleep schedules and road safety. The goals are to improve working conditions and decrease the risk of industrial accidents. Regulating a trucker's workload and amount of rest per 24-hour period is a good strategy for improving safety, but it is crucial to consider the periods preceding the beginning of work when evaluating the ability to drive.

European legislation has imposed regulations (EU 3820/85 and 3821/85) on the trucking industry to improve driver safety. In particular, the regulations limit the amount of time truckers are allowed to work during a 24-hour period to a maximum of 9 hours per day, with the possibility of working 10 hours per day, 2 days a week. After 6 consecutive working days, drivers are mandated to take a weekly rest period of at least 45 consecutive hours of freely disposed time (Section IV, Article 6). However, sleep loss is cumulative and European Economic Community law cannot regulate sleep behaviors during weekends. Recent findings show also that work load *per se* is not the main risk factor and fatigue is a poor predictor of performance decrement. This contradicts the vast majority of road safety messages and communication about driver's fatigue should be reconsidered. Health among occupational drivers also needs to be better investigated and sleep medicine needs to be promoted in the form of 'traffic medicine'.

Chronic daytime sleepiness is still under-diagnosed and obstructive sleep apnea syndrome is not sufficiently investigated nor treated in this vulnerable population of sedentary males. Health care, educational programs and work schedules integrating notions of sleep hygiene and sleep medicine could significantly improve industrial and road safety.

REFERENCES

1. Ohayon MM, Caulet M, Philip P, Guilleminault C, Priest RG. How sleep and mental disorders are related to complaints of daytime sleepiness. Arch Int Med 1997; 157: 2645–52.
2. Connor J, Whitlock G, Norton R, Jackson R. The role of driver sleepiness in car crashes: a systematic review of epidemiological studies. Accid Anal Prev 2001; 33: 31–41.
3. Young T, Palta M, Dempsey J, et al. The occurrence of sleep-disordered breathing among middle-aged adults. N Engl J Med 1993; 328(17): 1230–5.
4. Mitler MM, Carskadon MA, Czeisler CA, et al. Catastrophes, sleep and public policy: concensus report. Sleep 1988; 11: 100–9.
5. Peden M, Scurfield R, Sleet D, et al. World Report on Road Traffic Injury Prevention. Geneva: World Health Organization, 2004.
6. Hakkanen H, Summala H. Sleepiness at work among commercial truck drivers. Sleep 2000; 23: 49–57.
7. Summala H, Mikkola T. Fatal accidents among car and truck drivers: effects of fatigue, age, and alcohol consumption. Hum Factors 1994; 36(2): 315–26.
8. NTSB. Factors That Affect Fatigue in Heavy Truck Accidents. Washington, DC: National Transportation Safety Board, 1995.
9. Pack AI, Pack AM, Rodgman E, et al. Characteristics of crashes attributed to the driver having fallen asleep. Accid Anal Prev 1995; 27(6): 769–75.
10. Philip P, Taillard J, Quera-Salva MA, Bioulac B, Åkerstedt T. Simple reaction time, duration of driving and sleep deprivation in young versus old automobile drivers. J Sleep Res 1999; 8: 9–14.
11. Philip P, Taillard J, Sagaspe P, et al. Age, performance and sleep deprivation. J Sleep Res 2004; 13(2): 105–10.
12. Philip P, Sagaspe P, Moore N, et al. Fatigue, sleep restriction and driving performance. Accid Anal Prev 2005; 37(3): 473–8.
13. Åkerstedt T. Shift work and disturbed sleep/wakefulness. Occup Med 2003; 53: 89–94.
14. NTSB. Grounding of the US Tankship Exxon Valdez on Bligh Reef, Prince William Sound near Valdez, Alaska, March 24, 1989. Washington, DC: National Transportation Safety Board. Maritime Accident Report 1990; NTSB/MAR-90/04.
15. Philip P, Ghorayeb I, Stoohs R, et al. Determinants of sleepiness in automobile drivers. J Psychosom Res 1996; 41(3): 279–88.
16. Philip P, Taillard J, Guilleminault C, et al. Long distance driving and self-induced sleep deprivation among automobile drivers. Sleep 1999; 22(4): 475–80.
17. Philip P, Taillard J, Leger D, et al. Work and rest sleep schedules of 227 European truck drivers. Sleep Med 2002; 3(6): 507–11.
18. Mitler MM, Miller JC, Lipsitz JJ, Walsh JK, Wylie CD. The sleep of long-haul truck drivers. N Engl J Med 1997; 337(11): 755–61.
19. Stutts JC, Wilkins JW, Scott Osberg J, Vaughn BV. Driver risk factors for sleep-related crashes. Accid Anal Prev 2003; 35(3): 321–31.
20. Tucker P, Folkard S, Macdonald I. Rest breaks and accident risk. Lancet 2003; 361(9358): 680.
21. Aldrich MS. Automobile accidents in patients with sleep disorders. Sleep 1989; 12(6): 487–94.
22. Teran-Santos J, Jimenez-Gomez A, Cordero-Guevara J. The association between sleep apnea and the risk of traffic accidents. Cooperative Group Burgos-Santander. N Engl J Med 1999; 340(11): 847–51.
23. George CF, Smiley A. Sleep apnea and automobile crashes. Sleep 1999; 22(6): 790–5.
24. Stoohs RA, Bingham LA, Itoi A, Guilleminault C, Dement WC. Sleep and sleep-disordered breathing in commercial long-haul truck drivers. Chest 1995; 107(5): 1275–82.
25. George CF. Reduction in motor vehicle collisions following treatment of sleep apnoea with nasal CPAP. Thorax 2001; 56(7): 508–12.
26. Leveille SG, Buchner DM, Koepsell TD, et al. Psychoactive medications and injurious motor vehicle collisions involving older drivers. Epidemiology 1994; 5(6): 591–8.
27. Barbone F, McMahon AD, Davey PG, et al. Association of road-traffic accidents with

benzodiazepine use. Lancet 1998; 352(9137): 1331–6.

28. Hemmelgarn B, Suissa S, Huang A, Boivin JF, Pinard G. Benzodiazepine use and the risk of motor vehicle crash in the elderly. J Am Med Assoc 1997; 278(1): 27–31.

29. Hu PS, Trumble DA, Foley DJ, Eberhard JW, Wallace RB. Crash risks of older drivers: a panel data analysis. Accid Anal Prev 1998; 30(5): 569–81.

30. Hauser RA, Gauger L, Anderson WM, Zesiewicz TA. Pramipexole-induced somnolence and episodes of daytime sleep. Mov Disord 2000; 15(4): 658–63.

31. Howard ME, Desai AV, Grunstein RR, et al. Sleepiness, sleep-disordered breathing, and accident risk factors in commercial vehicle drivers. Am J Respir Crit Care Med 2004; 170(9): 1014–21.

32. Léger D. The cost of sleep-related accidents: a report for the National Commission on Sleep Disorders Research. Sleep 1994; 17(1): 84–93.

33. Sassani A, Findley LJ, Kryger M, et al. Reducing motor-vehicle collisions, costs, and fatalities by treating obstructive sleep apnea syndrome. Sleep 2004; 27(3): 453–8.

CHAPTER 10

Medico-legal aspects of sleep disorders

John Shneerson

Legal implications arise not only from sleep disorders, but also from problems with normal sleep, such as sleep deprivation, and the effects of drugs and alcohol on sleep.[1] The scientific understanding and medical knowledge of sleep and its disorders are developing rapidly but there is relatively little awareness of this among the general public, and the legal framework often fails to take sleep into account. There are many differences among the laws of different countries, but the principles discussed in this chapter are broadly similar in most Western jurisdictions and are transferable from one country to another (Table 10.1).

The actions carried out as a result of abnormalities of sleep or medical disorders of sleep may lead to either criminal or civil charges, but very often similar actions go unprosecuted. Violent behavior during sleep for instance may be long standing and the regular bed partner may come to regard this as normal or acceptable, but if it is inflicted on a stranger, who happens to be sleeping close by, a prosecution may result.

In criminal cases the onus is on the claimant to show 'beyond all reasonable doubt' that the defendant committed the act. This is taken to be approximately greater than a 90% probability. In civil cases, however, the standard of proof is to show that the defendant committed

Table 10.1 Common sleep-related legal situations

Claim	Charge
• Defendant claims to be asleep	– Assault – Manslaughter – Murder – Sexual assault – Rape – Indecent exposure – Theft – Driving offences
• Defendant claims abnormal state of awareness	– Theft – Sexual assault – Rape
• Claimant claims to be asleep	– Sexual assault – Rape
• Defendant claims to be awake	– Driving and other transportation offences – Work-related accidents
• Sleep disorders claimed to be due to an accident	– Insomnia – Excessive daytime sleepiness

the act 'on the balance of probability'. This is taken as more likely than not, or greater than 50% probability.

DEFENDANT CLAIMS TO BE ASLEEP

The defence usually relies on establishing that the act took place during an **automatism**. In English law to be found guilty requires not only a demonstration that the defendant carried out the act, but also that there was conscious knowledge of what was being done. Conversely, an automatism is behavior that is involuntary and of which the subject has no awareness.[2–4] Partially or reduced awareness of the action is not sufficient to fulfill the criteria for an automatism. This includes any movement of limbs or body completely uncontrolled by the mind and it implies that the subject did not know the nature of the act or that it was wrong. Lack of memory of the episode is not equivalent to an automatism and the defence that he or she could not control the impulse to carry out the act is also not accepted as an automatism.

The propensity to carry out activities in an automatism is usually due to a combination of an inherent tendency, plus specific trigger factors.[5–7] The law, however, unlike medicine, identifies two distinct types of automatism. *Sane automatism* implies that there was a trigger for the actions, that this trigger was external to the subject, and that the action was not due to any disease of the mind. This external event includes, for instance, a head injury, drugs, or an animal sting which initiated the action. The defence of a drug-induced sane automatism only succeeds if the drug was taken for medical purposes and not for pleasure or intoxication. If a sane automatism is accepted by the Court the subject is found not guilty of the offence and discharged.

Insane automatism implies that there is an internal cause for the action, which may for instance be epilepsy, diabetes, or a psychiatric disorder such as schizophrenia or depression. The legal implication of an internal cause or disease of the mind is that recurrence of the activity is more likely than if it were due to an external event, such as a head injury, which is less likely to recur. There is therefore a continuing danger to the public, and if an insane automatism is accepted by the Court the subject may be sentenced to detention in a mental hospital for custodial care and treatment.

There are three main types of offence in which an automatism may be claimed.

Sleep violence leading to assault, manslaughter, or murder

Physical activity during sleep is normally confined to brief jerky movements of the limbs in rapid eye movement (REM) sleep, and co-ordinated whole body movements usually at the transition from one sleep stage in non-REM (NREM) sleep to another or to wakefulness. The intense motor inhibition characteristic of REM sleep prevents the complex mental activity of dreams and nightmares from being physically enacted.

There is a wide range of sleep disorders in which movements occur, such as the restless legs syndrome, but in which violence is rarely, if ever, reported. Some conditions, however, lead to aggressive movements, which can be interpreted as being directed toward the bed partner or nearby sleeper. While very often these events do not lead to any prosecution, particularly if they are frequent and long standing and the regular partner has become adapted to them, occasionally they may lead to prosecution, especially if they are particularly violent, lead to injury or death, and if the victim is unused to the defendant's actions.

Medical conditions causing sleep violence

Sleep walking (somnambulism) Sleep walking is due to incomplete arousal to wakefulness from the deeper stages of NREM sleep (stages 3 and 4) leading to a condition in which motor activity, especially walking occurs but in the absence of any awareness. Sleep walking is commonest in children, but around 20% continue to walk as adults and this comprises 1–2% of the adult population. There is often a family history.[8] Sleep walking arising for the first time in adults is uncommon, and there is usually a readily detectable cause or significant psychopathology. Sleep walking may be triggered by any factor that promotes arousal from sleep,[9] such as a noisy sleep environment, pain, stress, fever or other sleep disorders, such as obstructive sleep apneas, which fragment the sleep pattern. It is also triggered by alcohol consumption and is more common after sleep deprivation, presumably because this induces more pronounced stages 3 and 4 NREM sleep from which arousal is less likely to be complete. Central nervous system depressant drugs, such as hypnotics, antipsychotics,[10] and tricyclic antidepressants may have similar effects.

The affected person characteristically walks from his or her bed and carries out complex activities such as walking downstairs, and may open the front door, or even drive a motor vehicle. Injuries resulting from, for example, falling down stairs or through windows are well recognized,[11] and although the sleep walker usually allows him- or herself to be put back to bed without resistance, any attempt at restraint or wakening may trigger a sudden act of violence.[12,13] This is presumably because the restraint causes a confusional arousal with disorientation, and a desire to escape. There is usually little or no recall of the episode and the person falls asleep readily afterwards. Sleep walking is most common towards the end of the first stage 3 and 4 NREM sleep episode, which is usually around 1 hour after sleep onset.

Confusional arousal This, like sleep walking, is due to a partial arousal from the deeper stages of NREM sleep (stages 3 and 4) to wakefulness. It is most common in children, but readily occurs in adults, especially with forced awakening, for instance, when sleep is disturbed by the bed partner or the ringing of a telephone bell. The trigger factors such as sleep deprivation, shift work, and sedative drugs are similar to those that initiate sleep walking, and their timing in the first third of the night is similar to sleep walking.

Sleep terrors These are commonest in children but may also occur in adults. Like sleep walking and confusional arousals they occur at the transition from stages 3 and 4 NREM sleep to wakefulness, but they are associated with more marked autonomic activity such as signs of fear or panic, sweating, dilated pupils, rapid respiratory and heart rates, increased muscle tone, and often frenetic activity. There is no recall of the event or of any dream content, but there may be a sensation of intense fear as if the affected person is coming out of a faint or frightening near death situation.

Post-traumatic stress disorder This condition follows either a military or civilian traumatic event and is characterized by repetitive intrusive thoughts, flashbacks, and 'nightmares' related to the episode. These patients are often restless sleepers and awaken suddenly from the 'nightmares' with violent movements. These episodes arise either from REM or usually stages 1 and 2 NREM sleep and are most common between 12.00 a.m. and 3.00 a.m., in contrast to typical nightmares which occur later in the night. There is often a recall event related to the trauma, although this may be disguised or generalized.

REM sleep behavior disorder This is characterized by vivid aggressive dreams associated with abnormal movements arising from REM sleep. It is commonest in older people, particularly men, and while it may be triggered by drugs, such as antidepressants, particularly venlafaxine, it is often due to a degenerative neurological disorder, such as parkinsonism.[14] It is usually a chronic problem, but can occur acutely with drug intoxication, such as alcohol, or acute withdrawal of REM sleep suppressant drugs, such as amphetamines and antidepressants.

The dreams usually have an aggressive and violent content, and involve being threatened, or confronted by unfamiliar people or animals, leading the affected person to react by fleeing or fighting back. There is close concordance between the dream content and the type of physical activity observed.[15] Actions such as kicking, punching, running, and jumping may be present with exploratory or aggressive behavior. Either the afflicted or the bed partner may be injured, and restraint is resisted. Violence can be intense, particularly if the bed partner is misinterpreted by the defendant as an assailant.

Status dissociatus This causes similar activities to those seen in the REM sleep behavior disorder. It is due to more widespread degeneration in the sleep control mechanisms.

Narcolepsy Violence during sleep is rare, but may occur during hypnagogic hallucinations (pre-sleep dreams) if the subject perceives a threat and misinterprets the bed partner as the aggressor.

Obstructive sleep apneas Obstructive sleep apneas are due to transient closure of the upper airway during sleep associated with repetitive arousals. This fragmentation of sleep leads to excessive daytime sleepiness, but at the moment of each arousal the subject may only be partially aware of his or her surroundings. This reduced awareness may be combined with complex motor behavior. Violence may occur particularly if arousal occurs during REM sleep and is associated with dream-like hallucinations, but it can occur without these.[16]

Epilepsy Nocturnal epilepsy is commonest either early in the night, particularly in stages 1 and 2 NREM sleep, or 1–2 hours before or after the transition from sleep to wakefulness in the morning. Violence during epileptic seizures is uncommon,[17] but may occur with nocturnal frontal lobe seizures, which often invoke complex and aggressive behavior, and occasionally with temporal lobe epilepsy. It is more common, however, in post-ictal states in which there is reduced awareness of the environment, particularly after temporal lobe seizures.[18]

Psychogenic causes Dissociative disorders are associated with violence during sleep.[19] These

Table 10.2 Features of sleep-related violence

- Lack of motivation. No evidence of personal animosity or potential personal gain from the violence
- No evidence for premeditation of the action
- Amnesia for the event with no recall of any relevant activity
- Remorse or guilt following discovery of the action
- No attempt to conceal the crime
- Self reporting to the police or other authority

episodes occur after 30–90 seconds of wakefulness during which the subject appears behaviorally to be asleep. These subjects have often experienced previous abuse and re-enactment of this forms part of the violence.

Legal aspects

To succeed with the defence of automatism due to a sleep disorder it is essential initially to establish whether the subject was awake or asleep and whether there was any awareness of the actions. Each of the various sleep disorders which can lead to violence in a state of automatism has specific features as described above, but in all of them the characteristics listed in Table 10.2 are usually present.

In sleep walking, confusional arousals, and sleep terrors the specific features shown in Table 10.3 are usually present, and the features of the REM sleep behavior disorder are listed in Table 10.4.

By contrast, violence occurring during wakefulness, in which the perpetrator may be feigning to be asleep, often has a motive and there is evidence of premeditation. Remorse is uncommon after the event.

Investigations of sleep architecture using techniques such as polysomnography may show specific features of individual disorders.[20–22] These could include, for instance, loss of muscle atonia during REM sleep in REM sleep

Table 10.3 Features of violence due to sleep walking, confusional arousals and sleep terrors

- Family history or personal history of one or other of these types of arousal disorder
- The activity occurs in the first third of the night, usually around one hour after falling asleep
- Trigger factors such as sleep deprivation, stress, forced awakening, due to environmental causes, or alcohol are present

Table 10.4 Features of violence in REM sleep behavior disorder

- Association of the physical activity with the violent content of the dreams
- Older age
- Usually male
- Evidence of neurodegenerative disorders (e.g., Parkinson's disease) or ingestion of relevant medication (e.g., venlafaxine)

behavior disorder, and long duration of stages 3 and 4 NREM sleep with frequent microarousals to wakefulness in sleep walking, confusional arousals, and sleep terrors. Other conditions such as obstructive sleep apneas and narcolepsy can usually be identified with polysomnography or multiple sleep latency tests.

Once the presence of a sleep disorder and its specific type has been established the next step is to evaluate whether this was self-induced or not. The ingestion of alcohol or medication for other than purely medical reasons, and specifically for the purposes of intoxication or pleasure, renders the defence of automatism non-viable. The taking of alcohol, which in the past may have induced sleep walking, would render murder during a further sleep walking episode after alcohol intake indefensible on the basis of an automatism.

If the episode is sleep related and not self-induced and the defence for automatism is accepted the Court has to decide whether this is sane or insane. There has been considerable legal confusion about this and the distinction, which dates back to the nineteenth century when relatively little was known about psychiatry and neurological disorders, is hard to reconcile with modern medical practice.

In sleep walking, confusional arousals, and sleep terrors there is no evidence that the subject can act out any conscious or subconscious intent. Although the brain and spinal cord enable the subject to walk and carry out other semi-purposeful activities, there is no evidence that the mind is awake.[23,24] It is, as far as is known, in a state of normal sleep. Sleep walking is therefore not a disease of the mind, but a sleep disorder in which the motor and mental aspects of sleep are dissociated. Sleep walkers do not show any features of a disease of the mind during wakefulness. For these reasons sleep walking is best regarded as a sane rather than insane automatism.

Sexual assault and rape

The charge of sexual assault or rape rests on the claimant demonstrating that the activity was non-consensual. This may be because the victim was unable to give consent through being asleep, intoxicated with alcohol or drugs, or both, or unconscious for some other reason (see below), or because the defendant engaged or attempted to engage in sexual activity while the victim was awake, but withheld consent. The defence in this situation rests on showing that the defendant's actions amounted to an automatism (see above) due to a sleep disorder.

Medical conditions causing sexual assault and rape

Sleep walking A sleep walker may leave his or her bed or bedroom and walk into the bedroom of another person. His or her actions may then be interpreted as sexually orientated, but during the sleep walking episode itself there is no awareness of actions of this type, and erections, which are not a feature of NREM sleep, are rarely present. At the end of the sleep walking episode, however, there may be a confusional arousal in which the subject is partially aware of his or her situation and in which sexual approaches may be made.

Sexsomnia This is a rarely reported, but probably quite common, disorder which is more frequent in males than females.[25–28] It usually appears in early adult life. Sexual intercourse is usually attempted and often achieved, while the subject has no awareness, or subsequent recall of this. If the sexual activity occurs with children there may be an allegation of sexual abuse.[29] Following the episode there may be feelings of guilt, shame or embarrassment.

There is usually history of other behavioral disorders in sleep, such as sleep walking and often a family history of this as well. The sexual activity may be triggered by sleep deprivation or sleep fragmentation due to for instance obstructive sleep apneas, alcohol, or stress.

Kleine–Levin syndrome This rare disorder is associated with intermittent episodes of excessive daytime sleepiness, often with a temporarily increased appetite, personality changes, and sexual hyperactivity, which may be compulsive.

Dissociative states Sexual activity is usually related to previous abuse situations. These disorders need to be distinguished from sexual approaches during wakefulness during the night, but with no recall admitted subsequently. This type of activity is almost always carried out by males rather than females.

Legal aspects

The defendant may claim that the assault did not take place and that the accusation is fabricated, or that the victim dreamt or imagined the assault, but if it is accepted that it did take place the defence of automatism can be used, similarly to sleep violence.[30]

The same general features are present with a sexual assault during sleep as with sleep violence in that the defendant should have no recall of the episode and would not be expected to conceal any evidence.[31,32] Sexual assault and rape are uncommon in sleep walking except in the confusional arousal stage at the end of a sleep walking episode, and occur early in the night. In sexsomnia the sexual activity may occur at any time during the night. The episode may be prolonged for greater than 30 minutes and it is unusual for the subject to walk out of the bedroom. It is commonest in young adults with a previous history of sleep walking or sleep talking.

INDECENT EXPOSURE

Indecent exposure is well recognized to occur in sleep walkers who sleep in the nude.[33] It only occasionally leads to charges, depending on the situation in which it occurs. The defence is usually that of an automatism.[34,35] There is no recall of the episode.[36] The presence of an erection at the time of the exposure makes it less likely to be due to sleep walking, because this arises from NREM rather than REM sleep and it is primarily in the latter that erections during sleep occur.

Other offences

Automatism while sleep walking has been used as a defence against charges of theft.[37] Automatism is a valid defence against driving offences if it can be established that driving took place while sleep walking[13] or other comparable sleep disorders.

DEFENDANT CLAIMS ABNORMAL STATE OF AWARENESS

The defence of claiming that criminal activities were carried out in an abnormal state of awareness due to a sleep disorder is similar to that of claiming that it is due to an automatism. This defence has been used following prosecution for recurrent shoplifting in a subject with narcolepsy[38] and for murder, probably due to a confusional arousal.[39] A lowered state of awareness due to increased sleepiness was alleged. Narcolepsy is also associated with dreams occurring during wakefulness (hypnagogic and hypnopompic hallucinations) which closely simulate reality.[40] These may lead to false accusations, such as being sexually assaulted and misinterpretation of reality.[41]

Sleep deprivation causes a variety of neuropsychological as well as motor abnormalities. Not only does the level of alertness and concentration fall, but the subject becomes easily distractible and hallucinations due to altered perceptions of reality may arise. These may be visual, but can also be auditory. There is also a reduction of the visual field and of the ability to search this for important features. These changes have important implications for assessing the accuracy of witnesses in criminal investigations who may inappropriately maintain confidence in reporting events, omit aspects of incidents, and misinterpret what occurred.[42]

CLAIMANT CLAIMS TO BE ASLEEP

The commonest situation in which the claimant claims to be asleep, but the defendant awake, is in the claim for sexual assault or rape. The victim claims that consent could not be given because she, or occasionally he, was not aware or awake at the time of the activity. The defendant may claim that the episode never took place or that the claimant was sufficiently aware to give consent or at least to indicate that it was not withheld. The situation may be complicated if the victim is intoxicated with alcohol or drugs, or both, in which case the act may still be non-consensual, but only partly related to sleep and partly to the intoxication.

There may be witnesses or other contemporary evidence regarding the activity which may suggest whether or not the victim consented, but this may be difficult since if the victim was asleep, intoxicated, or unconscious during the act, there may be no outward signs of rejecting the sexual advances, and this may be mistaken for co-operating with them. If the claimant was asleep there should be no recall of the episode. In practice the situation is often less clear cut with the words and actions of the victim being interpreted by the defendant as giving consent and the onset of sleep preventing the victim from rejecting the activity. This is then followed by an accusation of sexual assault or rape.

While the physical stimulation associated with sexual assault may be insufficient to wake the claimant from sleep, rape is more likely to do so except in certain situations in which the victim may not waken. Younger people are more difficult to waken from sleep than older adults and arousal becomes progressively more difficult as the deeper stages of NREM sleep are entered. Stages 3 and 4 NREM sleep are particularly prominent around 1 hour after sleep onset, whereas, unless there is significant sleep deprivation or a sleep disorder, only the lighter stages of NREM sleep are present immediately after sleep onset. At this time awakening would be expected to occur more readily with any form of physical stimulation. Similarly, later in the night there is less stages 3 and 4 NREM sleep and more REM sleep, from which it is easier to awaken, and any sort of assault is likely to occur with recall of the event by the claimant at this time of the night.

The ingestion of sedative drugs and alcohol makes it more difficult for the claimant to waken, and the duration of this effect will depend on the dose and timing of the drug as well as its duration of action, and whether or not it has been used chronically. The victim may have taken the sedative drug intentionally or unknowingly, as with drug-facilitated sexual assault with, for instance, sodium oxybate (gamma hydroxybutyrate, Xyrem),[43] flunitrazepam (Rohypnol),[44] or temazepam.

DEFENDANT CLAIMS TO BE AWAKE

The commonest situation is where the claimant has to establish that the defendant was asleep or sleepy enough to cause an accident. Accidents may occur at work, but most prosecutions involve transportation. This may be by road, rail, sea, air, or even with space travel, but the medical aspects and legal principles are common to each.

It is estimated that 1–3% of all road traffic accidents are due to driver drowsiness[45] and perhaps 10% of serious accidents and 20% of motorway accidents in the UK. There are now more fatal accidents related to driver sleepiness than to driving with a blood alcohol concentration above the legal limit. These accidents typically involve males under the age of 30 who are driving alone. They appear to be poor at recognizing the degree of their sleepiness.[46]

It may be difficult to assess whether or not an accident is due to driver drowsiness, but these accidents are typically single vehicle accidents, occurring at night, particularly between 2.00 a.m. and 6.00 a.m. even though there is the least amount of traffic at this time, and between 2.00 p.m. and 4.00 p.m.[47] These are the times when the tendency to sleepiness is greatest. These accidents are often fatal because the driver fails to take any avoiding action and there are no skid marks because of failure to brake to avoid impact.

The sleepy driver may be observed to change speed due to intermittent loss of muscle activity in the leg controlling the accelerator. Shunting accidents at traffic lights and roundabouts are frequent, and the driver often weaves or changes lanes and may even veer off the road into oncoming cars or static objects. Articulated lorries may jack-knife if the driver suddenly over-reacts by making a corrective steering action on regaining alertness after a lapse of concentration or a microsleep.

It is common for drivers to be unaware of the road for several miles before an accident. This may be a normal reaction to concentrating on other things, but may be due to microsleeps or light sleep in which the driver is able to retain some control of the vehicle. The sleepy driver often has a glazed expression, with a reduced blinking frequency and impaired responsiveness to external stimuli, together with a loss of peripheral vision.

As sleepiness increases, the ability to concentrate deteriorates, particularly in monotonous driving situations such as on motorways, and accidents become more likely. If sleepiness is severe there may be hallucinations due to intrusion of REM sleep into wakefulness and a failure to scan the visual field for important features.

There are large inter-individual differences in the effects of sleep deprivation on driving performance. Many people can manage with around 5 hours sleep each night as long as they are motivated and interested in driving and deficits in attention can be improved by effort and caffeine.

Medical causes

Excessive sleepiness may be due to insufficient duration of sleep (sleep deprivation, sleep restriction), impaired quality of sleep (sleep fragmentation), or a hypersomnia in which there is a disorder of sleep control leading to increased sleepiness during the day despite an adequate duration of sleep at night (Table 10.5).

Most road traffic accidents due to excessive sleepiness are caused by drivers who have had insufficient sleep. Those who are chronically mildly sleep deprived are more vulnerable to additional acute episodes of sleep loss, for instance due to working long hours or shift work. This is particularly important after the first night of shift work when the subject may have been awake for more than 24 hours before attempting to drive home.

Insufficient sleep is a risk particularly for commercial drivers who have to meet deadlines or make emergency deliveries involving driving at night, shift work, or long driving times. The comfortable driving cabs and power steering of modern commercial vehicles make driving

Table 10.5 Common causes of excessive sleepiness

- Sleep deprivation
- Sleep fragmentation
  - Obstructive sleep apneas
  - Restless legs syndrome
  - Poor sleep environment
- Circadian rhythm disorders
  - Shift work
  - Delayed sleep phase syndrome
  - Advanced sleep phase syndrome
- Neurological disorders
  - Narcolepsy
  - Klein-Levin syndrome
  - Myotonic dystrophy
  - Encephalitis
  - Idiopathic hypersomnia
  - Brain injuries
- Drugs

easier and less stimulating. European Union regulations limit heavy goods vehicle and bus driving to not more than 9 hours continuously without a rest period in any 24 hours and for not more than 56 hours each week. There are no regulations concerning taxi drivers' hours of work.

Medical disorders causing excessive sleepiness also predispose to road traffic accidents. The risk of these is increased about sixfold with obstructive sleep apneas.[48,49] Sedative drugs and alcohol also accentuate sleepiness, especially following sleep restriction and if there is an underlying sleep disorder. The effect of a single drink of alcohol at times when the circadian rhythm facilitates sleep (2.00–6.00 a.m. and 2.00–4.00 p.m.) may be the equivalent of two or three taken at 10.00 a.m. when alertness is maximal.

Sedative drugs not only cause sleepiness, but also impair vision, co-ordination, cognitive function, the perception of risk, and the important aspects of memory, such as anticipation of exits from motorways. The effects of sedative medication vary according to the nature of the drugs, the dose, time of ingestion, and the duration of action, as well as previous shift work or sleep deprivation, age and individual vulnerability. Examples of sedative drugs that predispose to road traffic accidents are benzodiazepines and related drugs, barbiturates, antidepressants, opiates, antihistamines, dopamine receptor agonists, alcohol, and cannabis. A roadside test is available for alcohol, but not for any other drugs.

Legal aspects

Drivers of motor vehicles or users of potentially hazardous machinery have a responsibility not to cause harm to those around them. The question arises as to whether it would be reasonable for the driver to foresee the danger from driving while sleepy, or falling asleep.[50] After an accident drivers often fail to recall that they were sleepy beforehand or that they fell asleep, but sleepiness in young adults is recognized at the time, at least in the laboratory situation, even if subsequent recall is lost. In other words sleep does not happen without any warning of drowsiness and the driver therefore has a duty of care not to continue to drive while sleepy.

Sleepiness itself is, however, difficult to measure. Objective laboratory tests such as the multiple sleep latency tests or maintenance wakefulness test have been used in normal persons and those with sleep disorders, but are not applicable to the roadside situation. Driving simulators, vigilance tests, divided attention tests, tracking tests, cognitive and perception tests and reaction times, both simple and complex, have been used to assess a driver's ability to drive safely, but none has proved satisfactory. It is therefore difficult to assess accurately how sleepy the driver was, or was likely to have been, at the time of the accident except from analysis of the sleep patterns before the accident and the behavior at the time of the accident.

It could be argued that at the moment of falling asleep the driver is no longer acting voluntarily and cannot be held responsible for any subsequent acts. This defence of automatism has failed because it has been held that drivers were responsible for allowing themselves to fall into this state of automatism knowingly, because prior to falling asleep they chose to continue driving while feeling sleepy. Similarly, if sleep is induced through taking alcohol or a sedative drug the defence of automatism would fail, but if alcohol or a sedative drug was unknowingly added to a drink and caused sudden loss of awareness the defence of automatism would probably be upheld. The defence of automatism should stand if sleep walking can be established as the cause of the driving (see above). If, however, the sleep walking was induced by drugs or alcohol knowingly taken there would be no valid defence.

In addition to not driving while sleepy, the individual also has a duty to notify the licensing authority, which in the UK is the Driver and Vehicle Licensing Agency (DVLA), about the diagnosis of any medical disorder that may increase sleepiness and might cause difficulty with driving. These include conditions such as obstructive sleep apneas, but narcolepsy has to be notified on diagnosis irrespective of the severity of the symptoms. The regulations concerning self-notification vary considerably among different countries and in the USA among different states,[51] although certain principles appear to be common to many countries.

The physician has a duty to inform the patient that he or she should notify the relevant licensing authority and the insurance company of any sleep disorder that may impair the ability to drive. The doctor's role is not to make these notifications except in exceptional circumstances, when the duty to society as a whole outweighs the duty of confidentiality to the individual, because of the size of the risk of an accident and the patient's failure to notify the authorities.

The employer also has a duty of care to the employee if the work pattern may lead to excessive sleepiness while driving.[52,53] This occurs with shift work, and particularly driving home after a long overnight shift. The state of prosecution of employers in this situation is uncertain, but charges of corporate manslaughter or similar allegations may be made if a driver causes death in an accident which was due to sleepiness attributable to the working conditions. Employers should make arrangements for employees to nap after shift work or have alternative arrangements for them to return home without having to drive.

SLEEP DISORDER IS CLAIMED TO BE DUE TO AN ACCIDENT

Accidents leading to litigation, such as brain injuries, can cause a variety of sleep abnormalities.[54]

Insomnia

This may be due to pain or other symptoms directly related to the trauma, anxiety, depression, post-traumatic stress disorder, a delayed sleep phase syndrome or non-24-hour sleep–wake rhythm, which is often associated with a deterioration in vision caused by the accident. The postconcussion syndrome also leads to insomnia, which is often transient.

It may be difficult to attribute insomnia after a brain injury precisely to any one of the possible causes or to assess how much is functional and how much is organic, but the insomnia and fatigue that is associated with it may significantly hinder rehabilitation after the injury.

Excessive sleepiness

Medical conditions

Sleepiness may be due to the following consequences of a brain injury.

Post-traumatic hypersomnia This is thought to be due to widespread damage to the sleep–wake control mechanisms. It usually follows a brain injury sufficiently severe to cause coma initially. The excessive sleepiness may improve for over a year, but recovery is often incomplete. Frequent and prolonged naps during the day with subalertness between them are often associated with a prolonged nocturnal sleep episode.[55] The clinical features are similar to those of idiopathic hypersomnia, apart from the history of brain injury.

Sleep apneas Central sleep apneas may be caused by damage to the respiratory control mechanisms, and obstructive sleep apneas are frequently seen after brain injuries.[56,57] It is uncertain, however, how frequently these were present before the incident only recognized afterwards. Secondary results of the brain injury, such as weight gain, may also predispose to obstructive sleep apneas.

Narcolepsy This may follow brain injury, particularly if there is loss of consciousness initially. It may be a result of injury to any part of the head. It is usually apparent immediately after the injury or within a few weeks or months.[58] The HLA type (DQB1*0602), which is present in around 95% of Caucasians with idiopathic narcolepsy, is only present in around 50% of those following brain injury.[59]

Klein–Levin syndrome This is commoner in males than females and usually occurs in adolescence or early adult life. Episodes of daytime sleepiness are associated with a voracious nonselective appetite and often with sexual disinhibition and psychological changes. These features probably represent fluctuating hypothalamic or thalamic inflammation which may result from a brain injury.[60] The condition tends to gradually improve.

Periodic limb movements in sleep These have been linked with brain injuries, but, like obstructive sleep apneas, it is uncertain how frequently they were present before the injury, but unrecognized.[61]

Circadian rhythm disorders The circadian control of sleep can be disturbed by brain injury. A delayed sleep phase syndrome is common[62] and the impairment in vision may lead to a non-24-hour sleep–wake cycle because of failure of light to entrain the circadian rhythm.[63]

Drugs Drugs required following brain injuries, such as antiepileptic drugs and those needed for psychiatric disturbances, may cause sedation.

Legal aspects

It is important to establish objectively whether or not the subject is sleepy. Continuous actigraphic movement monitoring for 2–3 weeks will give useful information regarding the rest and activity patterns, but it often necessary for the victim to undergo polysomnography. This will demonstrate the sleep onset REM sleep of narcolepsy, obstructive or central sleep apneas, periodic limb movements during sleep and other causes of excessive sleepiness. Multiple sleep latency tests during the day may show the sleep onset REM sleep of narcolepsy and the shorter sleep latency associated with this condition and with other disorders that cause excessive sleepiness.

It is important to assess whether there was any pre-existing sleep disorder causing sleepiness or any factor which might have predisposed to the abnormalities found after the injury. Impairment in sleep hygiene due to maladaptive behavior patterns following the injury, such as resting in bed for much of the day, may also present as excessive sleepiness after a brain injury.

Excessive sleepiness should be distinguished from fatigue, which is common after brain injuries, and in which there may be both mental and physical tiredness. Fatigue may persist throughout the day or occur after minor exertion or mental effort. The tiredness is, however, not associated with a need for sleep. This post-brain injury fatigue may be disabling and, like excessive sleepiness, may hinder rehabilitation, but it should be distinguished from true excessive sleepiness, as it has different causes and treatment.

REFERENCES

1. Shneerson JM. Sleep Medicine: a Guide to Sleep and its Disorders. Oxford: Blackwell Publishing, 2005.
2. Fenwick P. Somnambulism and the law: a review. Behav Sci Law 1987; 3: 343–57.
3. Mahowald MW, Schenck CH. Medical-legal aspects of sleep medicine. Neurol Clin 1999; 17(2): 215–34.
4. Mahowald MW, Schenck CH. Parasomnias: sleepwalking and the law. Sleep Med Rev 2000; 4(4): 321–39.
5. Moldofsky H, Gilbert R, Lue FA, MacLean AW. Forensic sleep medicine: violence, sleep, nocturnal wandering. Sleep-related violence. Sleep 1995; 18(9): 731–9.
6. Ohayon MM, Caulet M, Priest RG. Violent behavior during sleep. J Clin Psychiatry 1997; 58(8): 369–76.
7. Cartwright R. Sleepwalking violence: a sleep disorder, a legal dilemma, and a psychological challenge. Am J Psychiatry 2004; 161: 1149–58.
8. Guilleminault C, Moscovitch A, Leger D. Injury, violence and nocturnal wanderings. Am J Forensic Psychiatry 1995; 16(4): 33–46.
9. Raschka LB. Sleep and violence. Can J Psychiatry 1984; 29: 132–4.
10. Scott AIF. Attempted strangulation during phenothiazine-induced sleep-walking and night terrors. Br J Psychiatry 1988; 153: 692–4.
11. Guilleminault C, Leger D, Philip P, Ohayon MM. Nocturnal wandering and violence: review of a sleep clinic population. J Forensic Sci 1998; 43(1): 158–63.
12. Broughton R, Billings R, Cartwright R, et al. Homicidal somnambulism: a case report. Sleep 1994; 17(3): 253–64.
13. Schenck CH, Mahowald MW. A polysomnographically documented case of adult somnambulism with long-distance automobile driving and frequent nocturnal violence: parasomnia with continuing danger as a noninsane automatism? Sleep 1995; 18(9): 765–72.
14. Comella CL, Nardine TM, Diederich NJ, Stebbins GT. Sleep-related violence, injury and REM sleep behavior disorder in Parkinson's disease. Neurology 1998; 51(2): 526–9.
15. Schenck CH, Bundlie SR, Ettinger MG, Mahowald MW. Chronic behavioral disorders of human REM sleep: a new category of parasomnia. Sleep 1986; 9(2): 293–307.
16. Nofzinger EA, Wettstein RM. Homicidal behavior and sleep apnea: a case report and medicolegal discussion. Sleep 1995; 18(9): 776–82.
17. Borum R, Appelbaum KL. Epilepsy, aggression, and criminal responsibility. Psychiatr Serv 1996; 47: 762–3.
18. Guilleminault C, Moscovitch A, Léger D. Forensic sleep medicine: nocturnal wandering and violence. Sleep 1995; 18(9): 740–8.
19. Agargun MY, Kara H, Ozer OA, et al. Sleep-related violence, dissociative experiences, and childhood traumatic events. Sleep Hypnosis 2002; 4(2): 52–7.
20. Broughton RJ, Shimizu T. Sleep-related violence: a medical and forensic challenge. Sleep 1995; 18(9): 727–30.
21. Cartwright R. Sleep-related violence: does the polysomnogram help establish the diagnosis? Sleep Med 2000; 1: 331–5.
22. Mahowald MW, Bundlie SR, Hurwitz TD, Schenck CH. Sleep violence–forensic science implications: polygraphic and video documentation. J Forensic Sci 1990; 35(2): 413–32.
23. Gilmore JV. Murdering while asleep: clinical and forensic issues. Forensic Rep 1991; 4: 455–9.
24. Oswald I, Evans J. On serious violence during sleep-walking. Br J Psychiatry 1985; 147: 688–91.
25. Shapiro CM, Trajanovic NN, Fedoroff JP. Sexsomnia – a new parasomnia? Can J Psychiatry 2003; 48(5): 311–17.
26. Guilleminault C, Moscovitch A, Yuen K, Payares D. Atypical sexual behavior during sleep. Psychosom Med 2002; 64: 328–36.
27. Alves R, Aloe F, Tavares S. Sexual behavior in sleep, sleepwalking and possible REM behavior disorder: a case report. Sleep Res Online 1999; 2(3): 71–2.
28. Shapiro CM, Fedoroff JP, Trajanovic NN. Sexual behavior in sleep: a newly described parasomnia. Sleep Res 1995; 25: 367.
29. Schenck CH, Mahowald MW. An analysis of a recent criminal trial involving sexual misconduct with a child, alcohol abuse and a successful sleepwalking defence: arguments supporting two proposed new forensic categories. Med Sci Law 1998; 38(2): 147–52.
30. Rosenfeld DS, Elhajjar AJ. Sleepsex: a variant of sleepwalking. Arch Sex Behav 1998; 27(3); 269–78.
31. Mangan MA. A phenomenology of problematic sexual behavior occurring in sleep. Arch Sex Behav 2004; 33(3): 287–93.

32. Fenwick P. Sleep and sexual offending. Med Sci Law 1996; 36(2): 122–34.

33. Thomas TN. Sleepwalking disorder and Mens Rea: a review and case report. J Forensic Sci 1997; 42(1): 17–24.

34. Buchanan A. Sleepwalking and indecent exposure. Med Sci Law 1991; 31(1): 38–40.

35. Bowden P. Letter to the Editor. Sleepwalking and indecent exposure. Med Sci Law 1991; 31(4): 359.

36. Schenck CH, Mahowald MW. Letter to the Editor. Sleepwalking and indecent exposure. Med Sci Law 1992; 31(1): 86–7.

37. Legal Correspondent. Sleepwalking and guilt. Br Med J 1970; 186.

38. Zorick FJ, Salis PJ, Roth T, Kramer M. Narcolepsy and automatic behavior: a case report. J Clin Psychiatry 1979; 40: 194–7.

39. Ovuga EBL. Murder during sleep-walking. East African Med J 1992; 69(9): 533–4.

40. Szucs A, Janszky A, Hollo G, Migleczi PH, Halasz P. Misleading hallucinations in unrecognised narcolepsy. Acta Psychiatr Scand 2003; 108: 314–17.

41. Hays P. False but sincere accusations of sexual assault made by narcoleptic patients. Med Leg J 1992; 60(4): 265–71.

42. Blagrove M, Akehurst L. Effects of sleep loss on confidence-accuracy relationships for reasoning and eyewitness memory. J Exp Psychol Appl 2000; 6(1): 59–73.

43. Fuller DE, Hornfeldt CS, Kelloway JS, Stahl PJ, Anderson TF. The Xyrem® Risk Management Program. Drug Safety 2004; 27(5): 293–306.

44. Simmons MM, Cupp MJ. Use and abuse of flunitrazepam. Ann Pharmacotherapy 1998; 32: 117–19.

45. Laube I, Seeger R, Russi EW, Bloch KE. Accidents related to sleepiness: review of medical causes and prevention with special reference to Switzerland. Schweiz Med Wochenschr 1998; 128: 1487–99.

46. Reyner LA, Horne JA. Falling asleep whilst driving: are drivers aware of prior sleepiness? Int J Leg Med 1998; 111: 120–3.

47. Horne J, Reyner L. Vehicle accidents related to sleep: a review. Occup Environ Med 1999; 56: 289–94.

48. American Thoracic Society. Sleep apnea, sleepiness, and driving risk. Am J Respir Crit Care Med 1994; 150: 1463–73.

49. McNicholas WT, Krierger J. Public health and medicolegal implications of sleep apnea. Eur Respir J 2002; 20: 1594–609.

50. Jones CB, Dorrian J, Rajaratnam SMW. Fatigue and the criminal law. Ind Health 2005; 43: 63–70.

51. Pakola SJ, Dinges DF, Pack AI. Driving and sleepiness. Review of regulations and guidelines for commercial and noncommercial drivers with sleep apnea and narcolepsy. Sleep 1995; 18(9): 787–96.

52. Ellis E, Grunstein RR. Medico-legal aspects of sleep disorders: sleepiness and civil liability. Sleep Med Rev 2001; 5(1): 33–46.

53. Rajaratnam SMW. Legal issues in accidents caused by sleepiness. J Human Ergol 2001; 30: 107–11.

54. Shneerson J. Excessive sleepiness after brain injury. ACNR 2005; 5(3): 17–18.

55. Guilleminault C, Faull KF, Laughton M, van den Hoed J. Posttraumatic excessive daytime sleepiness: a review of 20 patients. Neurology 1983; 33: 1584–9.

56. Webster JB, Bell KR, Hussey JD, Natale TK, Lakshminarayan S. Sleep apnea in adults with traumatic brain injury. A preliminary investigation. Arch Phys Med Rehabil 2001; 82: 316–21.

57. Castriotta RJ, Lai JM. Sleep disorders associated with traumatic brain injury. Arch Phys Med Rehabil 2001; 82: 1403–6.

58. Maccario M, Ruggles KH, Meriwether MW. Post-traumatic narcolepsy. Military Med 1987; 152: 370–1.

59. Lankford DA, Wellman JJ, O'Hara C. Posttraumatic narcolepsy in mild to moderate closed head injury. Sleep 1994; 17: S25–8.

60. Will RG, Young JPR, Thomas DJ. Kleine–Levin syndrome: report of two cases with onset of symptoms precipitated by head trauma. Br J Psychiatry 1988; 152: 410–12.

61. Masel BE, Scheibel RS, Kimbark T, Kuna ST. Excessive daytime sleepiness in adults with brain injuries. Arch Phys Med Rehabil 2001; 82: 1526–32.

62. Patten SB, Lauderdale WM. Delayed sleep phase disorder after traumatic brain injury. J Am Acad Child Adolesc Psych 1992; 31: 100–2.

63. Boivin DB, James FO, Santo JB, Caliyurt O, Chalk C. Non 24-hour sleep–wake syndrome following a car accident. Neurology 2003; 60: 1841–3.

CHAPTER 11

Insomnia: impact on work, economics, and quality of life

Damien Léger

Insomnia is a common complaint which is reported by the adult population throughout the world.[1,2] Despite its high prevalence, insomnia remains largely unrecognized by health professionals as a disease entity, principally because it is more frequently viewed as a symptom of other more primary pathological conditions. Another barrier to a clear conceptualization of insomnia is that it is often difficult for patients and for health professionals to understand when it is severe enough to require treatment. Further, there is still insufficient knowledge about the management of insomnia. In the last decade several consensus meetings about the recognition, diagnosis, and treatment of insomnia have been held,[3–8] all of them emphasizing the seriousness of insomnia's impact on public health and of the need to appreciate its consequences for work, economics, and quality of life.

The aim of this chapter is to identify some of the effects of insomnia on work and daily life which underscore the seriousness of the condition as a public health issue. Another objective is to point out what is definitely known about the condition and which areas merit further investigation to properly assess insomnia's public health impact. The first part therefore deals with the definition and recognition of insomnia, while the second part concentrates on the consequences of insomnia for work, economics, and quality of life.

PART 1: RECOGNITION AND DIAGNOSIS OF INSOMNIA

DEFINITION OF INSOMNIA

In terms of clinical practice and of epidemiology, chronic insomnia is usually defined based on the criteria of the *Diagnostic and Statistical Manual of Mental Disorders* (DSM-IV)[9] or of the *International Classification of Sleep Disorders* (ICSD)[10] which are:

- difficulty in falling asleep (sleep initiating insomnia), the occurrence of nocturnal awakenings with difficulties getting back to sleep (sleep maintenance insomnia), an early morning awakening (sleep offset insomnia), or a non-refreshing or non-restorative sleep, and often some combination thereof;
- at least three times a week for at least one month;
- insomnia produces clinically significant distress or impairment in social, occupational, or other important areas of daytime functioning.

More recently an American Academy of Sleep Medicine Work Group[8] also proposed research diagnostic criteria for insomnia disorder.

- One or more of the following sleep-related complaints: (1) difficulty initiating sleep; (2)

difficulty maintaining sleep; (3) waking up too early; or (4) sleep that is chronically non-restorative or poor in quality.

- The above sleep difficulty occurs despite adequate opportunity and circumstances for sleep.
- At least one of the following forms of daytime impairment related to the night-time sleep difficulty is reported by the individual: (1) fatigue/malaise; (2) attention, concentration, or memory impairment; (3) social/vocational dysfunction or poor school performance; (4) mood disturbance/irritability; (5) daytime sleepiness; (6) motivation/energy/initiative reduction; (7) proneness for errors/accidents at work or while driving; (8) tension headaches, and/or gastrointestinal symptoms in response to sleep loss; and (9) concerns or worries about sleep.

Insomnia may be primary or secondary to a variety of disorders, environmental factors and/or comorbidities. Identifying and treating potential underlying conditions are priorities in the management of insomnia.

PRIMARY INSOMNIA

Primary insomnia is an intrinsic sleep disorder that is characterized by the presence of insomnia for at least one month.[8–10] Primary insomnia is a condition which:

- does not occur exclusively during the course of another sleep disorder such as sleep-disordered breathing, periodic limb movements, restless leg syndrome, narcolepsy, parasomnia or circadian rhythm disorder;
- does not occur in the course of another mental or psychiatric disorder or, if it does, it shows some independence from the temporal course of the mental or psychiatric condition;
- is not due to the direct physiologic effect of a general sleep disruptive medical condition, or if it does occur in the presence of such a condition, its temporal course shows

some independence from that condition's temporal course;
- is not due to a substance or treatment abuse or withdrawal, nor to a physical/environmental factor.

A common mechanism accounting for the persistence of insomnia is conditioned (learned or psychophysiological) insomnia. It begins usually with an episode of acute situational insomnia, secondary to a stressor such as jet-lag, pain, illness, or medication (insomnia precipitating factors). Then the patient associates the bed with not sleeping and becomes hyperaroused at night. This in turn produces a strategy of coping which has the effect of perpetuating the insomnia (insomnia perpetuating factors).[11] Individual differences in the vulnerability to sleep disturbances may constitute a continuum from vulnerability to transient or episodic insomnia through overt chronic primary insomnia.[12] Ruminating about not being able to sleep plays a major role.

SECONDARY INSOMNIA

Insomnia is frequently associated with a variety of other conditions including sleep disorders, mental or physical disorders, toxicological or environmental factors and in these circumstances insomnia may be more properly viewed as a symptom. It is the role of the practitioner to carefully check all these conditions before considering insomnia as a primary disorder.

Almost all sleep disorders disturb sleep seriously enough to induce a complaint of insomnia or poor sleep. Sleep apnea affects 5–10% of the general population. It increases with age and with the body mass index. It causes arousals and awakenings during all stages of sleep. Patients usually complain of non-restorative sleep rather than of real insomnia. Restless leg syndrome, which affects 5–10% of the general population, may impact sleep initiation and maintenance. Restless leg syndrome may also occur comorbidly with sleep apnea. Circadian rhythm disorders are linked to a dysfunction of the biological clock, due to an internal condition (delayed or advanced phase syndromes) or secondary to the underexposure of the retina to light (blindness), or misalignment between external and endogenous rhythms (shift workers, jet-lag). Circadian rhythm disruptions in turn may induce sleep onset insomnia, early morning awakening, frequent arousals and daytime sleepiness. Narcolepsy and parasomnias are also frequently associated with poor sleep.

Mental disorders or comorbidities are commonly associated with insomnia. Ohayon et al.[13] surveyed the general population and found among insomniacs that 30.1% and 23% had previously sought help for anxiety and depression, respectively. Similarly, in primary care patients with severe insomnia, a high prevalence of psychiatric diagnoses was found: 21.7% of severe insomniacs had depression, 7.2% neurosis/personality disorders, 10.2% acute psychological distress, 4.6% alcohol or drug abuse, 5.6% psychosomatic disorders, and 1% psychosis.[14]

Studies of specific populations reveal strong correlation between complaints of sleep disturbances and a variety of medical conditions including pain, and disorders of the cardio-respiratory, musculoskeletal, and central nervous systems.[15] Several endocrine and gastrointestinal disorders are also associated with sleep disruption. Nocturnal gastrointestinal reflux episodes, for instance, may arise during sleep and induce abrupt arousals.[16] A large number of medications and toxic agents (alcohol, drugs) can also impact sleep continuity.

Environmental factors may also induce sleep disruption and fragmentation even in good sleepers. Noise is one of the most common. Recently, the World Health Organization office of environment and health has considered insomnia as one of the major health effects of noise exposure.[17] Low or high temperature, altitude, and light also have an influence on sleep continuity.

DURATION OF INSOMNIA: TRANSIENT OR CHRONIC

The duration of a patient's complaint has important implications. The ICSD defines acute or transient insomnia as persisting for no greater than one week and subacute or short-term insomnia as lasting from one week to three months.[10] Both are considered adjustment sleep disorders and are associated with a reaction to an identifiable stressor. Transient insomnia usually disappears with the reduction of, or adaptation to, the stressor. However, it may also be the foundation of a long-term condition. The individual's emotional and behavioral responses to the first episodes of transient insomnia seem to play an important role in the course of the disease.[11,12,18] Therefore, early identification and management of insomnia may play a role in the prevention of long-term insomnia. Insomnia is considered to be chronic if it lasts more than one[9] to three months.[10] From our experience, we believe that one month is a reasonable period to begin to talk of 'chronic insomnia' and six months to one year a convenient period to observe public health (work and economics) consequences of insomnia. Retrospective studies indicate that about 80% of severe insomniacs have had the problem for greater than one year, with approximately 40% reporting greater than five year duration.[13,19] Longitudinal studies suggest that 30–80% of moderate-to-severe insomniacs show no significant remission over time.[6,19,20]

SEVERITY OF INSOMNIA

There is no clear consensus on the definition of severe insomnia. Although clinicians frequently encounter complaints in this regard it is probably insufficient to develop definitions of the disorder based on self-assessments made by patients. Many studies have observed that a large number of so-called 'severe insomniacs' did not consult any practitioner for years about their sleep problem. Chronic duration or nightly frequency may be a criterion of severity. The magnitude of the impaired daytime functioning may also represent a basis for assessing severe insomnia. In several studies which were focussed on the daytime consequences of insomnia, we have considered reports of at least two symptoms of poor sleep according to the DSM-IV definition of insomnia as fulfilling the definition of severe insomnia.[21–23]

PART 2: PUBLIC HEALTH CONSEQUENCES OF INSOMNIA

EPIDEMIOLOGY

Insomnia has to be clearly defined if we want to know accurately its prevalence in the general population. The early surveys inquired about sleep disorders over the lifetime and found as much as 90% of subjects complaining of poor sleep.[24] These data are confusing and more recently the DSM-IV or ICSD definitions of insomnia have been more often applied in epidemiological settings. Several large samples have been studied in the last decade. In 2002, Ohayon and Smirne[25] conducted a study with a representative sample population of 3970 individuals aged 15 years or older in the UK: insomnia symptoms were reported by 27.6% of the sample. Sleep dissatisfaction was found in 10.1% and insomnia disorder diagnoses in 7% of the sample. The use of sleep-enhancing medication was reported by 5.7%. In an epidemiological study, Léger et al.[21] surveyed a representative sample of the French population that included 12 778 individuals and found that 19% reported having insomnia while 9% had symptoms of severe insomnia (at least two symptoms of insomnia according to the DSM-IV definition). In a general population survey of 3000 subjects in Japan, Kim et al.[26] found a prevalence rate of 21.4% for insomnia. In a recent 2004 study in the USA, the National Sleep Foundation surveyed a representative sample of 1506 subjects over 18 years of age and found that 21% of the sample had insomnia according to the ICSD definition, but that only 9% had insomnia and daytime sequelae.[27] In a compilation of recent studies made in 2002, Ohayon[1] concluded that around one adult in three in the general population had symptoms of insomnia. However, only 16–21% had insomnia symptoms at least three times a week, of which from 13% to 17% qualified their trouble as important or major, and from 9% to 13% had insomnia and daytime consequences. To our knowledge, there is still no epidemiological study using the new research criteria.[8]

Sociodemographics

Almost all studies show an increasing prevalence of insomnia with age and a sex ratio in favor of women.[1–7] In their sample of 12 778, Léger et al.[21] found that severe insomnia was almost twice as prevalent among women as among men (12% vs. 6.3%; $p < 0.0001$). Older people usually had more severe complaints than younger ones. In a representative sample ($n = 5622$) of the general population of France aged 15 years or older, Ohayon and Lemoine[28] found that the prevalence of insomnia was twice as frequent in those of 65 years of age or older compared with persons younger than 45 years. Moreover, in this last study, 47.1% of those above 65 years reported three symptoms of insomnia compared with 32.2% for the group under 44 years old ($p < 0.001$). However, younger persons (under 45 years) and females reported significantly more daytime sequelae of insomnia than older persons (above 65 years) and males.

Only a few studies have attempted to examine the link between perceived job stress and the prevalence of insomnia. An exception was a survey study by Nakata et al.[29] of 1161 male white-collar employees of a Japanese electric equipment company. Among the 23.6% of the workers who had insomnia symptoms, those with high intragroup conflict (odds ratio

[OR] = 1.6), or high job dissatisfaction (OR = 1.5) had a significantly increased risk of insomnia after adjusting for multiple confounding factors. Limited employment opportunities, a poor physical environment, and low coworker support also were weakly associated with a risk of insomnia among workers.

Insomnia is also generally more prevalent in persons of low socioeconomic status,[30] although a number of exceptions to this generalization have been found. In France, for instance, the prevalence of insomnia was greatest among white-collar group respondents (20.8%).[21] A trend was also found toward lower rates of insomnia in senior executives, those in liberal professions, and in the farmers' group. Doi et al.,[31] in a cross-sectional study including 4868 daytime white-collar workers in Japan, similarly showed that poor sleep was significantly more prevalent in the white-collar group (30–45%) than in the general working population. Recently, Gellis et al.[32] have investigated the likelihood of insomnia and insomnia-related health consequences among a sample of at least 50 men and 50 women in each age decade from 20 to 80+ years old and of different socioeconomic status.[32] Results indicate that individuals of lower personal and household education are significantly more likely to experience insomnia, even after researchers accounted for ethnicity, gender, and age. Additionally, individuals with fewer years of education, particularly those who had dropped out of high school, experienced greater subjective impairment because of their insomnia.

Seeking help and access to treatments

Insomniacs, even severe cases, do not always seek help for treatment. An early Gallup study of insomniacs found that only 5% had ever visited a physician to discuss specifically their sleeping problem, and that only 21% had ever taken a prescription medication for sleep.[24] In France, 53% of severe insomniacs versus 27% of other patients with occasional sleep problems reported that they had ever visited a doctor specifically for insomnia (p < 10-4).[22]

A number of individuals with sleep disorders attempt to deal with their problem by nonmedical means, for example, by using non-prescription drugs, watching television, reading, or drinking alcohol to promote sleep.[1] In a survey of a representative sample of 2181 adults aged 18–45 years in the Detroit area, Johnson et al.[33] found that 13.3% had used alcohol as a sleep aid in the past year and 10.1% an over-the-counter medication. Fifteen per cent of those who had used alcohol as a sleep aid did it for at least one month; however, the duration of use was short for the majority of users (less than one week). Only 5.3% had used a prescription medication. In another survey, however, it was found that 10.8% of French adults regularly used prescription medication to promote sleep.[34] Recently, a consecutive sample (n = 700) of adults in the USA attending non-emergency primary care appointments were screened for sleep problems. A follow-up mailed survey then assessed insomnia symptoms, daytime impairment, beliefs about sleep, medication use, sleepiness and fatigue, and medical help-seeking.[35] It was found that 52% of patients with probable insomnia had reported discussing this with a physician. Multivariate logistic regression analyses indicated that discussing one's probable insomnia with a physician was independently associated with having a greater number of medical conditions (OR = 2.19 [95% CI, 1.13 to 4.22]), being more highly educated (OR = 1.67 [95% CI, 1.11 to 2.51]), sleeping less per night (OR = 0.71 [95% CI, 0.52 to 0.96]), and greater perceived daytime impairment due to insomnia (OR = 2.07 [95% CI, 1.06 to 4.03]).

Diagnosis of insomnia is not always followed by treatment. In Germany, a Nationwide Insomnia Screening and Awareness Study (NISAS-2000) found that close to 50% of all patients with insomnia did not receive a prescription for a specific insomnia therapy.[36]

Natural history

There are very few data on the natural history of insomnia. Severe insomnia seems to be more persistent than mild insomnia. Katz and McHorney[20] reassessed two years later a group of 3445 patients with insomnia: 83% of patients with severe insomnia remained so categorized, compared with 59% of patients with mild insomnia. Hohagen et al.[19] also showed that four months after a first survey, 87% of patients who initially reported a sleep complaint still had one. According to Mendelson et al.,[37] 88.2% of patients continue to report sleep problems five years after the onset. Predisposing, precipitating, and perpetuating factors contribute to the natural history of insomnia in patients presenting variable vulnerability.[12,38] In a recent study of 345 patients evaluated for insomnia at a sleep disorders clinic in Quebec, Bastien et al.[39] identified several specific precipitating factors related to the onset of insomnia. The most common of these were events related to family, health, and work/school. Sixty-five per cent of precipitating events had a negative valence. These events differed with the age of onset of insomnia but not with the gender of participants.

Comorbidity with depression and anxiety

Insomnia is associated with a variety of medical and psychiatric conditions. For many it is usually more intuitively comfortable to infer that insomnia is due to medical problems rather than being a comorbid condition with psychiatric disease. Nevertheless, depression and anxiety are estimated to occur comorbidly in 35–60% of chronic insomniacs.[1,4–7,13,14,38] Several longitudinal studies have shown that insomnia may represent a substantial and statistical risk for the development of depressive disorders.[40–42] However, there is actually increasing support for the suggestion that the coexistence of these two disease types is based on a common underlying pathology rather than being two correlated but separate disease states. In order to clarify public health consequences due to primary insomnia alone, it seems, however, important to clearly identify insomniacs with psychiatric diseases in the design of the studies.

DAYTIME CONSEQUENCES OF INSOMNIA

Even though there is broad consensus on the fact that daytime impact is a major criterion in the definition of insomnia,[7–9] the precise nature of this impact remains subject to debate. In a review of insomnia and daytime functioning, Riedel and Lichstein[43] suggested that the lack of objective findings in the literature might be explained by (a) a focus on variables which do not suggest impairment (rather than areas of actual impairment), and (b) methodological problems (such as non-homogeneous groups of subjects), which may have hidden actual differences between insomniacs and good sleepers. Daytime sleepiness has received the most attention but it is becoming clear that a large number of insomniacs are not sleepy during the day.[44,45] Bonnet and Arand[45] have even used multiple sleep latency tests to demonstrate that insomniacs were more alert in the daytime than good sleepers. However, the absence of an objective somnolence deficit does not mean that insomniacs are not impaired during the daytime.

Riedel and Lichstein[43] also recommended using objective measures of work performance (absenteeism, promotion, etc.) to clarify the impact of insomnia on daytime functioning. Insomnia is not a visible handicap in the workplace and it is difficult for insomniacs to explain to their colleagues and managers that they have had a poor night and that they need to rest. Insomniacs have to face a regular work load and they often complain of difficulties in their professional life.[37,46,47] However, there are few data assessing the true impact of insomnia on daily work. This is a crucial point to try to evaluate the impact of insomnia on absenteeism and other work measures in a real setting.

Absenteeism

In economic and epidemiological studies, overall measures of the respondent's health appeared to be the most important covariate of absenteeism. Paringer[48] was one of the first to demonstrate that health variables were more strongly associated with absenteeism than economic ones. In a large, cross-sectional, national probability sample of 1308 workers in the USA, Leigh[49] demonstrated that complaining of insomnia was the most predictable factor for absenteeism from among 36 variables. In a study comparing 80 insomniacs at work to 135 good sleepers, it was found that insomniacs had double the control rate of absenteeism.[22] Lavie also found a higher rate of absenteeism in insomniacs, as well as a higher rate of work accidents, and hypothesized that coworkers of the missing insomniacs were more exposed to accidents due to their work overload[50].

However, these preliminary studies were based on general population samples: insomnia was not always clearly defined and the groups of insomniacs were heterogeneous. Moreover, the absenteeism data were mainly based on the patients' self-reports and not on objective data. In a recent study Léger et al.[51] specifically surveyed the absenteeism of a group of insomniacs at work compared to a matched group of good sleepers and found that insomniacs showed almost twice as much absenteeism as the good sleepers. The difference between insomniacs and good sleepers was particularly high for managers (OR=2.29) and women (OR=2.31). We believe that this study is of particular interest because (a) we dealt with objective rather than subjective data on absenteeism, (b) insomnia was defined according to international classifications, (c) patients with depression and anxiety were excluded, (d) participants were all full-time workers and representative of the active population in the area and (e) patients

with chronic disease (which may interfere with sleep) and pregnant women were excluded from the study. Hence, in the group studied here, it seems more probable that significant differences between insomniacs and good sleepers reflect the impact of insomnia itself, rather than the effects of comorbidities.

Other occupational characteristics

The most original study on this point was conducted by Johnson et al.[52] who demonstrated that insomniacs in the navy were slower at work and had poorer career advancement than good sleepers. The difficulty of comparing the respective work contents of insomniacs and good sleepers was a major concern in the discussion of these results.

Insomniacs' impairment at the workplace has been assessed by very few authors. Lavie, in a large and detailed study of the lifestyle, health, sleep, and work habits of 1502 employees, concluded that sleep habits directly affect the workplace.[50] They showed that workers with daytime fatigue had significantly more complaints of somnolence during work breaks than other workers (14.2% vs. 3.5%, $p < 0.001$), a higher frequency of napping at work (16.8% vs. 1.4%, $p < 0.0001$), and significantly less job satisfaction.[50] However, this study was not directly focussed on insomnia but on sleep disorders. In a study comparing 240 severe insomniacs (SI) to 391 good sleepers (GS), Léger et al.[22] have explored work consequences of insomnia.[22] Fifteen per cent of SI versus 6% of GS ($p < 0.001$) reported having made errors at work over the previous month, which could have resulted in serious consequences. For 6% of SI versus 2% of GS, errors had occurred more than once during the previous month ($p = 0.0032$). Twelve per cent of insomniacs versus 6% of GS reported being late to work during the previous month (not significant). Moreover, 18% of SI versus 8% of GS ($p = 0.0004$) felt that they had exhibited poor efficiency at work. Thirteen per cent of SI versus 9% of GS reported difficulties completing complicated tasks at work (not significant). In a recent work, Daley et al.[53] questioned 930 adults from the province of Quebec about sleep and professional consequences. Reduced productivity was assessed by the visual analogue scale. Thirty-five per cent of insomniacs versus 9.8% of the good sleepers group reported reduced productivity. These preliminary findings need to be followed up by further studies using similarly precise methodologies that compare insomniacs to good sleepers who work in the same field.

Accidents

The impact of sleep disorders on automobile accidents is a crucial issue from a public health point of view. Public authorities and the media are actually closely informed concerning the risk of sleepiness at the wheel during the night and about the effects of sleep debt and sleep pathologies (sleep apnea, hypersomnia) on accidents (see Chapters 9 and 16). However, there are very few data on the risk of accidents due exclusively to insomnia.

Insomnia may increase the risk of accidents in several ways, including sleep deprivation, lack of attention, and side effects from hypnotic medications which people use to treat the disorder. Motor vehicle accidents (MVA) and work accidents (WA) have been mainly observed. In the French study mentioned earlier, comparing 240 severe insomniacs (SI) to 391 good sleepers (GS),[22] WA were eight times more common over the past 12 months in SI (8%) than in GS (1%) ($p=0.0150$), with an average number of 0.07 ($\pm$ 0.25) accidents per SI versus 0.01 ($\pm$ 0.11) per GS ($p=0.0550$). There was, however, no statistical difference for MVA over the past 12 months between the groups (9% vs. 10%). The authors explained the discrepancy between WA and MVA by the fact that SI may have avoided driving or driven shorter distances: 65.8% of SI versus 72.5% of GS drove a car ($p=0.012$). Lavie[50] also showed a higher rate of WA in insomniacs (in their lifetime) than in GS (52.1% vs. 35.6%, $p<0.01$). The rate of MVA

due to fatigue (5% vs. 2%, not significant) was slightly but not significantly increased in insomniacs. Daley et al.[53] did not find similarly a different rate of MVA in the last six months between insomniacs and good sleepers, in a group of 930 adults in Quebec. However, 23.5% of drivers reporting an accident felt that insomnia had played an important role in the event. Moreover, 39.5% of participants saw a link between their sleep difficulties and other types of accidents ($p<0.001$).

Regarding the effects of drug treatments on driving ability, it is usually admitted that long-term half-life hypnotics (medium to long-term benzodiazepines and antihistamines) may induce a risk of accident, while driving, in the morning and a risk of falls at night in the elderly. In Europe, the vast majority of hypnotics are bottled with labels warning of the possible risk of accidents due to the treatment. There is, however, little published on the effects of common hypnotics on driving ability. Partinen et al.[54] have recently performed a double-blind, randomized, placebo-controlled, three-treatment, three-period, cross-over study investigating the effects of zolpidem (10 mg) and temazepam (20 mg) versus placebo in 18 insomniacs, in real-life conditions on driving performance. After polysomnography at baseline and each treatment night, patients underwent a STISIM driving simulator test 5.5 hours after drug intake at 7.30 a.m. on the next morning. There were no differences between treatments for the primary outcome measure (mean time to collision; baseline: 0.120 s, P: 0.124, T: 0.118, Z: 0.124; $p\geq0.12$ for all pairwise comparisons). No differences were recorded for speed deviation and reaction time to tasks for the various treatments; however, lane position deviation was greater after administration of zolpidem in comparison to both placebo and temazepam ($p=0.025$ and 0.05, respectively). The investigators strongly warned patients not to take hypnotics in the evening if they intended to drive an automobile early the next morning. Using a mathematical model, Menzin et al.[55] calculated the potential effects of sleep medications on motor vehicle accidents and costs, and applied the model to typical highway conditions in France. They used the model of standard deviation of a vehicle's lateral position (SDLP), and hypothesized that compared with zaleplon, the use of zopiclone over 14 days in France would be expected to result in 503 excess accidents per 100 000 drivers.

HEALTH STATUS AND HEALTH CARE USE

Several studies have looked at the links between insomnia and general health status. Although insomnia appears to be associated with poorer health status, it is difficult to know whether insomnia is the result of the poorer health status or its cause. Poor health leads to an increase in the use of medical services. This includes visits to doctors and other health professionals, intake of medications, and the number and duration of hospitalizations.

Weyerer and Dilling[56] found an average annual consultation rate among mild and moderately severe insomniacs significantly higher than those without sleep disorders (10.61 and 12.87 consultations per year, respectively, vs. 5.25 per year for good sleepers). They also reported a hospitalization rate of 21.9% (severe insomniacs) vs. 12.2% (good sleepers). Lavie[50] also found a higher rate of hospitalizations for insomniacs as did Kales et al.,[57] who found an annual hospitalization rate of 15.7%. In the Léger et al.[22] study, 18% of SI and 9% of GS had been hospitalized during the previous 12 months ($p=0.0017$), with an average of 0.17 (± 0.40) hospitalizations for SI versus 0.11 (± 0.45) hospitalizations for the GS (NS). The average duration of stay in hospital was 1.19 (± 3.45) days for SI versus 0.76 (± 3.83) days for the GS (NS). Fifty-nine per cent of SI and 49% of GS had undergone a medical evaluation in the previous six months ($p=0.0138$) with an average of 2 (± 3.6) evaluations for SI versus 1.2 (± 2.2)

for GS ($p=0.0198$). Severe insomniacs had had more blood studies (48% vs. 34%, $p=0.0005$) and radiological procedures (17% vs. 10%, $p=0.0142$) than good sleepers; they also had more outpatient visits and used more medication (particularly cardiovascular, central nervous system, genitourinary, and gastrointestinal medications) than good sleepers (see Table 11.1). However, there was no difference in the use of analgesic medications, despite the fact that 46% of insomniacs versus 29% of good sleepers ($p<0.001$) said they were particularly sensitive to pain. This is an important point, as pain may be an obvious cause of sleep disturbance. Kales et al.[57] have reported that poor mental and physical health were far more prevalent among insomniacs than controls. Recently, Katz and McHorney[42] calculated the odds ratio (OR) between chronic diseases and complaints of insomnia. Severe insomnia was strongly linked to current depression (OR=8.2), as well as to congestive heart failure (OR=2.5), obstructive airway disease (OR=1.6), and prostate problems (OR=1.6). Darko et al.[58] showed, in a prospective study, that fatigue and sleep disturbance were frequent symptoms of advanced human immunodeficiency virus (HIV) infection and emphasized the important alerting value of these complaints. Finally, the fact that insomnia can be a risk factor for psychiatric diseases and alcoholism[3,7,33] was also conclusively demonstrated by Katz et al.[57]

These findings have two implications. First, insomnia seems to be associated with poorer health status; indeed, insomniacs should be evaluated for psychiatric and somatic disorders. Second, although we cannot conclude whether insomnia is the cause of or the result of worsened health status, insomniacs are clearly at increased risk for certain diseases and a higher use of medical services. Many of the findings reported to be consequences of insomnia are actually correlates. Until a cause–effect relationship is established, correlate or comorbidity may be more accurate terms to describe the relationship between insomnia and poor medical status.

Table 11.1 Health and absenteeism due to sickness in insomniacs[a]

	Severe insomniacs (SI)	Good sleepers (GS)	Odds ratio	95% confidence interval
A: % of subjects visiting health professionals within 2 months of study	**240 = 100%**	**391 = 100%**		
% of subjects with at least 1 visit overall	82	68	2.15	1.43–3.25*
To general practitioner	71	54	2.07	1.45–2.96*
To specialists	30	29	1.05	0.73–1.52
To other health professionals	15	8	2.05	1.19–3.52*
B: % of subjects regularly on medications at survey time	**236 = 100%**	**387 = 100%**		
% of subjects on at least 1 drug	67	44	2.59	1.82–3.68*
Cardiovascular	37	27	1.57	1.09–2.25*
Beta-blockers	23	19	1.28	0.84–1.93*
Phlebotropics	14	5	3.15	1.68–5.92*
Antiarrhythmics & anticoagulants	11	5	2.4	1.25–4.64*
Other treatments:				
Urogenital	12	7	1.79	0.99–3.24*
Gastrointestinal	11	4	3.07	1.52–6.24*
Vitamins and minerals	11	4	3.07	1.52–6.24*
Glucose and lipid metabolism	2	4	0.54	0.17–1.6
Musculoskeletal	7	4	1.93	0.89–4.16
Hormones	3	2	1.45	0.47–4.46
Respiratory	3	1	2.93	0.76–12.02
Ophthalmology	2	1	2.07	0.48–9.27

(continued)

Table 11.1 (continued)

	Severe insomniacs (SI)	Good sleepers (GS)	Odds ratio	95% confidence interval
C: Absenteeism due to sickness within previous 12 months	**80 = 100%**	**135 = 100%**		
% of subjects involved	31	19	1.91	0.96–3.78**
% of subjects with 1 leave of absence	19	13	1.50	0.67–3.38**
% with 2 leaves of absence	9	4	2.55	0.69–9.65
% with 3 leaves of absence	1	0		
% with >3 leaves of absence	2	2	1.13	0.13–8.52
Average number of leaves of absence:				
Total group ± SD	0.48 ± 1.60	0.24 ± 0.67		NS
Average duration of one leave of absence (days)				NS
Total group ± SD	5.38 ± 15.40	3.62 ± 15.23		

[a]From the 1598 responders to questionnaire Q 2538 individuals were identified as severe insomniacs and were pulled out from the total group. Using responses to questions on anxiety and depression, a segment of these two subgroups that had positive responses were eliminated from further tabulation. A further review of the non-severe insomniacs without anxiety and depression was done and this subgroup was subdivided in 'mild insomniacs' and 'good sleepers'. The latter subgroup ($n = 391$) was compared to the severe insomniacs without anxiety and depression ($n = 240$). For further details, see text.

P-value is comparison between severe insomniacs and good sleepers: *$p < 0.01$; **$p < 0.05$.

SD; standard deviation: NS, not significant.

Source: Léger et al.[22]

Costs of insomnia

At this time there is very little documentation of the economic consequences of insomnia. The National Commission of Sleep Disorders Research (NCSDR) in the USA estimated the direct cost of insomnia in 1990 to be $15.4 billion, extrapolating from available data.[59] However, in the judgment of the Commission, 'the absence of hard epidemiological data makes it impossible to calculate the precise cost of sleep disorders, but some data do exist to show that the costs are substantial'. In a 1988 study carried out for the NCSDR, Léger[60] examined the cost of accidents related to sleep disorders in the USA and estimated this to be between $43.15 billion and $56.02 billion. Stoller[61] made an estimate of the total cost of insomnia for 1988 in the USA, based on a literature review of the economic costs and effects associated with insomnia. Her estimate of this cost was from $92.5 billion to $107.5 billion.

All consensus reports agree that a full appreciation of the social and economic costs of insomnia is limited by the lack of socioeconomic data on the issue. Areas where information is needed include insomnia-related use of health care services. Another factor complicating an accurate assessment of the problem is the degree of overlap between insomnia and many somatic and psychiatric diseases. We have tried to summarize the work that has been accomplished in the field and emphasized what should be done to improve an understanding of the economic consequences of insomnia.

The economic impact of insomnia can be divided into direct costs, indirect costs, and related costs. *Direct costs* of insomnia are charges for medical care or self-treatment that are borne by patients, government, organized health care providers, or insurance companies. *Indirect costs* refer to patient- and employer-borne costs that result from insomnia-related morbidity and mortality. *Related costs* are those which can be rationally associated with the illness, such as the cost of property damage resulting from accidents associated with insomnia.

Direct costs of insomnia

Direct costs of insomnia include outpatient visits, sleep recordings, and medications specifically indicated for insomnia. There is very little knowledge about costs of this kind. In 1999, Walsh and Engelhardt[62] estimated, on 1995 values basis, the direct costs of insomnia to be $13.93 billion, which consisted of health care services ($11.96 billion, including nursing), home care ($10.9 billion), and medications/substances used for treatment ($1.97 billion). Léger et al.[34] also made a similarly based estimate of the direct costs of insomnia in France in 1995 at $2.067 billion divided mainly between $1.75 billion for outpatient visits and $310.59 million for substances used for insomnia treatment. It was of particular interest to observe the low cost of sleep centers in this estimate: $1.75 million. In both estimates, the cost of these prescriptions was very little compared with other costs. However, the direct costs related to sleep disorders evaluation by practitioners seem to be a small part of the total cost of insomnia.

Indirect costs of insomnia

The indirect costs of insomnia are the potential consequences of insomnia on society, such as health problems, professional consequences (loss of productivity, and absenteeism), and accidents. The only estimate of the cost of accidents related to sleep disorders ($46–52 billion in 1988) was more focussed on sleepiness at the wheel than on insomnia.[60] As mentioned earlier, Johnson et al.[52] demonstrated among navy recruits that insomniacs were slower at work and had poorer career advancement than good sleepers. Based on this last mentioned study, Stoller[61] estimated the loss in productivity due to insomnia in the USA to be $41.1 billion in 1988. The cost of absenteeism among nonmanagerial personnel was estimated to be about $143 per day, or more than $57 billion per year.

Discussion about the costs of insomnia

With the exception of the estimates provided in these few studies, the total costs of insomnia remain largely unknown and thus it is difficult to have a clear understanding of insomnia's economic impact. Studies on insomnia's direct costs have been made only in two countries,[34,61] and it is difficult to apply these results to other parts of the world. The studies on indirect costs are based on hypotheses and limited sample sizes and their generalizability will need to be confirmed by larger studies with more representative samples. The same amount of insomnia may not necessarily have the same impact in different countries and there is a need for cross-cultural studies to better understand the daily economic impact of insomnia around the world.[30] Future studies might try to adopt standardized economic measures such as the gross national product to facilitate comparisons between countries.

Quality of life and insomnia

Few investigations have specifically assessed the impact of insomnia on quality of life (Qol). Most studies in this area have dealt with the impact of cancer on insomnia and Qol, although other investigations have explored the effects of sleep impairment on Qol in the context of diabetes, depression, Parkinson's disease, chronic renal diseases with hemodialysis, patients with HIV, or chronic psychiatric diseases. Qol is also sometimes used to evaluate pharmacologic and non-pharmacologic treatments of insomnia.

Assessment of the daytime consequences

The World Health Organization's consensus report on sleep and health strongly recommends more studies on the Qol of insomniacs.[4] Surprisingly, there are relatively few works specifically devoted to the subject.[23,63–66]

The SF-36, a very widely used scale in Qol,[67] was first used for insomnia research in a survey designed to document the prevalence of insomnia and its impact on Qol,[63] which showed that individuals with insomnia reported lower Qol scores. This association remained significant after controlling for demographic variables and comorbid conditions.

Zamitt et al.[64] used several instruments to evaluate the impact of insomnia on Qol in a sample of 261 insomniacs compared to a control group of 101 good sleepers. Insomniacs were recruited by advertisements and fulfilled the DSM-IV criteria for insomnia. Individuals fulfilling criteria of having irregular sleep patterns, sleep apnea, restless leg syndrome, periodic limb movement disorders, a history of psychiatric illness, alcohol or substance abuse, epilepsy and HIV were excluded from the study. The investigators used the SF-36 and the Qol inventory, a 31 items questionnaire specifically designed for the study that included aspects related to sleep, cognitive function, daytime performance, social and family relationships, and health. The authors showed a significant difference between the two groups ($p < 0.0001$, MANOVA) on all eight SF-36 subscales. Insomniacs reported more health concerns related to limits on physical activity, more interference with normal social activities due to physical or emotional problems, more bodily pain, poorer general health, less vitality, more emotional difficulties, and more mental health problems than the good sleepers' group. Using the Qol inventory they also found a significant impact on the Qol of insomniacs. The authors suggested that the SF-36 can be used to assess differences between patients with insomnia and healthy controls, and that the SF-36 may have clinical utility as a measure of insomnia-associated impairment.

Léger et al.[23] also used the SF-36 to evaluate the quality of life of three matched groups of 240 severe insomniacs, 422 mild insomniacs, and 391 good sleepers selected from the general population. They eliminated from the original group those meeting DSM-IV criteria for anxiety and depression. They found that severe insomniacs had lower scores on eight dimensions of the SF-36 than mild insomniacs and good sleepers. Mild insomniacs also had lower scores in the same eight dimensions than good sleepers. However, the mental health status and the emotional state were worse in severe and mild insomniacs than in good sleepers. This result demonstrates a clear inter-relation between insomnia and emotional state, despite the fact that those with DSM-IV criteria for anxiety and depression had been eliminated. The authors concluded that SF-36 was sensitive to the severity of insomnia and seemed to be a reliable instrument to assess the impact of insomnia on Qol.

Shubert et al.[65] found the same kind of relationship between the severity of insomnia and decreased Qol in a group of 2800 elderly patients (aged from 53 to 97 years) by means of telephone interview, as part of a five-year follow-up examination of the Epidemiology of Hearing Loss Study. Participants were asked about symptoms of poor sleep. A response of 'often' or 'almost always' was coded as positive for an insomnia trait. The SF-36 was administered to assess Qol of these patients: 26% of the population reported one insomnia trait, 13% reported two, and 10% reported three. The eight domains of the SF-36 were significantly decreased as the number of insomnia traits increased. The authors concluded that insomnia is common among older adults and is associated with a decreased Qol.

Idzikowski[66] discussed the concept of Qol applied to sleep and introduced the view that short sleep is not necessarily deleterious, but that abnormally shortened or fragmented sleep can reduce an individual's Qol. Katz and McHorney[42] finally demonstrated that insomnia by itself affects the Qol of patients suffering from chronic illness. Insomnia was severe in 16% and mild in 34% of these patients. Differences between patients with mild insomnia versus no insomnia showed small-to-medium decrements across SF-36 subscales ranging from 4.1 to 9.3 points (on a scale of 100)

and for severe insomnia from 12.0 to 23.9 points. Insomnia appeared in this study to be an independent factor of a worsened Qol to almost the same extent as chronic conditions such as congestive heart failure and clinical depression.

Quality of life in the treatment of insomnia

Goldenberg et al.[68] and Léger et al.[69] showed in questionnaire studies that the drug zopiclone improved the Qol of insomniacs (on professional, relational, sentimental, domestic, leisure, and safety aspects) to an extent which was not significantly different from that of good sleepers. Baca et al.[70] also showed in a questionnaire study that zolpidem improved patients' Qol in four major areas: social support, general satisfaction, physical and psychological well-being, and absence of work overload/free time. However, to the best of our knowledge no extensive survey has compared the effects of several hypnotics with well-validated Qol instruments. Regarding non-pharmacologic therapies, Quesnel et al.[71] have shown the efficacy of cognitive-behavioral therapy in insomnia in 10 women treated for non-metastatic breast cancer. They found an improvement of sleep assessed by polysomnography and at the global and cognitive subscales of the QLQ-C30.

Insomnia affects the daily lives of patients. However, it is often difficult to evaluate its impact and the efficacy of treatments. Qol measurement seems to be a good means for better understanding the complaints of insomniacs regarding their day-to-day functioning. Several studies have shown the sensitivity of the SF-36 in evaluating the impact of insomnia by itself or in relation with other associated chronic diseases. We also recommend more accurate Qol tools specifically designed for insomnia should be developed.

HD-16: a specifically designed quality of life scale for insomniacs

For many chronic diseases, a disease-focussed Qol instrument has been shown to be useful for

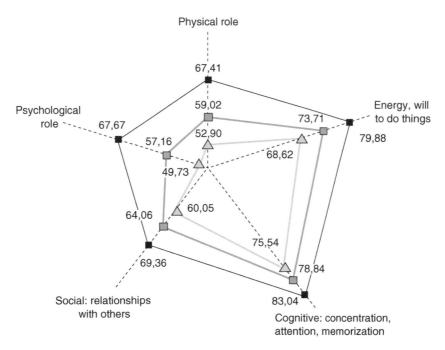

Figure 11.1 HD-16: a specifically designed insomnia quality of life scale among three groups. ▲ = good sleepers; ■ = mild insomniacs; ◆ = severe insomniacs.

accurately evaluating insomnia's impact on the daily lives of patients and to show the efficacy of some treatments. In the field of insomnia itself, there is a need for specific instruments to better encompass the Qol of patients. This is why HD-16, an insomnia questionnaire specifically designed for insomniacs, has been proposed.[72] Based on interviews with severe insomniacs, a 43-item questionnaire on Qol has been developed and tested in one group of 240 severe insomniacs, in one group of 422 mild insomniacs, and in one group of 391 good sleepers. A development program evolving through 10 steps led to the construction of a specific Qol scale. Five dimensions were validated as both relevant and independent from each other: physical role, psychological role, social relationships with others, cognitive (concentration, attention, memorization), and motivational energy. Sixteen out of the 43 items initially tested were found to significantly differentiate the various subgroups of

poor and good sleepers. Based on the 16 items selected, Léger and colleagues called the scale the Hotel Dieu 16 (HD-16). The score's specificity (correlation score: 0.36) and reliability (Cronbach coefficient alpha = 0.78) were verified. The results in the three groups are shown in Figure 11.1.

EPILOGUE

Millions of people around the world suffer from insomnia. In addition to its disruptive influence on quality of sleep, insomnia also deeply affects the daily lives of patients. The economic impact of insomnia on society appears enormous, although a need is recognized to improve survey methodologies and to use standardized economic measures for more effective country-to-country comparisons. There is also an increasing amount of evidence linking insomnia to several severe public health concerns including obesity, diabetes, depression, and cardiovascular diseases.

There is a major need for education of doctors and information of the general public about sleep and insomnia management. This author considers that combined therapies emphasizing both pharmacologic and non-pharmacologic treatments offer the best promise for helping patients in the daily management of chronic insomnia.

REFERENCES

1. Ohayon MM. Epidemiology of insomnia: what we know and what we still need to learn. Sleep Med Rev 2002; 6: 97–111.
2. Soldatos CR, Allaert FA, Ohta T, Dikeos DG. How do individuals sleep around the world? Results from a single-day survey in ten countries. Sleep Med 2005; 6: 5–13.
3. Roth T, Hajak G, Ustun TB. Consensus for the pharmacological management of insomnia in the new millenium. Int J Clin Pract 2001; 55: 42–52.
4. World Health Organization. Insomnia: an international consensus conference report, Versailles, 13–15 October 1996. WHO Publications MSA/MDN/98.2, 1998, 55 p. Geneva: WHO.
5. Buysse DJ. Diagnosis and assessment of sleep and circadian rhythm disorders. J Psychiatr Pract 2005; 11: 102–15.
6. Kupfer DJ, Reynolds CF. Management of insomnia. N Engl J Med 1997; 336: 341–6.
7. Schenck CH, Mahowald MW, Sack RL. Assessment and management of insomnia. J Am Med Assoc 2003; 19: 2475–9.
8. Edinger JD, Bonnet MH, Bootzin RR, et al. Derivation of research diagnostic criteria for insomnia: report of an American Academy of Sleep Medicine Work Group. Sleep 2004; 27: 1567–96.
9. Diagnostic and Statistical Manual of Mental Disorders, 4th edn: DSM-IV. Washington, DC: American Psychiatric Association, 1994.
10. Diagnostic Classification Steering Committee. International Classification of Sleep Disorders: Diagnostic and Coding Manual. Rochester, MN: American Sleep Disorders Association; 1990.
11. Morin CM, Rodrigue S, Ivers H. Role of stress, arousal and coping skills in primary insomnia. Psychosom Med 2003; 65: 259–67.
12. Drake C, Richardson G, Roehrs T, Scofield H, Roth T. Vulnerability to stress-related sleep disturbance and hyperarousal. Sleep 2004; 27: 285–91.
13. Ohayon MM, Caulet M, Priest RG, Guilleminault C. DSM-IV and ICSD-90 insomnia symptoms and sleep dissatisfaction. Br J Psychiatry 1997; 171: 382–8.
14. Hohagen F, Rink K, Kappler C, et al. Prevalence and treatment of insomnia in general practice. A longitudinal study. Eur Arch Psychiatry Clin Neurosci 1993; 242: 329–36.
15. Pilowski I, Cettenden I, Townley M. Sleep disturbance in pain clinic patients. Pain 1985; 23: 27–33.
16. Shoenut JP, Yamashiro Y, Orr WC, et al. Effects of severe gastroesophageal reflux on sleep stage in patients with a peristaltic esophagus. Dig Dis Sci 1996; 41: 372–6.
17. World Health Organization Regional Office for Europe. European technical meeting on sleep on health, Bonn, Germany, 2004. eneva: WHO.
18. Edinger JD, Stout AL, Hoelscher TJ. Cluster analysis of insomniac's MMPI profiles: relation of sub-types to sleep history and treatment outcome. Psychosom Med 1988; 50: 77–87.
19. Hohagen F, Kappler C, Schramm E, et al. Sleep onset insomnia, sleep maintaining insomnia and insomnia with early morning awakening–temporal stability of subtypes to a longitudinal study on general practice attendees. Sleep 1994; 17: 551–4.
20. Katz DA, McHorney CA. Clinical correlates of insomnia in patients with chronic illness. Arch Intern Med 1998; 159: 1099–107.
21. Léger D, Guilleminault C, Dreyfus JP, Delahaye C, Paillard M. Prevalence of insomnia in a survey of 12 778 adults in France. J Sleep Res 2000; 9: 35–42.
22. Léger D, Guilleminault C, Bader G, Levy E, Paillard M. Medical and socio-professional impact of insomnia. Sleep 2002; 25: 625–9.
23. Léger D, Scheuermaier K, Philip P, Paillard M, Guilleminault C. SF-36: evaluation of quality of life in severe and mild insomniacs compared with good sleepers. Psychosom Med 2001; 63: 49–55.

24. National Sleep Foundation (NSF). Sleep in America. Princeton, NJ: Gallup Organization, 1991.

25. Ohayon MM, Smirne S. Prevalence and consequences of insomnia disorders in the general population of Italy. Sleep Med 2002; 3: 115–20.

26. Kim K, Uchiyama M, Okawa M, Liu X, Ogihara R. An epidemiological study of insomnia among the Japanese general population. Sleep 2000; 23: 41–7.

27. National Sleep Foundation (NSF). Sleep in America 2004. Gallup Organization. Available: www.sleepfoundation.org/about/index.php [accessed August 18 2006].

28. Ohayon MM, Lemoine P. Daytime consequences of insomnia complaints in the French general population. L'Encephale 2004; xxx: 222–7.

29. Nakata A, Haratani T, Takahashi M, et al. Job stress, social support, and prevalence of insomnia in a population of Japanese daytime workers. Social Sci Med 2004; 59: 1719–30.

30. Walsh JK. Clinical and socioeconomic correlates of insomnia. J Clin Psychiatry 2004; 65(Suppl 8): 13–19.

31. Doi Y, Minowa M, Tango T. Impact and correlates of poor sleep quality in Japanese white-collar employees. Sleep 2003; 26: 467–71.

32. Gellis LA, Lichstein KL, Scarinci IC, et al. Socioeconomic status and insomnia. J Abnorm Psychol 2005; 114: 111–18.

33. Johnson EO, Roehrs T, Roth T, Breslau N. Epidemiology of alcohol and medication as aids to sleep in early adulthood. Sleep 1998; 21: 178–86.

34. Léger D, Levy E, Paillard M. The direct costs of insomnia in France. Sleep 1999; 22(Suppl 2): 5394–401.

35. Aikens JE, Rouse ME. Help-seeking for insomnia among adult patients in primary care. J Am Board Fam Pract 2005; 18: 257–61.

36. Wittchen HU, Krause P, Hofler M, et al. NISAS-2000: the 'Nationwide Insomnia Screening and Awareness Study'. Prevalence and interventions in primary care. Fortschr Med Orig 2001; 119: 9–19.

37. Mendelson WB, Garnett D, Linnoila M. Do insomniacs have impaired daytime functioning? Biol Psychiatry 1984; 19: 1261–3.

38. Drake CL, Roehrs T, Roth T. Insomnia causes, consequences, and therapeutics: an overview. Depression and Anxiety 2003; 18: 163–76.

39. Bastien CH, Vallieres A, Morin CM. Precipitating factors of insomnia. Behav Sleep Med 2004; 2: 50–62.

40. Ford DE, Kamerow DB. Epidemiological study of sleep disturbances and psychiatric disorders. An opportunity for prevention? J Am Med Assoc 1989; 262: 1479–84.

41. Chang PP, Ford DE, Mead LA, Cooper-Patrick L, Klag MJ. Insomnia in young men and subsequent depression. The Johns Hopkins Precursors Study. Am J Epidemiol 1997; 146: 105–14.

42. Katz DA, McHorney CA. The relationship between insomnia and health-related quality of life in patients with chronic illness. J Fam Pract 2002; 51: 229–35.

43. Riedel BW, Lichstein KL. Insomnia and daytime functioning. Sleep Med Rev 2000; 4: 277–98.

44. Stepanski E, Zorick F, Roehrs T, et al. Daytime alertness in patients with chronic insomnia compared with asymptomatic control subjects. Sleep 1988; 11: 54–60.

45. Bonnet MH, Arand DL. Activity, arousal, and the MSLT in patients with insomnia. Sleep 2000; 23: 205–12.

46. Schneider-Helmert D. Twenty-four hour sleep/wake function and personality patterns in chronic insomniacs and healthy controls. Sleep 1987; 11: 54–60.

47. Manocchia M, Keller S, Ware JE. Sleep problems, health-related quality of life, work functioning and health care utilization among the chronically ill. Quality of Life Research 2001; 10: 331–45.

48. Paringer L. Women and absenteeism: health or economics? J Econom Business 1985; 37: 123–7.

49. Leigh P. Employee and job attributes and predictors of absenteeism in a national sample of workers: the importance of health and dangerous working conditions. Social Sci Med 1991; 33: 127–31.

50. Lavie P. Sleep habits and sleep disturbances in industrial workers in Israel: main findings and some characteristics of workers complaining of daytime sleepiness. Sleep 1981; 4: 147–58.

51. Léger D, Massuel MA, Comet D and the SISYPHE group. Consequences of insomnia on professional activity in the Paris Region. Sleep 2004; 27: A270.

52. Johnson LC, Spinweber CL, Gomez SA, Matteson LT. Daytime sleepiness, performance, mood, nocturnal sleep: the effect of

benzodiazepine and caffeine on their relationship. Sleep 1990; 13: 121–35.

53. Daley ME, LeBlanc M, Morin CM. The impact of insomnia on absenteeism, productivity and accidents rate. Sleep 2005; 28: A247.

54. Partinen M, Hirvonen K, Hublin C, Halavaara M, Hiltunen H. Effects of after-midnight intake of zolpidem and temazepam on driving ability in women with non-organic insomnia. Sleep Med 2003; 4: 553–61.

55. Menzin J, Lang KM, Levy P, Levy EA. General model of the effects of sleep medications on the risk and cost of motor vehicle accidents and its application to France. Pharmacoeconomics 2001; 19: 69–78.

56. Wereyer S, Dilling H. Prevalence and treatment of insomnia in the community: results from the Upper Bavarian field study. Sleep 1991; 14: 392–8.

57. Kales JD, Kales A, Bixler EO, et al. Biopsychobehavioral correlates of insomnia. Clinical characteristics and behavior correlates. Am J Psychiatry 1984; 141: 1371–6.

58. Darko DF, McCutchan JA, Kripke DF, Gillin JC, Golshan S. Fatigue, sleep disturbance, disability, and indices of progression of HIV infection. Am J Psychiatry 1992; 149: 514–20.

59. National Commission on Sleep Disorders Research. Wake up America : a national sleep alert, vol 1. Executive Summary and Executive Report of National Commission of Sleep Disorders Research. Washington, DC: US Government Printing Office, 1993.

60. Léger D. The cost of sleep related accidents: a report for the National Commission of Sleep Disorders Research. Sleep 1994; 17: 84–93.

61. Stoller MK. Economic effects of insomnia. Clinical Therapeutics 1994; 16: 263–87.

62. Walsh JK, Engelhardt CL. The direct economic costs of insomnia in the United States for 1995. Sleep 1999; 22(Suppl 2): S386–S93.

63. Hatoum HT, Kong SX, Kania CM, Wong JM, Mendelson WB. Insomnia, health-related quality of life and healthcare resource consumption. A study of managed-care organisation enrolees. Pharmacoeconomics 1998; 6: 629–37.

64. Zammitt GK, Weiner J, Damato N, Sillup JP, McMillan CA. Quality of life in people with insomnia. Sleep 1999; 22: S379–85.

65. Schubert CR, Cruickshanks KJ, Dalton DS, Klein BE, Klein R, Nondahl DM. Prevalence of sleep problems and quality of life in an older population. Sleep 2002; 25: 889–93.

66. Idzikowski C. Impact of insomnia on health-related quality of life. Pharmacoeconomics 1996; 10(Suppl 1): 15–24.

67. Russel IT. The SF-36 health survey questionnaire: an outcome measure suitable for routine use in the NHS. Br Med J 1993; 306: 1440–4.

68. Goldenberg F, Hindmarch J, Joyce CRB, et al. Zopiclone, sleep and health related quality of life. Hum Psychopharmacol 1994; 9: 245–52.

69. Léger D, Janus C, Pellois A, Quera-Salva MA, Dreyfus JP. Sleep, morning alertness and quality of life in subjects treated with zopiclone and in good sleepers. Study comparing 167 patients and 381 good sleepers. Eur Psychiatry 1995; 10(Suppl 3): 99–102.

70. Baca E, Estivill E, Hernandez B, Lopez JS on behalf of Castivil group. Quality of life in insomnia: influence of zolpidem. J Sleep Res 2002; 11(Suppl 1): 10.

71. Quesnel C, Savard J, Simard S, Ivers H, Morin C. Efficacy of cognitive-behavioral therapy for insomnia in women treated for nonmetastatic breast cancer. J Consult Clin Psychol 2003; 71: 189–200.

72. Léger D, Scheuermaier K, Raffray T, et al. HD-16: a new quality of life instrument specifically designed for insomnia. Sleep Med 2005; 6: 191–8.

CHAPTER 12

Public health impact of insomnia and low-cost behavioral interventions

Meagan Daley, Simon Beaulieu-Bonneau and Charles M Morin

Insomnia is an important health problem that affects significant numbers of people and can have serious consequences.[1,2] While it is the most prevalent of sleep disorders, individuals often go undiagnosed and thus untreated for many years, often resorting to self-help remedies such as alcohol, over-the-counter medications, natural products and untested treatments in the interim, the effectiveness of which is dubious if not deleterious.[3] Chronic difficulties initiating and maintaining sleep are often associated with psychosocial and occupational impairments such as daytime fatigue, mood disturbances, performance impairments, and reduced quality of life, all of which are costly on a number of levels, both to the individuals as well as to society.[4–7] This chapter provides an overview of insomnia, with a focus on the public health and socioeconomic impact of the disorder and with a presentation of low-cost behavioral interventions available to patients.

DEFINITION OF INSOMNIA

Insomnia complaints are heterogeneous in nature, and involve reduced quality, duration, or efficiency of sleep. Patients may present difficulties in initiating sleep (sleep onset insomnia), staying asleep because of frequent or prolonged awakenings during the night, or waking up too early in the morning without being able to go back to sleep (sleep maintenance insomnia). The object of the complaint can also refer to non-restorative or poor quality sleep leading to daytime fatigue, loss of energy, distress, or social, occupational, or functional impairment. These different types of insomnia are not mutually exclusive as one patient may present simultaneously difficulties in initiating and maintaining sleep. Insomnia may be situational, as in periods of stressful life-events, episodic, with recurring periods of disturbed sleep, or persisting over months or years.[8,9]

Three major classification systems exist to aid in the diagnosis of insomnia: the *International Classification of Sleep Disorders*,[10] the *International Classification of Diseases-10*,[11] and the *Diagnostic and Statistical Manual of Mental Disorders-IV* (DSM-IV).[12] The emphasis on frequency, severity, and duration of symptoms varies according to the nosology used. (See Edinger[13] and Ohayon[14] for a discussion of the use of these classification systems.) Although insomnia may be a syndrome in itself, it is most commonly encountered as a symptom of a medical, psychiatric, or other sleep disorder. For example, it can be caused by pain, alcohol, or drug abuse, or be due to the use of certain medications (e.g., bronchodilators, beta-blockers, or antidepressants) or to the pathophysiology of numerous medical conditions (e.g., hyperthyroidism or fibromyalgia). Psychological and behavioral factors such as stress, hyperarousal, faulty beliefs about sleep, or poor sleep habits are often the mediating variables that contribute to the development and maintenance of insomnia.

PREVALENCE AND RISK FACTORS

Estimates of the prevalence of this disorder vary according to the operational definition used. For example, when symptoms such as difficulty falling asleep or maintaining sleep (either during the night or early in the morning) are considered, insomnia prevalence is estimated at around a third of the population. If other symptoms such as dissatisfaction with sleep quality/quantity or daytime consequences are considered, this figure is reduced by at least half. Strict application of DSM-IV criteria leads to the most conservative prevalence estimate of between 4.4% and 6.4%. Ohayon[14] provides a review of the epidemiology research and the definitions used.

Several demographic, psychosocial, and health variables have been associated with insomnia complaints. Surveys have consistently found higher rates of insomnia complaints among women,[14,15] older adults[16–19] and individuals who are unemployed, separated or widowed, living alone and/or homemakers.[1,18] While women appear to be about 1.5 times more likely to suffer from insomnia, it is unclear whether this rate reflects true differences or rather gender differences in reporting and/or sleep perception. A wide array of medical ailments is also associated with insomnia. These include respiratory, heart, and gastrointestinal difficulties,[20,21] asthma, arthritis, headaches, ulcers, and high blood pressure,[22] and early death.[23,24]

In addition, it would appear that insomnia breeds insomnia. A study of possible risk factors for insomnia revealed that, from among variables such as health problems, gender, obesity, snoring and socioeconomic status, the strongest predictor of insomnia was reports of insomnia in the period 10–12 years preceding evaluation.[15] In the Ford and Kamerow study,[1] 31% of individuals reporting insomnia at first interview reported continued insomnia at one-year follow-up. Family history has also been demonstrated to be a risk factor in several studies. For example, in a study by Bastien and Morin,[25] 26.6% of participants were found to have at least one relative with insomnia complaints. This familial relationship was the strongest for individuals reporting the following: sleep onset insomnia, primary insomnia, or early age of onset. Dauvilliers et al.[26] corroborated and extended this study by including a control group and by looking at first-degree relatives and their insomnia diagnoses. They found an even higher familial incidence – 73% for individuals with primary insomnia – with mothers being the family member most likely to have insomnia. The relative contribution of genetics and environment has yet to be elucidated.

Epidemiological, cross-sectional, and longitudinal evidence indicate a high rate of comorbidity between sleep disturbances and psychopathology (for review, see Morin and Ware[27] or Benca et al.[28] for a meta-analysis of sleep and psychiatric disorder research based on electroencephalographic readings). This is no surprise given that sleep disturbance is a diagnostic criterion or a clinical feature in several psychiatric disorders, particularly anxiety (e.g., generalized anxiety disorder) and affective disorders (e.g., major depression). In practice, it is not always easy to distinguish between primary insomnia and insomnia secondary to psychiatric disorder, a reality that is particularly problematic when attempting to estimate the costs of insomnia. Many authors have emphasized the importance of using standardized classification tools to clearly distinguish the two groups and facilitate appropriate treatment planning.

IMPACT OF INSOMNIA

The impact of insomnia on individuals and society can be felt on a number of levels, including decreased quality of life, difficulties with social and occupational functioning, and increased risk of developing psychological problems. Increased health care use, public safety concerns and economic costs are also issues associated with the disorder.

Quality of life

A number of studies describe the negative impact insomnia can have on health-related quality of life. In particular, several authors have used the Medical Outcomes Study Short Form Health Survey[29] (SF-36) and found significantly lower scores on measures of cognitive function and on multiple domains including social, emotional, and physical functioning in adult insomniacs as compared to controls.[7,30] Similar results have been found in elderly insomnia sufferers[31] and in managed-care organization enrollers.[32] Katz and McHorney[33] found that insomniacs with chronic illnesses had lower quality of life scores than good sleepers, even after controlling for anxiety, depression and medical illness. (See Léger et al.[34] for further discussion of quality of life in insomnia.)

Functional impairment

Insomnia can also have a serious impact on various aspects of daytime functioning, including work performance and accidents. One study estimates that individuals reporting poor sleep miss at least five more days of work per year than good sleepers.[35] Other preliminary descriptive studies also suggest that insomnia sufferers have higher absenteeism rates[36] as well as lower work productivity, satisfaction, and performance levels,[35,37] and reduced promotions and access to upper pay scale ranges.[38] Similarly, difficulties on the job such as problems concentrating, memory, effectiveness,

decision making, and on-the-job accidents are also more frequent in individuals with sleep problems.[35,39] Finally, in a cross-sectional investigation of 1308 workers that looked at the relationship among various job characteristics, health factors, insomnia and absenteeism, Leigh[40] found that, from among 37 independent variables studied, insomnia came second only to being a mother with small children as far as its predictive value for absences from work. Of course, one can also see the possibility of a close correlation between being the mother of small children and having insomnia.

Various dimensions of cognitive function (e.g., attention, memory, reaction time) have been demonstrated to be associated with poor sleep. These decrements can produce serious consequences when individuals are carrying out tasks that require optimal cognitive function, such as driving. Aldrich[41] found that automobile accidents occur 2.5 times more frequently in individuals with insomnia than in those without. In a large-scale epidemiological study by Balter & Uhlenhuth,[42] the prevalence of motor vehicle or other serious accidents was four times more frequent in individuals reporting untreated insomnia than normal controls and insomniacs treated with medication. Elsewhere, it has been demonstrated that experiencing an average of 16 nights of poor sleep per month puts people at a three times greater risk of an accident than if they do not experience sleep difficulties.[35] Study methodologies and results are heterogeneous and therefore this issue requires further investigation. In addition, interpreting results is often complicated by the fact that the largest proportions of accidents related to sleep disorders happen to people suffering from narcolepsy and sleep apnea. As a result, the impact of insomnia alone on accident rates is less clear.

Sleepiness and fatigue appear to be directly responsible for some of these accidents. Individuals with insomnia are more than twice as likely as good sleepers to report fatigue as having been a factor in their motor vehicle accident (5% vs. 2%[2]) and more than 50% of night workers acknowledge having fallen asleep on the job at least once. Sleepiness has also been implicated in several major industrial accidents (e.g., Chernobyl nuclear accident), all occurring in the middle of the night. Although these accidents are probably related more to sleep deprivation than insomnia *per se*, it does highlight the potential impact of lack of sleep on public health and safety.

Mental health

Results from prospective research indicate that insomnia is a risk factor for the development of depression, anxiety disorder, and psychiatric problems in general.[1,43–46] Riemann and Volderholzer[47] reviewed eight longitudinal epidemiological studies looking exclusively at the link between insomnia and its predictive value for depression. The authors state that 'almost unambiguously' the presence of insomnia at baseline predicted an increased risk of depression at one- to three-year follow-up. While no causal link has been established, Hall and Platt[48] found global or partial insomnia to be one of the predictors of a severe suicide attempt. Despite some weaknesses in methodologies, the link between insomnia and suicide attempts, seriousness of attempts, and suicide completions has been identified by others as well,[49,50,51] albeit predominantly in psychiatric patients. Finally, several studies have identified an association between insomnia and the presence or development of drug or alcohol abuse or dependence.[1,43,46] While occult factors such as comorbid psychiatric or physical illness may also explain this relationship, it should not be discounted before being further investigated, especially given the potentially devastating effects of drug and alcohol abuse on individuals, families and society.

Health care resource use

Several studies suggest that insomnia sufferers have poorer general health and use health care services more frequently than good sleepers, even after controlling for higher levels of mood, anxiety, and medical illnesses.[1,5] Research also suggests higher hospitalization rates in insomniacs. When it comes to consultations related to sleep difficulties, surveys suggest that between 5% and 36% of insomnia sufferers have consulted a physician specifically for these problems, while 27% to 55% have discussed sleep problems with a physician in the course of a consultation for another problem.[4,52,53] Another study found that 32% of survey respondents with insomnia syndrome had consulted a health care practitioner at some time in their life.[3]

People with insomnia often use prescription medications, alcohol, or over-the-counter (OTC) products such as Nytol, Sominex, Unisom, analgesics, and cough and cold remedies in an attempt to improve their sleep. The 1991 Gallup[2] survey revealed that 40% of Americans with insomnia had self-medicated with OTC products or alcohol, with 20% having taken a prescription medication to help them sleep. Ohayon and Caulet[54] proposed more conservative prescription trends, suggesting that between 2% and 10% of people with insomnia use prescribed medication for their sleep difficulties. Of course, the definition of insomnia can influence these figures. A recent population-based survey of 2001 Quebec residents revealed that 36% of respondents with insomnia syndrome had used natural products, 33% had used prescribed medications, 11% had used alcohol, and 8% had used OTC products in the previous year. Smaller proportions had used alternatives such as massage therapy (10%) and acupuncture (2%).[3]

Johnson et al.[55] looked at the length of time during which substances were taken and found that 9% of OTC product users, 15% of alcohol users and 36% of prescription medication users had used these substances for a period exceeding one month.[55] The fact that a full two-thirds of this same group reported having an insufficient understanding of available treatments makes self-medication a potentially worrisome phenomenon. This is made particularly salient if we consider one study's findings which revealed that individuals with occasional insomnia consume alcohol as a sleep aid an average of 3.6 times a week, and that individuals with chronic insomnia complaints do so 6.8 times per week.[4] Finally, the elderly population, already over-represented for insomnia, are also important consumers of sedative, hypnotic, and anxiolytic drugs[56] and may be at increased risk of suffering from effects related to drug interactions. Research using a sample of Canadian elderly people suggests that almost 50% of this population use some kind of sleep aid, with 50% of these cases involving the use of an OTC product and 17% involving the use of a prescription medication. More data on long-term substance use and abuse are necessary.

COST OF INSOMNIA

The prevalence of insomnia and the apparent chronicity and morbidity of this condition lead to the important question: What are the costs associated with this condition? In fact, little research has been conducted to address this question. Probably in partial response to shrinking budgets, demands of third-party payers and increased pressure for accountability and accessibility of treatments, estimates of the economic burden of certain physical and mental illnesses have been produced, along with estimates of the costs associated with treating them. While cost research in mental health has been slower to evolve than cost research in physical health, some data do exist. For example, Dupont et al.[57] report that the overall cost of all mental disorders in the USA is about $204.4 billion per year, with anxiety disorders among the most costly at $65 billion. Furthermore, the costs associated with some psychological disorders, such as depression, anxiety and schizophrenia, have received considerably more research attention than insomnia, as a quick Medline or PsychInfo search will demonstrate (see Rush,[58] Hofmann

and Barlow,[59] and Goldstein,[60] respectively, for reviews of this literature).

Authors typically make reference to two broad categories of costs: direct and indirect. Direct costs refer to the value of all goods, services and other resources consumed as a result of the application of an intervention, as well as any present and eventual side effects or consequences of the intervention. Examples are medications and other products, tests (e.g., x-rays, sleep lab monitoring), consultations, transportation to and from consultations, and overhead costs. Resource use is the important factor, regardless of whether or not money is actually exchanged. Indirect costs typically refer to an illness-induced reduced capacity to work or to participate in other activities, or to the economic losses associated with death resulting from a given illness. Absenteeism and productivity losses on the job are most typically considered in this category. Table 12.1 contains a breakdown of the various types of direct and indirect costs to be considered in cost analyses (see Drummond et al.,[61] Miller and Magruder,[62] and Petitti[63] for in-depth discussions of cost analysis terms and methodology).

Research findings

The first estimates of direct costs associated with insomnia were based on data assembled for the National Commission on Sleep Disorder Research in the USA and were estimated at about $15.4 billion for the year 1990. Walsh and Engelhardt[6] later undertook another cost analysis with the goal of evaluating costs for 1995. The results of that study provide the most recent direct cost estimates available for the USA, viz. $13.9 billion. A breakdown of this figure can be found in Table 12.2, alongside the data contributing to a more conservative estimate that was provided by Chilcott and Shapiro,[64] viz. $1.79 billion. In fact, most existing estimates are based on different modes of interpreting predominantly the same databases and sources. The exception to this is the only

Table 12.1 Types of direct and indirect costs to include in cost analyses of treated and untreated insomnia

Cost category	Types of acts to be counted and valued
Direct costs	• Consultations (e.g., physicians, psychologists, social workers, homeopathy, acupuncture, light therapy) • Hospital or sleep clinic services • Institutionalization (due to insomnia: overheads, utilities, equipment, tests, etc.) • Transportation and child care (consultation driven) • Prescription medications (benzodiazepines, antidepressants, anxiolytics) • Over-the-counter products (antihistamines, melatonin, valerian, herbal products) • Alcohol (taken as a sleep aid)
Indirect or related costs	• Absenteeism • Reduced productivity (work or other activities) • Motor vehicle and other accidents • Medical and psychiatric expenses resulting from illness or mortality associated with insomnia • Insomnia-related accident damage costs • Quality of life • Psychological symptoms (depression, anxiety) • Lost productivity costs due to illness-caused premature death

European study on the direct costs of insomnia. This study, conducted by Léger et al.,[65] used a number of published surveys to estimate costs associated with outpatient visits to health care practitioners, sleep recordings and treatment by sleep specialists, and products, be they prescription or not, for inducing sleep. They arrived at a figure of about 10 million French francs (or about US $2 billion). Léger et al.'s[65] data are provided in Table 12.2 alongside the data from the two other studies that will be discussed further here.

The Walsh and Engelhardt[6] findings represent the most recent example of the research and methods used to date. To facilitate comprehension of the figures, the data sources used in this study will be briefly described. Data regarding physician visits were obtained from unpublished registers of the 1994 National Ambulatory Medical Care Survey (NAMCS).[66] This is a national (USA) probability sample survey of office visits to non-federally employed physicians. Information on primary complaints, diagnoses, and medications prescribed are available. Visits to psychologists, social workers, sleep specialist centers, and homes of multiple occupancy (HMOs) were estimated using extrapolation methods described in detail in the original article. Nursing home estimates were based on data from other studies[67,68] citing the importance of the elderly patient's sleep disruption in the caregiver's decision to seek nursing home placement. Based on these studies, the authors estimated that 20.4% of nursing home admissions were due to elderly persons' sleep problems. Prescription medication costs

Table 12.2 Breakdown of direct costs related to insomnia in the USA and France

	Costs (US$ millions for first two columns, US$ for third)		
	Chilcott & Shapiro[64a]	*Walsh & Engelhardt*[6a]	*Léger, Levy & Paillard*[65b]
Substances			
Prescription	455.3	809.92	245 866 680 (hypnotics)
			43 666 666 (anxiolytics)
Non-prescription	84.0	325.80	64 724 040 (OTCs)
Alcohol	574.6	780.39	
Melatonin		50.00	
Sub total	1113.9	1966.11	310 590 000
Services			
Nursing homes	7.0	10900.00	
Psychiatrists	116.4		200 787 870
Physicians	317.0	660.00	1 149 555 555
Psychologists	39.1	122.40	2 746 870
Social workers		75.30	
Sleep specialists	8.4	18.20	
Mental health facilities	108.6	153.00	
Hospitals	77.5	30.80	
Occupational health			402 181 810
Sleep specialist investigations			1 409 091
Sub total	674.0	11 960.70	1 756 681 091
Total	1787.9	13 926.81	2 067 271 100

[a]The annual expenditure by the US population on various services for the treatment of or related to insomnia. Dollar amounts are US$ million/year estimated for the year 1995.[6,64] [b]Direct costs of insomnia in France (1995) converted from franc to US$.

were obtained from two major databases: (a) the Retail/Provider Perspective Audit, and (b) the National Disease and Therapeutic Index. The first database contains information regarding purchases of medications (e.g., by drug stores, hospitals, HMOs, etc.), while the second tracks prescription patterns in a random sample of participating physicians. Data regarding non-prescription sleep aids were obtained by consulting a firm called Information Resources

regarding utilization of pre-identified products. Finally, costs associated with alcohol use were calculated by combining data obtained from different sources[5,69] on the prevalence of using alcohol as a sleep aid and multiplying the estimated frequency (number of nights) by a cost of $1.50 per night of alcohol use.

Using these sources, Walsh and Engelhardt[6] estimated the total direct costs associated with insomnia in 1995 in the USA to be about

$13.9 billion. Substances used for insomnia accounted for $1.96 billion (prescription medications = $809 million; non-prescription medications = $325 million; alcohol = $780 million; and melatonin = $50 million). Health care services used for insomnia made up the remainder of the total at $11.96 billion. The greatest expenditures were for outpatient physician visits ($660 million), psychologist visits ($122 million), mental health organizations ($153 million) and nursing home admissions due to sleep difficulties ($10.9 billion). This last figure is contested by some as being too liberal; however, the literature suggests that between 62% and 70% of caregivers place elderly persons in nursing home facilities at least in part because of sleep problems, and that if it weren't for these difficulties many elderly persons would be kept at home.[67,68] While transportation costs for visits to and from appointments are typically considered as direct costs, to our knowledge, no estimates exist for insomnia-related transportation costs.

The indirect costs associated with insomnia (i.e., absenteeism, reduced productivity, accidents) have been given only passing mention in the literature, their conspicuous absence most likely being due to several factors: first, these costs are more difficult to estimate and quantify; second, there is no single, definitive database from which to draw; and third, measurement of these variables is subject to interpretation bias as well as well-documented distortions of memory. Nonetheless, Stoller[70] attempted to quantify work-related deficits by combining data obtained in a study of workplace performance in navy servicemen[38] with her own insomnia prevalence estimate of 33% and a performance decrement estimate of 4%. Her calculations placed the monetary value of absenteeism and lost productivity at US$41.1 billion annually (at 1995 value). A per person estimate was attempted by Chilcott and Shapiro,[64] who suggest a decrease in work productivity due to insomnia of 10%. This amounts to $3000 per insomnia sufferer per year.

Stoller[70] also looked at a number of other indirect costs; she placed the cost of insomnia-related accidents at between $26.42 billion and $38.43 billion annually (based on 1988 accident rate figures, a 0.33 insomnia prevalence rate and the assumption that accidents occur two to three times more frequently in insomniacs). Finally, she also estimated insomnia-related alcoholism at between $8.5 and $11.6 billion, insomnia-related depression at $1 billion and insomnia-related accidents at about $26.5 to $38.6 billion. Her overall estimate of indirect costs is thus situated between $77.05 and $92.13 billion, a figure that Walsh and Engelhardt[6] suggest is inflated. Indeed, this figure is difficult to fathom if one accepts Dupont et al.'s[57] estimate of $204 billion for the overall cost of mental disorders. In fact Walsh (as cited in Walsh and Engelhardt[6]) suggests a overall estimate revised downward of between $30 and $35 billion (i.e., direct and indirect costs combined). While Stoller's[70] work has been viewed as a liberal estimate because of the high prevalence rate used, her data are still frequently used to describe the indirect economic consequences of insomnia.

It is clear that more prospective studies are required to evaluate the economic burden of insomnia. Furthermore, the research described above is an example of what is referred to as cost-of-illness or burden-of-illness research. This type of research is conducted in order to identify costs associated with an untreated disorder during a given time period.[62] To our knowledge, no *cost-effectiveness* study of insomnia treatment has been conducted thus far. Preliminary analysis has been conducted to describe the costs of treating insomnia with the newer hypnotic drugs such as zaleplon, zolpidem, and zopiclone versus the costs of treating with benzodiazepines; however, the research reported does not allow cost-effectiveness conclusions to be drawn, given the lack of direct comparison across medications in an individual study and the lack of adequate outcome measures. (See the systematic review and economic evaluation by Dündar et al.[71])

Cost-effectiveness analysis (CEA) is the model most frequently used in mental health, as it does not require that outcome variables of interest (e.g., improvement in sleep/depression/global functioning) be expressed in monetary terms; original measurement units may be maintained (see Drummond et al.[61] and Hargreaves et al.[72] for more). The end goal in conducting CEA is to obtain a cost-effectiveness ratio that expresses the costs relative to the health benefits of an intervention of interest. This is done by calculating the difference in cost between two interventions, and dividing it by the difference in their effectiveness measured using the same outcome instrument. In fact, CEA is the logical follow-up to a burden-of-illness study and produces the type of data that is increasingly required (e.g., by insurance companies) to justify the use of one therapy modality over another (i.e., which therapy can offer the best results at the lowest cost?). It should also be the kind of data that *practitioners* seek out and weigh when making treatment recommendations. Note that many studies make reference to 'cost-effectiveness' of a given treatment for a given disorder, without providing any actual cost data to support this claim. Until actual data are available, assumptions will continue to be made based on common sense and logic. The following section will provide an overview of various behavioral interventions available for insomnia as well as a discussion as to their likely cost-effectiveness.

PSYCHOLOGICAL INTERVENTIONS

Despite the high prevalence and burden of insomnia, only a minority of individuals with sleep disturbances receive treatment. The first line of treatment usually involves self-medication with herbal/dietary supplements, OTC sleep aids, or alcohol, although the risks and benefits of these products are not well documented.[3,4,18,55,73] When professional help is sought, it is usually with a general practitioner

and a prescribed hypnotic medication is often the only proposed recommendation. Although sleep medications are efficacious for short-term use, their long-term use is associated with risks of adverse effects, tolerance, and dependence. In addition, there is very limited evidence of long-term efficacy. Psychological interventions represent the other main approach in the treatment of insomnia and will be discussed in the following section.

Relaxation

Relaxation techniques represent the most widely used non-pharmacologic treatments for insomnia. The rationale behind their use is that individuals with insomnia often present high levels of arousal, both during the day and at night. This arousal, which can be physiologic (e.g., muscular tension) or cognitive (e.g., intrusive thoughts), may prevent sleep from occurring. Relaxation techniques are used to reduce hyperarousal and facilitate sleep; some of them target physiologic arousal (e.g., progressive muscle relaxation, biofeedback), while others target cognitive arousal (e.g., meditation, yoga, imagery training). Progressive muscular relaxation and biofeedback have received more scientific attention. However, the use of biofeedback for insomnia seems to be declining, primarily because of the time and equipment required. Regardless of the method, regular training is necessary and professional guidance may be helpful for an adequate use of the chosen technique.

Stimulus control

Stimulus control,[74] which is based on the theory of operant conditioning, was first developed in the early 1970s by Bootzin. Individuals with insomnia are typically apprehensive about bedtime, yielding to the gradual development of an association between the bed, bedroom and bedtime, on the one hand, and frustration, arousal and wakefulness, on the other hand. Stimulus control is a set of behavioral procedures designed to reassociate temporal (bedtime) and environmental (bed, bedroom) cues with rapid sleep onset, and establish a steady sleep–wake circadian rhythm by adopting a regular sleep schedule. Standard instructions include: (1) go to bed only when sleepy; (2) use the bed and bedroom only for sleep and sexual activity; (3) leave the bedroom when unable to sleep within 15–20 minutes, engage in a calming activity but avoid falling asleep, and return to bed only when sleepy again (this procedure is to be repeated as often as necessary during the night); (4) arise at the same time every morning regardless of the number of hours slept the night before; and (5) avoid napping during the day. Strict observation of all of these procedures is indispensable to benefit from stimulus control therapy.

Restriction of time in bed

This behavioral intervention is often called *sleep restriction*, but the term *restriction of time in bed* is more appropriate. People with insomnia commonly increase their time spent in bed in an effort to obtain more sleep. However, this strategy may have the opposite effect, yielding to fragmented and poor sleep, therefore perpetuating insomnia. The standard restriction procedure consists of curtailing time spent in bed to the actual sleep time. The use of a sleep diary is essential for the application of the restriction of time in bed. The first step is to estimate the average sleep time per night, preferably based on sleep diary data collected for at least one week. Then, a sleep window, with fixed bedtime and arising time, is determined in which the person can sleep or attempt to sleep. The duration of the sleep window corresponds to the estimated average nightly sleep time and can be adjusted weekly on the basis of sleep efficiency (ratio of total sleep time over time spent in bed×100). Typical guidelines indicate that the sleep window can be increased by about 20 minutes if sleep efficiency

reaches 85%, and decreased by about 20 minutes if sleep efficiency is below 80%. Changes in the sleep window can be applied in the evening or morning, depending on individual considerations (e.g., working hours, preferences). During the first weeks of implementation, restriction of time in bed usually induces a mild state of sleep deprivation, promoting more consolidated and efficient sleep, but also causing daytime sleepiness. For this reason, the sleep window should never be of less than five hours. Moreover, the procedure should be used with caution for people who engage in risky activities, such as truck driving or construction working.

Cognitive therapy

Individuals with insomnia often entertain faulty beliefs and dysfunctional attitudes about sleep and insomnia. These cognitions contribute to perpetuate insomnia by interacting with emotional distress and inappropriate behaviors. The objective of cognitive therapy for insomnia is to identify faulty beliefs and dysfunctional attitudes and replace them with more adapted alternatives in order to break the self-fulfilling nature of the insomnia vicious circle.[9] More specifically, the preferred method is cognitive restructuring, which uses several clinical techniques (e.g., attention shifting, reattribution training, decatastrophizing), and is widely used for a variety of conditions (e.g., depression, anxiety disorders, chronic illnesses). For individuals with insomnia, targets of cognitive restructuring include: (1) misattribution and amplification of the consequences of insomnia (e.g., 'Insomnia will have a serious impact on my health'); (2) unrealistic expectations regarding sleep (e.g., 'I must get eight hours of sleep every night'); (3) misconceptions about the causes of insomnia (e.g., 'It is normal to have insomnia because I am getting older'); (4) faulty beliefs about sleep-promoting behaviors (e.g., 'Trying to sleep as hard as I can is the best method to fall asleep'); and

(5) performance anxiety, which arises because of unsuccessful efforts to control the process of sleep. Cognitive therapy can also be useful to help individuals with insomnia cope with relapses or residual sleep difficulties persisting after the discontinuation of treatment.

Paradoxical intention

Paradoxical intention can be conceptualized as a form of cognitive restructuring principally aimed at performance anxiety, which can prevent sleep from occurring. Paradoxical intention consists of persuading the individual to engage in the apprehended activity: remaining awake. This strategy should reduce performance anxiety and favor sleep. However, therapeutic gains following paradoxical intention are quite variable from individual to individual, and they are inferior to those obtained with other psychological treatments.

Sleep hygiene

The main objective of sleep hygiene education is to inform about lifestyle and environmental factors that may have an impact, either positive or negative, on sleep. These factors are rarely sufficient to cause insomnia but they can exacerbate existing sleep difficulties. When used alone, sleep hygiene has limited benefits, but it should be incorporated in a multifaceted treatment to target environmental factors. Sleep hygiene recommendations include: (1) avoid stimulants (e.g., caffeine, nicotine) several hours before bedtime; (2) do not drink alcohol too close to bedtime, since it leads to fragmented sleep and early morning awakenings; (3) avoid heavy meals too close to bedtime; (4) avoid exercising in the late evening since it may alter sleep onset; on the other hand, exercising in the late afternoon or early evening can be sleep promoting; and (5) maintain a calm, dark, and comfortable environment in the bedroom to make it sleep inducing.

Multifaceted cognitive behavior therapy

The behavioral and cognitive interventions described above are often combined to maximize the benefits. Studies evaluating multifaceted cognitive behavior therapy (CBT) have demonstrated that, compared to single interventions, they yield comparable but not consistently superior benefits. Optimal multifaceted CBT would include stimulus control and/or sleep restriction, combined with a relaxation and cognitive restructuring component.[75]

EMPIRICAL SUPPORT FOR PSYCHOLOGICAL INTERVENTIONS

Since their early development in the 1950s, non-pharmacologic interventions for insomnia have received considerable scientific attention. Indeed, more than 100 studies have been published in the last 25 years to evaluate the efficacy of such interventions.[76] A recent review by a task force of the American Academy of Sleep Medicine[10, 77] analyzed the results of 48 clinical trials, including a total of more than 2000 participants, and two meta-analyses.[78,79] Another meta-analysis was published later, which compared behavioral and pharmacologic treatment outcomes.[80] The main conclusions of these publications are that: (1) between 70% and 80% of participants benefit from psychological interventions; (2) these interventions yield durable and reliable benefits with minimal adverse effects; (3) the short-term outcomes are similar to those observed in pharmacologic studies; and (4) they may be more cost-effective than pharmacotherapy on a long-term basis.

The American Academy's[10] review also evaluated the existing psychological interventions according to the criteria proposed by a task force of division 12 of the American Psychological Association for empirically validated psychological treatments.[81,82] Three types of interventions meet the Association's criteria for empirically supported treatments (i.e., stimulus control, progressive muscle relaxation, paradoxical intention) and three others meet the criteria for probably efficacious treatments (i.e., sleep restriction, biofeedback, multifaceted CBT). Insomnia treatment has also been discussed at length in a book on evidence-based interventions: *A Guide to Treatments that Work*.[83] Stimulus control, restriction of time in bed, relaxation, and CBT were all identified as effective treatments, while the benefits of sleep hygiene and paradoxical intention were less clearly demonstrated. Finally, there is increasing evidence showing that CBT treatment is well accepted by patients and is often preferred over pharmacologic interventions.[84]

LOW-COST INTERVENTIONS

Although they are empirically supported, psychological treatments for insomnia are still relatively unknown and under-used by health care practitioners.[85] Important barriers to more widespread use include the lack of information and poor dissemination of such interventions, the time and effort required to implement behavioral changes, and their limited availability in the health care system.[85] Therefore, there is a need to validate more readily accessible and cost-effective interventions and to quantify their cost-effectiveness in monetary terms. Self-help, Internet-based, and group interventions represent alternatives to reduce costs and maximize benefits for a large number of individuals with insomnia. The literature about the empirical evidence for these three treatment formats is summarized below.

Self-help interventions

Self-help interventions for insomnia represent a promising cost-effective alternative or complement to traditional therapist-guided treatments. Several studies have evaluated a minimal intervention for insomnia.[86–94] All were conducted with individuals having primary insomnia, except the study by Currie and colleagues,[88] which evaluated cognitive-behavioral interventions in recovering alcoholics. All but three studies[87,89,93] included a no-treatment or waiting list control group; three studies included a comparison condition in which the treatment was therapist driven.[87,88,91] Except for one study, which used only progressive muscle relaxation,[89] all others evaluated multifaceted treatments. For most of them, the core components included (1) educational materials about sleep, insomnia, good sleep hygiene practices; (2) behavioral recommendations about sleep scheduling (i.e., stimulus control, restriction of time in bed); (3) relaxation; and (4) psychological methods for changing beliefs and attitudes about sleep (e.g., cognitive restructuring). Table 12.3 presents the methodological characteristics of the empirical studies on self-help psychological treatment for insomnia.

Overall, results from these self-help treatment studies show significant improvement in several sleep variables for treatment conditions compared to control groups, with changes well maintained at three[90,91] and six month[3,87] follow-ups. Bastien et al.[87] found that self-help treatment with weekly telephone consultations yielded improvements comparable to those obtained with therapist-guided individual or group treatment. This result is not entirely consistent with those reported in a meta-analysis suggesting that therapist-guided treatments yield better outcomes than self-help interventions.[78] Another study involving a community sample revealed that a minimal intervention can be effective in alleviating a broad range of insomnia symptoms, ranging from mild difficulties to a chronic insomnia syndrome.[3] Currie et al.[88] demonstrated that recovering alcoholics had improved sleep following self-help CBT, although this format had less impact than the individual therapist-guided condition. Research suggests that certain variables may moderate treatment outcome. For example, one study found that treatment response was greater

Table 12.3 Methodological characteristics of 10 empirical studies on self-help treatment for insomnia

Reference	Sample	Conditions and treatment content	Treatment media
Alperson & Biglan[86]	n=29 (17–80 years old)	– Self-help treatment (Rel, SC) – Self-help treatment (Rel, in-bed activities) – Waiting-list control	Treatment manual
Bastien et al.[87]	n=45 (>18 years old)	– Self-help treatment with telephone consultations (SC, RTB, CT, SH, Inf) – Individual therapist-guided treatment (idem) – Group therapist-guided treatment (idem)	Treatment booklets
Currie et al.[88]	n=60 recovering alcoholics (18–70 years old)	– Self-help treatment with telephone support (SC, RTB, Rel, CT, Inf) – Individual therapist-guided treatment (idem) – Waiting-list control	Treatment manual
Gustafson[89]	n=22 (mean, 42 years old)	– Self-help treatment (Rel)	Audiotapes and treatment booklet
Mimeault & Morin[90]	n=54 (18–54 years old)	– Self-help treatment (SC, RTB, CT, SH, Inf) – Self-help treatment with telephone consultations (idem) – Waiting-list control	Treatment booklets
Morawetz[91]	n=141 (23–60 years old)	– Self-help treatment (SC, Rel, Inf) – Individual therapist-guided treatment (idem) – Waiting-list control	Audiotape and treatment manual
Morin et al.[92]	n=192 (18–77 years old)	– Self-help treatment (SC, RTB, CT, SH, Inf) – No-treatment control	Treatment booklets
Oosterhuis & Klip[93]	n=325 (15–86 years old)	– Self-help treatment (SC, Rel, SH, Inf)	Television and radio clips, booklet and audiotape

(continued)

167

Table 12.3 (Continued)

Reference	Sample	Conditions and treatment content	Treatment media
Riedel et al.[94]	n = 100 (> 60 years old)	– Self-help treatment; one insomnia condition, one good sleepers control condition (RTB, Inf) – Self-help treatment with therapist guidance; one insomnia condition, one good sleepers control condition (idem) – Waiting-list control	Videotape and treatment pamphlet
Ström et al.[95]	n = 81 (> 18 years old)	– Self-help treatment (SC, RTB, Rel, CT, SH, Inf) – Waiting-list control	Internet treatment program

This table was adapted from Vallières, Ouellet & Morin.[96] CT = cognitive therapy; Inf = educational information; Rel = relaxation; RTB = restriction of time in bed; SC = stimulus control; SH = sleep hygiene.

for younger persons relative to older ones[86] and another suggested that hypnotic medication users did not benefit as much from self-help treatment as unmedicated patients.[91] It has also been shown that minimal therapist guidance may enhance sleep improvements when compared to self-help-only conditions.[90,94]

Despite these promising results, a word of caution is needed. In fact, self-help interventions may not be indicated or recommended for all individuals with insomnia. This could be particularly true for people with more severe insomnia symptomatology, with comorbid medical or psychological conditions, or for chronic hypnotic users. These subgroups of individuals with insomnia might benefit from a more structured intervention involving therapist guidance.

Internet interventions

Internet-based interventions represent another low-cost format. They are similar to other self-help modalities, but may be more practical and readily accessible for some people. One randomized controlled trial evaluated an Internet-based treatment for insomnia[95] (see Table 12.3 for methodological characteristics). Results showed significant improvements for sleep parameters in the treatment group. However, the control group also improved on several variables, and the dropout rate was high (24%). Therefore, research is still needed to evaluate the feasibility and efficacy of the Internet as a medium in the treatment of insomnia.

Group therapy

Group therapy represents another way to reduce insomnia treatment costs, since only one therapist is required for groups typically averaging from 5 to 10 individuals. The group format has been evaluated in an approximately equal number of clinical trials as the individual format.[3] According to the meta-analysis by Morin et al.[78] individual therapy yielded significantly better improvements than group therapy for number of

awakenings, but not for the three other sleep-dependent variables (i.e., sleep-onset latency, total wake time, total sleep time). Moreover, as mentioned earlier, one study comparing self-help, individual, and group formats found similar benefits for the three conditions.[87] However, to our knowledge, it is the only study with a direct comparison of individual and group interventions. A recently published trial, comparing a group CBT with a self-help information condition as a control group, assessed the impact of early intervention on long-term clinical improvement, two issues of importance when considering a cost-effectiveness perspective.[97] After a one-year follow-up, the CBT group intervention produced clinically significant improvements on sleep variables, as well as reductions in dysfunctional beliefs and attitudes about sleep, and negative daytime consequences. This study reflects the potential benefits of a group therapy format.

CONCLUSIONS AND RECOMMENDATIONS

Insomnia is a prevalent problem that is under-diagnosed and under-treated. It has serious repercussions on individuals, affecting their quality of life, daytime functioning, and health. The costs to individuals and to society as a whole are therefore substantial. As discussed earlier, the vast majority of individuals with sleep complaints do not consult for their problem.[1] In addition, a significant number of individuals resort to insomnia treatments that have not been validated, including alcohol and OTC substances.

Despite the promising results of cognitive and behavioral treatments for insomnia, research is still needed to validate optimal interventions and make them more widely available.[98] In particular, studies should focus on long-term clinical improvement because of the chronic nature of insomnia and the risk of relapse. In addition, samples should be more representative of the entire insomnia continuum. Indeed, selection criteria often limit the composition of samples to severe chronic primary insomnia sufferers, missing a large number of individuals experiencing sleep difficulties who could benefit from an intervention (e.g., those with secondary insomnia, taking sleep-promoting medication, or not fulfilling all the established diagnostic criteria for chronic insomnia). Factors moderating treatment response should also be investigated to provide guidelines as to which treatment content and format are more suitable for which type of patient. Furthermore, optimization of cost-effective treatments has to involve better and more widespread treatment dissemination. In order to achieve this goal, treatment implementation methods must be developed within the primary health care systems.

It is also time to increase efforts to collect the data that will provide more accurate and reliable figures of the economic ramifications of insomnia.[98] In 1997, an International Workshop on Sleep and Health that addressed research and clinical perspectives emphasized that there is a paucity of research into the cost of untreated insomnia and the degree to which treatment may reduce these costs.[99] This is true, despite the possibility that psychologists may be reluctant to quantify the impact of insomnia in monetary terms, as much for ethical as for methodological knowledge considerations.

The following suggestions are thus offered for future cost research. First, 'burden of illness' research should be undertaken with the aim of describing indirect and direct costs incurred by individuals with varying degrees of insomnia symptomatology. Ideally, longitudinal, population-based research should be conducted that collects data on all forms of health care system and product utilization. A clear and comprehensive cost checklist should be used, based on guidelines set down by Gold et al.[100] Use of such a checklist in future insomnia treatment cost assessments would permit direct cost-effectiveness comparisons across different insomnia treatment modalities and would

enhance reliability. Cost-effectiveness research would use this same checklist, but would apply it when comparing costs across intervention modalities at pre- and post-treatment.

Simultaneously gathering sociodemographic information and data on variables such as depression, anxiety, stress, and general health could ultimately contribute to a better understanding of the relative relationship of insomnia and a multitude of other variables to costs. This is important information to obtain for outreach, education, and prevention programs. A longitudinal, population-based approach would also permit researchers to address some of the cost-calculating obstacles encountered thus far, especially as pertains to indirect costs; information concerning the day-to-day impact of insomnia in the workplace and on psychological, psychosocial, and health variables could be obtained and individuals could in fact be questioned directly as to the role insomnia played in various outcome variables such as accidents and work absences. Finally, a longitudinal approach would also facilitate the partitioning of costs where comorbidity is present. For example, if it were found that insomnia is a precursor to depression, then costs associated with depression could be attributable, in part, to insomnia. This methodology could be combined with the use of relevant administrative databases (e.g., private and public health care insurance sources, workplace records of absences, hospital databases, etc.) in order to cross-validate certain self-report data.

Future research needs to shift its focus to the negative impact of insomnia and to how effective treatment can reduce morbidity.[98] Furthermore, the time has come to hone evaluation techniques and begin producing research that not just describes the cost of this disorder but offers empirically based cost-effectiveness data. This is essential if we want to not only respond to the demands of an increasingly market-driven health care system, but, most importantly, also want to offer patients the best treatments available at the lowest cost possible.

Acknowledgment

Preparation of this chapter was supported in part by grants from the National Institute of Mental Health (MH60413) and by the Canadian Institutes of Health Research (MT42504).

REFERENCES

1. Ford DE, Kamerow DB. Epidemiologic study of sleep disturbances and psychiatric disorders. An opportunity for prevention? J Am Med Assoc 1989; 262: 479–84.

2. Gallup Organization. Sleep in America. Princeton, NJ: The Gallup Organization, 1991.

3. Morin CM, LeBlanc M, Daley M et al. Epidemiology of insomnia: prevalence, self-help treatments, consultations, and determinants of help-seeking behaviors. Sleep Med 2006; 7: 123–30.

4. Ancoli-Israel S, Roth T. Characteristics of insomnia in the United States: results of the 1991 National Sleep Foundation Survey. Sleep 1999; 22(Suppl 2): S347–53.

5. Simon GE, VonKorff M. Prevalence, burden, and treatment of insomnia in primary care. Am J Psychiatry 1997; 154: 1417–23.

6. Walsh JK, Engelhardt CL. The direct economic costs of insomnia in the United States for 1995. Sleep 1999; 22(Suppl 2): S386–93.

7. Zammit GK, Weiner J, Damato N, Sillup GP, McMillan CA. Quality of life in people with insomnia. Sleep 1999; 22(Suppl 2): S379–85.

8. Edinger JD, Bonnet MH, Bootzin RR, et al. Derivation of research diagnostic criteria for insomnia: report of an American Academy of Sleep Medicine work group. Sleep 2004; 27: 1567–88.

9. Morin CM, Espie CA. Insomnia: A Clinical Guide to Assessment and Treatment. 1st edn. New York: Kluwer Academic/Plenum, 2003.

10. American Academy of Sleep Medicine. International Classification of Sleep Disorders: Diagnostic and Coding Manual, 2nd edn. Rochester, MN: The American Academy of Sleep Medicine, 2005.

11. World Health Organization. The ICD-10 Classification of Mental and Behavioral Disorders: Diagnostic Criteria for Research, 10th revision edn. Geneva: The World Health Organization, 1992.

12. American Psychiatric Association. Diagnostic and Statistical Manual of Mental Disorders, 4th edn, text revision. Washington, DC: American Psychiatric Association, 2000.

13. Edinger JD. Classifying insomnia in a clinically useful way. J Clin Psychiatry 2004; 65(Suppl 8): 36–43.

14. Ohayon MM. Epidemiology of insomnia: what we know and what we still need to learn. Sleep Med Rev 2002; 6: 97–111.

15. Klink ME, Quan SF, Kaltenborn WT, Lebowitz MD. Risk factors associated with complaints of insomnia in a general adult population. Influence of previous complaints of insomnia. Arch Intern Med 1992; 152: 1634–7.

16. Bliwise DL, King AC, Harris RB, Haskell WL. Prevalence of self-reported poor sleep in a healthy population aged 50–65. Soc Sci Med 1992; 34: 49–55.

17. Foley DJ, Monjan AA, Izmirlian G, Hays JC, Blazer DG. Incidence and remission of insomnia among elderly adults in a biracial cohort. Sleep 1999; 22(Suppl 2): S373–8.

18. Mellinger GD, Balter MB, Uhlenhuth EH. Insomnia and its treatment, prevalence and correlates. Arch Gen Psychiatry 1985; 42: 225–32.

19. Vitiello MV. Sleep disorders and aging: understanding the causes. J Gerontol A Biol Sci Med Sci 1997; 52: M189–91.

20. Katz DA, McHorney CA. Clinical correlates of insomnia in patients with chronic illness. Arch Intern Med 1998; 158: 1099–107.

21. Vollrath M, Wicki W, Angst J. The Zurich study. VIII. Insomnia: association with depression, anxiety, somatic syndromes, and course of insomnia. Eur Arch Psychiatry Neurol Sci 1989; 239: 113–24.

22. Lavie P. Sleep habits and sleep disturbances in industrial workers in Israel: main findings and some characteristics of workers complaining of excessive daytime sleepiness. Sleep 1981; 4: 147–58.

23. Shapiro CM, Dement WC. ABC of sleep disorders. Impact and epidemiology of sleep disorders. Br Med J 1993; 306: 1604–7.

24. Wingard DL, Berkman LF. Mortality risk associated with sleeping patterns among adults. Sleep 1993; 6: 102–7.

25. Bastien CH, Morin CM. Familial incidence of insomnia. J Sleep Res 2000; 9: 49–54.

26. Dauvilliers Y, Morin C, Cervena K, et al. Family studies in insomnia. J Psychosom Res 2005; 58: 271–8.

27. Morin CM, Ware JC. Sleep and psychopathology. App Prev Psychol 1996; 5: 211–24.

28. Benca RM, Obermeyer WH, Thisted RA, Gillin JC. Sleep and psychiatric disorders. A meta-analysis. Arch Gen Psychiatry 1992; 49: 651–68.

29. Ware JE, Snow KK, Kosinski M, Gandek B. SF-36 Health Survey Manual and Interpretation Guide. Boston, MA: The Health Institute, New England Medical Center, 1993.

30. Leger D, Scheuermaier K, Philip P, Paillard M, Guilleminault C. SF-36: evaluation of quality of life in severe and mild insomniacs compared with good sleepers. Psychosom Med 2001; 63: 49–55.

31. Schubert CR, Cruickshanks KJ, Dalton DS, et al. Prevalence of sleep problems and quality of life in an older population. Sleep 2002; 25: 889–93.

32. Hatoum HT, Kong SX, Kania CM, Wong JM, Mendelson WB. Insomnia, health-related quality of life and healthcare resource consumption. A study of managed-care organisation enrollees. Pharmacoeconomics 1998; 14: 629–37.

33. Katz DA, McHorney CA. The relationship between insomnia and health-related quality of life in patients with chronic illness. J Fam Pract 2002; 51: 229–35.

34. Leger D, Scheuermaier K, Raffray T, et al. HD-16: a new quality of life instrument specifically designed for insomnia. Sleep Med 2005; 6: 191–8.

35. Schweitzer PK, Engelhardt CL, Hilliker NA, Muehlbach MJ, Walsh JK. Consequences of reported poor sleep. J Sleep Res 1992; 21: 260.

36. Jacquinet-Salord MC, Lang T, Fouriaud C, Nicoulet I, Bingham A. Sleeping tablet consumption, self reported quality of sleep, and working conditions. Group of Occupational Physicians of APSAT. J Epidemiol Community Health 1993; 47: 64–8.

37. Kupperman M, Lubeck DP, Mazonson PD, et al. Sleep problems and their correlates in a working population. J Gen Intern Med 1995; 10: 25–32.

38. Johnson LC, Spinweber CL. Good and poor sleepers differ in Navy performance. Mil Med 1983; 148: 727–31.

39. Leger D, Guilleminault C, Bader G, Levy E, Paillard M. Medical and socio-professional impact of insomnia. Sleep 2002; 25: 625–29.

40. Leigh JP. Employee and job attributes as predictors of absenteeism in a national sample of workers: the importance of health and dangerous working conditions. Soc Sci Med 1991; 33: 127–37.

41. Aldrich MS. Automobile accidents in patients with sleep disorders. Sleep 1989; 12: 487–94.

42. Balter MB, Uhlenhuth EH. New epidemiologic findings about insomnia and its treatment. J Clin Psychiatry 1992; 53(Suppl 34–39): discussion 40–2.

43. Breslau N, Roth T, Rosenthal L, Andreski P. Sleep disturbance and psychiatric disorders: a longitudinal epidemiological study of young adults. Biol Psychiatry 1996; 39: 411–18.

44. Chang PP, Ford DE, Mead LA, Cooper-Patrick L, Klag MJ. Insomnia in young men and subsequent depression. The Johns Hopkins Precursors Study. Am J Epidemiol 1997; 146: 105–14.

45. Roberts RE, Shema SJ, Kaplan GA, Strawbridge WJ. Sleep complaints and depression in an aging cohort: a prospective perspective. Am J Psychiatry 2000; 157: 81–8.

46. Weissman MM, Greenwald S, Nino-Murcia G, Dement WC. The morbidity of insomnia uncomplicated by psychiatric disorders. Gen Hosp Psychiatry 1997; 19: 245–50.

47. Riemann D, Voderholzer U. Primary insomnia: a risk factor to develop depression? J Affect Disord 2003; 76; 255–59.

48. Hall RC, Platt DE. Suicide risk assessment: a review of risk factors for suicide in 100 patients who made severe suicide attempts. Evaluation of suicide risk in a time of managed care. Psychosomatics 1999; 40: 18–27.

49. Fawcett J, Scheftner WA, Fogg L, et al. Time-related predictors of suicide in major affective disorder. Am J Psychiatry 1990; 147: 1189–94.

50. Paffenbarger RS, Lee IM, Leung R. Physical activity and personal characteristics associated with depression and suicide in American college men. Acta Psychiatr Scand 1994; 89: 16–22.

51. Robbins DR, Alessi NE. Depressive symptoms and suicidal behavior in adolescents. Am J Psychiatry 1985; 142: 588–92.

52. Ohayon MM, Caulet M, Priest RG, Guilleminault C. DSM-IV and ICSD-90 insomnia symptoms and sleep dissatisfaction. Br J Psychiatry 1997; 171: 382–8.

53. Ohayon MM, Hong SC. Prevalence of insomnia and associated factors in South Korea. J Psychosom Res 2002; 53: 593–600.

54. Ohayon MM, Caulet M. Psychotropic medication and insomnia complaints in two epidemiological studies. Can J Psychiatry 1996; 41: 457–64.

55. Johnson EO, Roehrs T, Roth T, Breslau N. Epidemiology of alcohol and medication as aids to sleep in early adulthood. Sleep 1998; 21: 178–86.

56. Morgan K, Clarke D. Risk factors for late-life insomnia in a representative general practice sample. Br J Gen Pract 1997; 47: 166–9.

57. DuPont RL, DuPont CM, Rice DR. The economic costs of anxiety disorders. In: Stein DJ, Hollander E, eds. Textbook for Anxiety Disorders. Washington DC: American Psychiatric Press Inc., 2002.

58. Rush AJ. Psychotherapy for major mood disorders: from efficacy to effectiveness. In: Miller NE, Magruder KE, eds. Cost-effectiveness of Psychotherapy: A Guide for practioners, researchers, and policymakers. New York: Oxford University Press, 1999: 211–23.

59. Hofmann SG, Barlow DH. The costs of anxiety disorders: implications for psychosocial interventions. In: Miller NE, Magruder KM, eds. Cost-effectiveness of Psychotherapy: A Guide for Practioners, Researchers, and Policymakers. New york: Oxford University Press, 1999: 224–34.

60. Goldstein MJ. Psychosocial treatments for individuals with schizophrenia and related disorders. In: Miller NE, Magruder KM, eds. Cost-effectiveness of Psychotherapy: A Guide for Practitioners, Researchers, and Policymakers. New york: Oxford University Press, 1999: 325–47.

61. Drummond MF, O'Brien B, Stoddard GL, Torrance GW. Methods for the Economic Evaluation of Health Care Programmes, 2nd edn. New York: Oxford University Press, 1997.

62. Miller NE, Magruder KM. Cost-effectiveness of Psychotherapy: A Guide for Practitioners, Researchers, and Policymakers. New york: Oxford University Press, 1999.

63. Petitti DB. Meta-Analysis, Decision Analysis, and Cost-Effectiveness Analysis: Methods for Quantitative Synthesis in Medicine, 1st edn. New York: Oxford University Press, 2000.

64. Chilcott LA, Shapiro CM. The socioeconomic impact of insomnia. An overview. Pharmacoeconomics 1996; 10(Suppl 1): 1–14.

65. Leger D, Levy E, Paillard M. The direct costs of insomnia in France. Sleep 1999; 22(Suppl 2): S394–401.

66. Schappert SM. National Ambulatory Medical Care Survey: 1994 summary. Adv Data 1996; 10: 1–18.

67. Pollak CP, Perlick D. Sleep problems and institutionalization of the elderly. J Geriatr Psychiatry Neurol 1991; 4(4): 204–10.

68. Sanford JR. Tolerance of debility in elderly dependants by supporters at home: its significance for hospital practice. Br Med J 1975; 3(5981): 471–73.

69. Gallup Organization. Sleep in America. Princeton, NJ: The Gallup Organization, 1995.

70. Stoller MK. Economic effects of insomnia. Clin Ther 1994; 16: 873–897; discussion 854.

71. Dündar Y, Dodd S, Strobl J, et al. Comparative efficacy of newer hypnotic drugs for the short-term management of insomnia: a systematic review and meta-analysis. Hum Psychopharmacol: Clin Exp 2004; 19: 305–22.

72. Hargreaves WA, Shumway M, Hu TW, Cuffel B. Cost-Outcome Methods for Mental Health, 1st edn. San Diego, CA: Academic Press, 1998.

73. Roehrs T, Roth T. Sleep, sleepiness, and alcohol use. Alcohol Res Health 2001; 25: 101–9.

74. Bootzin RR, Epstein D, Wood JM. Stimulus control instructions. In: Hauri PJ, ed. Case Studies in Insomnia. New York: Plenum, 1991: 19–28.

75. Morin CM, Hauri PJ, Espie CA, Spielman AJ, Buysse DJ, Bootzin RR. Nonpharmacologic treatment of chronic insomnia. An American Academy of Sleep Medicine review. Sleep 1999; 22: 1134–56.

76. Edinger JD, Wohlgemuth WK. The significance and management of persistent primary insomnia: the past, present and future of behavioral insomnia therapies. Sleep Med Rev 1999; 3: 101–18.

77. Morin CM, Bootzin RR, Buysse DJ, et al. Psychological and behavioral treatment of insomnia: (In progress) update of the recent evidence (1998–2004). Sleep (in press)

78. Morin CM, Culbert JP, Schwartz SM. Nonpharmacological interventions for insomnia: a meta-analysis of treatment efficacy. Am J Psychiatry 1994; 151: 1172–80.

79. Murtagh DR, Greenwood KM. Identifying effective psychological treatments for insomnia: a meta-analysis. J Consul Clin Psychol 1995; 63: 79–89.

80. Smith MT, Perlis ML, Park A et al. Comparative meta-analysis of pharmacotherapy and behavior therapy for persistent insomnia. Am J Psychiatry 2002; 159: 5–11.

81. Chambless DL, Hollon SD. Defining empirically supported therapies. J Consult Clin Psychol 1998; 66: 7–18.

82. Chambless DL, Baker MJ, Baucom DH, et al. Update on empirically validated therapies. II. Clin Psychol 1998; 5: 3–16.

83. Nowell PD, Buysse DJ, Morin CM, Reynolds CF 3rd, Kupfer DJ. Effective treatments for selected sleep disorders. In: Nathan PE, Gorman JM, eds. A Guide to Treatments That Work. New York: Oxford University Press, 2002: 593–609.

84. Vincent N, Lionberg C. Treatment preference and patient satisfaction in chronic insomnia. Sleep 2001; 24: 411–17.

85. Baillargeon L, Demers M, Gregoire JP, Pepin M. Study on insomnia treatment by family physicians. Can Fam Physician 1996; 42: 426–32.

86. Alperson J, Biglan A. Self-administered treatment of sleep onset insomnia and the importance of age. Behav Ther 1979; 10: 347–56.

87. Bastien CH, Morin CM, Ouellet MC, Blais FC, Bouchard S. Cognitive-behavioral therapy for insomnia: comparison of individual therapy, group therapy, and telephone consultations. J Consult Clin Psychol 2004; 72: 653–59.

88. Currie SR, Clark S, Hodgins D, el-Guebaly N. Randomized controlled trial of brief cognitive-behavioral interventions for insomnia in recovering alcoholics. Addiction 2004; 99: 1121–32.

89. Gustafson R. Treating insomnia with a self-administered muscle relaxation training program: a follow-up. Psychol Rep 1992; 70: 124–6.

90. Mimeault V, Morin CM. Self-help treatment for insomnia: bibliotherapy with and without professional guidance. J Consult Clin Psychol 1999; 67: 511–19.

91. Morawetz D. Behavioral self-help treatment for insomnia: a controlled evaluation. Behav Ther 1989; 20: 365–79.

92. Morin CM, Beaulieu-Bonneau S, LeBlanc M, Savard J. Self-help treatment for insomnia: a randomized controlled trial. Sleep 2005; 28: 1319–27.

93. Oosterhuis A, Klip E. Behavior therapy without therapists: treating the complaint of insomnia. Int J Health Sci 1993; 4: 27–32.

94. Riedel BW, Lichstein KL, Dwyer WO. Sleep compression and sleep education for older insomniacs: self-help versus therapist guidance. Psychol Aging 1995; 10: 54–63.

95. Ström L, Pettersson R, Andersson G. Internet-based treatment for insomnia: a controlled evaluation. J Consult Clin Psychol 2004; 72: 113–20.

96. Vallières A, Ouellet MC, Morin CM. Self-help treatment for insomnia. In: Hersen M, Sledge W, eds. Encyclopedia of Psychotherapy vol 2. San Diego, CA: Academic Press, 2002: 607–13.

97. Jansson M, Linton SJ. Cognitive-behavioral group therapy as an early intervention for insomnia: a randomized controlled trial. J Occup Rehabil 2005; 15: 177–90.

98. National Institutes of Health. State-of-the-science conference statement. Manifestations and management of chronic insomnia in adults. 2005; Available from: http: //consensus.nih.gov/ta/026/InsomniaDraftStatement061505.pdf. [accessed 2005, July 21]

99. Roth T, Costa e Silva JA, Chase MH. Sleep and health: research and clinical perspectives. Sleep 2000; 23: 52–3.

100. Gold MR, Siegel JE, Russell LB, Weinstein MC, eds. Cost-Effectiveness in Health and Medicine. New York: Oxford University Press, 1996: 176–209.

CHAPTER 13

Economic impact of sleep loss, sleepiness, and sleep disorders

Kin M Yuen and Clete Kushida

Sleep disturbances and sleep loss are often viewed as normal aspects of everyday life. In a globally connected system, advanced technology allows for frequent communication, and thus, interruptions in our daily lives. Since the turn of the last century, the general population has progressively reduced the amount of nocturnal sleep by about 20%. The 2000 Sleep in America Omnibus Poll by the National Sleep Foundation (NSF) revealed that 33% of American adults surveyed slept only 6.5 hours or less nightly during the working week.[1] Of those surveyed, 24% had difficulty getting up for work on two or more days per week, 58% had difficulty making decisions and solving problems.

The 2004 NSF poll revealed that children in the USA are similarly impacted by insufficient sleep. Of the 1st to 5th graders, 24% of these children were reported to get 'less than enough sleep' by their parents or caregivers.[2] Children were also reported to consume caffeinated beverages. Twenty-six per cent of all parents/caregivers surveyed stated that their child drinks one or more caffeinated beverages daily. Of all older school-aged children, 33% drink one or more caffeinated beverages per day, with 8% drinking two or more daily. Twenty-eight per cent of younger school-aged children and

18% of preschoolers typically drink one or more caffeinated beverages per day (Figure 13.1). It is certainly disconcerting that children may be consuming caffeinated beverages as a counter-measure for the effects of insufficient night-time sleep.

What effects does sleep deprivation incur in society? What impact does chronic sleep loss produce economically? These key questions and others will be addressed in this chapter.

SLEEP LOSS

Sleep loss is typically the result of voluntary sleep deprivation due to work or family commitments, or due to intrinsic factors (e.g., sleep disorders) or extrinsic factors (e.g., environmental noise). Despite the fact that excessive daytime sleepiness (EDS) is the inevitable result of sleep loss, many Americans fail to recognize the effects of daytime sleepiness. In NSF's poll in 1997 6% of those surveyed considered daytime sleepiness a serious problem, and 14% stated their sleepiness was moderately serious. It is clear that the consequences of sleep loss are being minimized by the public, which leads to the question: *How much sleep does one actually need before untoward effects are seen?*

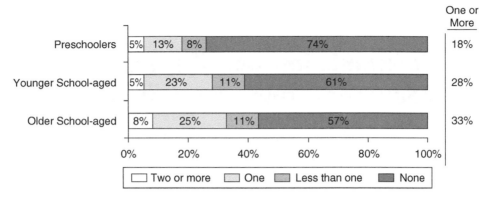

Figure 13.1 Children's caffeine consumption according to the 2004 Sleep in America Poll based on children of 3 years or older answering: preschoolers, $n=383$; younger school-aged; $n=383$; older school-aged, $n=252$. (Reproduced with permission of the National Sleep Foundation.[2])

Normal sleep

The adage of getting eight hours of sleep per night has been widely quoted as the optimal sleep duration, but total sleep time is highly dependent on age. Despite years of observations of the sleep of infants, children, and adults, only recently were normative data published for total sleep duration per 24 hours for these groups.[3,4] Using some of these recent data, it is now possible to estimate, for example, that a preschooler age 5 years who obtains 11 hours of nocturnal sleep is within the 50th percentile of his peers. (see Figure 13.2). Likewise, we are finally able to glimpse how different stages of life and gender may impact one's sleep. Recent studies show that women's menstrual cycle, state of pregnancy, and menopause all have potential adverse effects on their sleep.[5–13] Purportedly, although women have more preserved 'deep sleep' (stages 3 and 4 sleep), they are more likely to have subjective complaints about sleep in their 60s.[14–16] Nonetheless, both genders are likely to lose slow-wave sleep with age.[3]

Despite these population data, how do we know if we sleep enough? Most people who sleep 'enough' feel 'well rested' as they awaken from their sleep. There is no current standard to evaluate the degree of being 'well rested'. However, in other disciplines, such as sports medicine, for example, when athletes are not in peak performance, there are measurable parameters for correlation. Military operations have also developed performance measures to examine optimal effectiveness of their crew. In sleep medicine, we usually define what is not optimal or 'insufficient' as having daytime symptoms of sleepiness.

ASSESSMENT OF SLEEPINESS

Measurements for individuals

One helpful clinical tool is a sleep diary, which a person uses to estimate total amount of sleep on a daily, weekly, or monthly basis. By using a diary, the cumulative insufficient amount of sleep is seen as a possible explanation for daytime symptoms. These daytime symptoms may include excessive sleepiness, fatigue, irritability, moodiness, memory or concentration lapses, incoordination, or difficulty learning new tasks.[17] However, other more generalizable tools are needed to compare degrees of sleepiness.

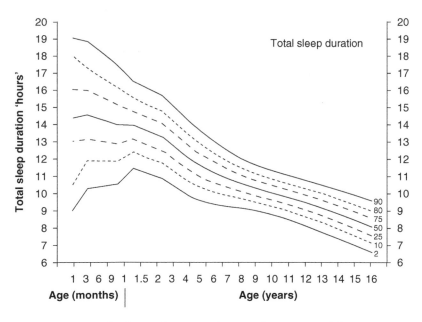

Figure 13.2 Normative total sleep duration from infancy to adolescence. (Adapted from Iglowstein et al.[4] and reproduced with permission.)

Instruments have been developed to capture individual differences and responses to sleepiness. Besides non-validated visual analog scales, the Stanford Sleepiness Scale (SSS) was among the earliest subjective instruments used to quantify sleepiness. The subject chooses one of seven descriptions of his/her current state, varying from 'feeling active' to 'almost in reverie'.[18] Similarly, the Karolinska Sleepiness Scale contains predominantly descriptions of sleepiness corresponding to a numeric scale of 1–9, where 1 = extremely alert and 9 = extremely sleepy.[19] A more widely used questionnaire is the Epworth Sleepiness Scale (ESS). The person rates the chance of dozing, from 0 to 3, under eight real-life circumstances. The higher the score, the more subjectively sleepy the person is. The maximum score is 24, minimum is 0, and a score above 10 is considered to indicate EDS.[20–33]

However, these subjective instruments have been criticized for lacking correlation with objective measures (e.g., multiple sleep latency test [MSLT]).[34,35] But a recent study based on factor analysis of the general population (sample size of 1562) revealed that there are gender differences in perceived daytime sleepiness and sleepy behavior in active or passive situations. The evaluations included self-reported sleepiness (13-item survey), ESS, sleep habits, SSS, and MSLT results from a subset of 145 subjects. Women are more likely to report feeling sleepy, but less likely to report falling asleep in either acceptable (such as watching television), or inappropriate (such as during conversation) circumstances.[36] Beside female gender, worse perceived sleepiness factor-based scores were also significantly related to younger age, higher sleep debt, and worse SSS scores. Conversely, male gender, older age, and worse MSLT scores were correlated with worse sleep propensity in both active and passive conditions. The authors suggested that self-reported, subjective daytime sleepiness and propensity to sleepy behavior are valid measures of different facets of sleepiness, and should be included in research.

Subsequently, more objective measures such as the multiple sleep latency test (MSLT) and maintenance of wakefulness test (MWT) were developed to quantify the degree of daytime sleepiness in individuals.[37–40] While the MSLT provides four or five standardized scheduled 'naps' of 20 minutes each to observe the average time it takes a person to fall asleep, the MWT tends to measure the ability of someone to stay awake in 20- or 40-minute naps. Cognitive and performance measures have also been instrumental in evaluating individual responses to sleep loss. Examples include psychomotor vigilance task (PVT),[41] driving performance (Steer Clear),[42,43] pupillometric alertness level test (ALT),[44–46] and other performance tasks such as those measuring serial reaction time, logical reasoning, serial subtraction, and multitask performance. These various tests have been used to measure lapses of concentration. Opinions differ among academicians as to how accurately these measures reflect the individual's degree of sleepiness. Additionally, actigraphy and polysomnography have been utilized to evaluate the amount and stages of the individual's sleep, respectively.

Other measures of sleepiness may be indirect, for example, the portion of caffeine one consumes to maintain wakefulness. Sanchez-Ortuno et al.[47] explored the association between sleep duration and daily caffeine intake in a 'French middle-aged working population'. The total sleep time and time in bed of employees of the National Electricity and Gas Company were analyzed against their daily caffeine consumption, and no significant relationship was found. Since caffeine is widely abused, with individuals having markedly different response to its effects and consuming non-standardized 'cup sizes', caffeine consumption is not often quantified for estimation of individual or societal sleepiness.

Other consequences of sleepiness from an individual's perspective generally impact social functioning. To the extent each person fails to meet social commitments such as not appearing for appointments, absences or tardiness for school/work, curtailing outdoor activities, and restricting driving, it is difficult to quantify except for absenteeism. Recent instruments have been developed to quantify the effects that specific diseases and disorders have on health-related quality of life. These scales have generally attempted to capture elements of physical, mental health, and aspects of social functioning. Examples are the generic scales, which include the medical short form (SF-36),[48–50] and the Functional Status Outcomes Questionnaire[51,52] which has been applied in patients with obstructive sleep apnea (OSA). Others are more disease specific, such as the Calgary Sleep Apnea Quality of Life Index for OSA.[53–55]

Irritability, depressive symptoms and anxiety are often reported by sleep-deprived individuals, and are measurable by depression and anxiety scales. One example is the Beck Depression Inventory,[56,57] which is a two-page, 21-item questionnaire that patients complete regarding their mood state over the previous week. The Hamilton Anxiety Scale,[58] a 14-item questionnaire, and Zung's Self-Rating Anxiety Scale,[59] a 20-item form, can be completed easily. Nonetheless, there are no normative data to define what is an 'acceptable' range for someone who is sleep deprived but not clinically depressed or anxious.

Measurements for population

On a larger scale, tools are available that measure the effects of sleep loss in economic terms. As alluded to previously, absenteeism has often been analyzed. Work-related accidents, traffic accidents, and shift work error rates are examples of quantifiable measures that capture elements of inattention, incoordination, and effects of mind-altering substances or all of these factors. The contribution of sleep loss in creating such errors and accidents has been estimated, and will be discussed below. Generally, when culpability may be in question, estimations tend to be biased to minimize blame in workplace or traffic accidents.

Major accidents such as the Exxon Valdez, Three Mile Island, and the Space Shuttle Challenger disasters have been reported to result from operator error because of sleep deprivation.[60] Daytime sleepiness is very common. In 1994, Ohayon et al.[61] estimated that 5.5% of the representative sample of 4972 subjects reported severe daytime sleepiness, and an additional 15.2% had moderate daytime sleepiness in Montreal, Quebec. The Australian study by Howard et al.[62] has estimated that the risk of motor vehicle accidents doubled for the sleepiest 5% of drivers (assessed by the ESS and Functional Outcomes of Sleep Questionnaire, odds ratio [OR]=1.91, p=0.02 and OR=2.23, p<0.01, respectively) and the risk of multiple accidents increased by 2.5 times (OR=2.67, p<0.01 and OR=2.39, p=0.01), after adjusting for established risk factors.[62] McConnell et al.[63] found similar results.

In 1999, the Council on Scientific Affairs of the American Medical Association[64] estimated that sleepiness was a causative factor in 1% to 3% of all US motor vehicle crashes: 'About 96% of sleep-related crashes involve passenger vehicle drivers and 3% involve drivers of large trucks'. The contributing risk factors included 'youth, shift work, alcohol and other drug use, over-the-counter and prescription medications, and sleep disorders'. Gander et al.[65] in New Zealand analyzed a sample of 5534 current drivers and found that besides younger age, higher average weekly driving hours, never/ rarely getting enough sleep (OR=1.26, 95% CI: 1.06–1.49), and self-report of any chance of dozing in a car while stopped in traffic (ESS question 8, OR=1.52, 95% CI: 1.15–2.02) were independent risk factors for motor vehicle accidents.

In a special report for the National Commission on Sleep Disorders Research (NCSDR) in 1994, Léger[66] estimated that the total cost of accidents in the USA attributable to sleepiness in 1988 was between $43.15 billion and $56.02 billion. The costs of *all* motor vehicle accidents ($70.2 billion), work-related accidents ($47.1 billion), home-based accidents ($17.4 billion) and public accidents ($10.9 billion) were $143.4 billion. Since motor vehicle accidents resulted in 49 000 deaths and 1 800 000 disabling injuries, Leger calculated a total cost of $70.2 billion. He used the 'human capital approach' to estimate potential earnings loss during disability, or lifetime earnings in a fatality, which was incorporated in the total cost. Medical expenses, insurance administration, and property damage from motor vehicle accidents were also included in the estimates.

Loss of productivity is another useful economic means to estimate the effects of sleep deprivation. In 1995, Kuppermann et al.[67] administered a cross-sectional survey at a San Francisco Bay Area telecommunications firm. Of 588 employees who worked for a minimum of six months, 30% reported currently experiencing sleep problems; they reported worse functioning and well-being in areas of general health, cognitive functioning, energy, more work-related problems (decreased job performance and lower satisfaction, increased absenteeism), and a greater likelihood of comorbid physical and mental health conditions than the respondents who did not have sleep problems. They also demonstrated a trend toward higher medical expenditures.

Similar results were discovered from 74 respondents in a randomly selected sample of 94 subjects in a Japanese study. Shimizu et al.[68] found that in one year ending in September 2000, sickness from cold symptoms and sleep loss was the most common reported cause of low productivity.

Furthermore, Philip et al.[69] also studied employees of the French National Gas and Electricity Board in a one-year period. Of 1105 participants, 6.7% reported severe subjective daytime somnolence of three days or more a week and 30% had at least one sickness-related absence. Importantly, there was a strong association between subjective daytime somnolence and sickness absence, which remained significant even after adjustment for potential confounding variables (age, sex, employment grade, sleep symptoms and self-reported diseases). For those that experienced EDS of ≥3 days per week, they had an OR of 2.2 (95% CI: 1.3–3.8) to incur absence as a result of sickness. Thus, sleepy workers had a higher rate of absenteeism, resulting in lower productivity.

Melamed and Oksenberg[70] had similar findings in an Israeli population among 532 non-shift daytime workers at eight industrial plants. Of the workers studied, 22.6% had EDS, which moreover was chronic: 96.3% had persistent daytime sleepiness for ≥2 years, and 56% for ≥10 years. The EDS was associated with doubling the risk (OR=2.23, 95% CI: 1.30–3.81) of sustaining a work injury, even after controlling for possible confounders, including factory category, job, and environmental conditions. However, it has been difficult to reliably estimate the monetary contribution from loss of productivity.

Health utilization is another means to measure the burden of under-diagnosis and the benefit of treatment for a particular disorder. Economic measures provide a framework for the discussion of alternative or competing resource allocation. Although the aforementioned studies alluded to increases in health utilization, few current studies were able to isolate portions incurred secondary to sleepiness from other causes versus those caused by sleep disorders. Thus, the section below will discuss further the published data of the economic impact of common sleep disorders.

ECONOMIC IMPACT OF COMMON SLEEP DISORDERS

The most common cause of EDS is sleep loss or deprivation. Hublin et al.[70] found in a survey that up to a third of adults experienced sleepiness due to partial sleep deprivation, and approximately 7% of the middle-aged adults have EDS secondary to sleep disorders. The Sleep Heart Health Study constitutes one of the largest ongoing populations ever examined. In 6440 participants of this study, Kapur et al.[71] demonstrated that there was an association between subjective complaints of daytime sleepiness, inadequate sleep time and insomnia, objective measures of sleep-disordered breathing, and an increase in an indirect measure of health care utilization via a modified chronic disease score (CDS). The CDS tabulated one year's pharmacy data based on the staff–homes of multiple occupancy (HMO) model at the Group Health Cooperative in Seattle, Washington State. The subjects with the highest quartile of EDS as measured by the ESS (>11) had an 11% increase in health utilization as compared to the lowest quartile. It is remarkable that subjects who did not have significant sleep-disordered breathing, but had feelings of sleepiness and fatigue, also demonstrated 18–20% higher health utilization. Thus, the role of sleep fragmentation or sleep loss in the socioeconomic impact from sleep disorders cannot be underestimated.

Obstructive sleep apnea

Obstructive sleep apnea (OSA) affects 4% of middle-aged men, and 2% of women aged 30–60 years.[72] The prevalence rate of asthma is similar.[73] Among minority groups, African-Americans, and the elderly, the prevalence rate is likely higher as obtained from recent literature.[60,74–78]

Prospective studies have well demonstrated an association between untreated moderate-to-severe levels of OSA and hypertension, congestive heart failure, arrhythmias, myocardial infarction, pulmonary hypertension, cor pulmonale, and stroke after adjusting for confounding factors such as obesity.[79–82] Recent literature also suggested an association between OSA and pre-eclampsia and observed adverse fetal outcome.[83–86] The increased health care costs have only been estimated for a small proportion of these consequences. Thus far, there has not been any systemic evaluation of economic impact resulting from the reduced concentration, memory, alertness, task performance or depressed mood associated with OSA.[87–90]

Although recent studies have confirmed the decrements in quality of life of patients suffering from mild-to-moderate OSA, with minor exceptions, health economic evaluations are yet to be performed based on such findings.[91,92] Admittedly, it is difficult to capture the monetary value of higher divorce rates and higher levels of irritability that were found in patients with OSA.[93,94]

Patients diagnosed with OSA were found to have a higher rate of traffic and occupational accidents.[95] Teran-Santos et al.[96] reported on 102 subjects who were long-haul truck drivers, in Burgos or Santander, Spain. Those with an AHI > 10 exhibited six times the odds (OR: 6.3) of having a car accident as compared to 152 case-matched controls after adjusting for alcohol consumption, body mass index, age, previous MVI, years of driving, use of sedative medications, visual acuity and sleep schedule.[96–99] Ulfberg et al.[100] found higher occupational accident rates among heavy snorers in Sweden. Of 704 consecutive patients studied, and 580 age-matched controls, male heavy snorers were twice as likely to have occupational accidents as compared to age-matched controls, whereas female heavy snorers had a threefold increase.

Similarly, health care utilization increases have been estimated for OSA patients. Costs are often separated into direct and indirect costs. Direct costs typically consist of hospitalization costs, physician fees, laboratory fees, and costs of medical treatments/medications. Direct non-medical costs can include costs of using transportation to and from the medical facility. Indirect/opportunity costs incurred with the death of a patient or while the individual is undergoing treatment are often expressed as days lost from work and reduced productivity. The so-called 'intangible costs' are the monetary values associated with pain and suffering.

Mostly, direct costs of health care utilizations of OSA patients have been reported. Indirect costs, productivity loss including sick days and costs of absenteeism, and costs of transportation have not yet been tabulated for OSA, though these have been reported in the few studies described above for sleepiness.

The National Commission on Sleep Disorders Research was the first to publish the estimated direct medical cost of sleep apnea at US $275 million in 1990.[101] More recently, direct medical cost analyses have been published by the group in Manitoba, Canada, and Puget Sound, Washington. Ronald et al.[102] analyzed the direct costs of physician claims and the number of hospital admissions for OSA patients in the Canadian Manitoba governmental health agency database. They found that of 181 patients (145 men, 36 women) with untreated OSA that were studied they had utilized health care at twice the rate of controls up to 10 years before diagnosis. The most significant increase in physician claims was noted up to three years before diagnosis. The total physician claims were $686 365 (Canadian) with a mean of $3792 per patient, whereas controls generated $356 376 with a mean of $1969 per patient. OSA patients had almost a twofold increase in hospitalizations compared with controls over the 10-year period: 1118 nights (6.2 per OSA patient), and 676 nights (3.7 per control patient). The total expenditure for the OSA patients exceeded their controls by $771 989 ($1 804 365 for OSA patients, and $1 032 376 for the controls) over 10 years prior to diagnosis.

The same group of investigators[103] subsequently reported that the annual physician claims of 344 male OSA patients and 1324 matched controls were significantly less at two years after diagnosis than the year before diagnosis: Canadian $174 (32.4 standard error [SE]) versus $260 (35.7 SE). There were 499 fewer physician contacts, and 151 fewer ordered medical tests (electrocardiogram, radiological evaluations, hypothyroid screen, and lipid tests). Hospital stays also decreased from 1.27

(0.25 SE) days per patient per year at one year before diagnosis to 0.54 (0.14 SE) days per patient per year. Of the 344 patients, 282 were 'adhering' to continuous positive airway pressure (CPAP) treatment, 62 were not. The treatment group's physician claims peaked at one year before diagnosis, and soon began to decline after diagnosis. The treatment group's hospital stays also decreased from 1.25 (0.28 SE) days per patient per year at one year before diagnosis to 0.53 (0.14 SE) days per patient per year. The health care utilization of the non-adherent group remained high throughout the five years before diagnosis, and 'this cost changed little over time'.

Kapur et al.[104] also found a twofold increase in direct medical costs of 238 consecutive cases of moderate-to-severe sleep-disordered breathing patients as compared to 476 controls matched for age, gender, and body mass index at the Group Health Cooperative (GHC)-HMO model of Puget Sound, Washington. The mean annual medical cost was $2720 for OSA cases prior to diagnosis, and $1384 for controls (1996 dollar value). The mean annual costs in OSA patients were higher than found in primary care patients with depressive and anxiety disorders ($2390) and much higher than primary care patients without depressive and anxiety disorders ($1397). The OSA patients were further stratified by CDS, and appeared to have a higher chronic disease burden compared to their controls one year before diagnosis. The medical costs were found to be directly related to the severity of OSA after adjusting for age, gender, and obesity. Therefore, beside obesity as a possible confounder in increasing health care utilization, OSA appeared to contribute independently to an increase in medical costs.

Based on a previous published report of under-diagnosis of moderate-to-severe OSA,[105] and epidemiological data of OSA prevalence in middle-aged adults, the authors estimated that $3.4 billion per year was attributable to untreated OSA.

Pediatric obstructive sleep apnea

Obstructive sleep apnea affects our children as well. In a special report generated by the Section on Pediatric Pulmonology, Subcommittee on Obstructive Sleep Apnea Syndrome after literature review from 1966–2000, Schechter[106] stated in *Pediatrics* that estimates of OSA prevalence in the pediatric population ranged from 0.7% to 10.3%. Among children with learning difficulties, some are affected by undiagnosed sleep disorders. The combined OR for neurobehavioral abnormalities in snoring children compared with controls is 2.93 (95% CI: 2.23–3.83). But despite case series that documented decreased somatic growth in children with OSA, right ventricular dysfunction and systemic hypertension, the risk of growth and cardiovascular problems could not be quantified from the published literature.

However, Gozal[107] was able to capture an improvement in academic performance in children suspected of OSA in 1998. Two hundred and ninety seven 1st graders who ranked on the bottom 10th percentile of academic performance, were screened with a questionnaire, a single night of pulse oximetry recording, and transcutaneous carbon dioxide level for suspected OSA. Of the fifty-four children, 18.1% were identified for intervention. The 24 children who underwent tonsillectomy and adenoidectomy showed improvements of their mean grades from 2.43 (0.17 SEM) to 2.87 (0.19 SEM) during the subsequent year. The 30 children in the control group whose parents elected no intervention showed no significant change in grades: 2.44 (0.13) to 2.46 (0.15). Again, though no monetary value can be attached, this demonstrated convincingly that treatment of pediatric OSA has positive effects that elude economic terms.

One study, nevertheless, was able to demonstrate an increase in health utilization in Israel.[108] Of 287 consecutive children with OSA, there was at least a twofold increase in utilization of health care services compared to 149 controls one year before diagnosis. The high-cost contributors were hospital days, medications, and emergency room visits. Patients with untreated OSA have many more sleepiness-related motor vehicle accidents as compared to a control group.

Health economic evaluations

For most health economic evaluations, which include cost–benefit, cost-effectiveness and cost–utility analyses, one begins by adopting a base-case scenario. The various perspectives used include individual, payer's, health system, or societal. Frequently, the human capital and willingness to pay approaches are helpful means to evaluate costs or benefits of interventions. The human capital approach estimates a person's lifetime earnings. For example, a life saved at age 55 years by an intervention equals 10 years of expected earnings gained. Similarly, a life lost through an intervention or inaction would generate the loss of the same earnings potential. The 'willingness to pay' approach asks a person to place a monetary value on his/her own life. An example is to estimate wage premiums to work in risky occupations.

Aside from estimations of accidents rate and the National Commission on Sleep Disorders Research report, these valuations of human life have not been widely used in sleep medicine. Critics often objected that patients' preferences for certain outcome of treatment have not been taken into consideration. Thus, in cost-effectiveness and cost–utility analyses, patient preferences are captured in 'utilities'. Perfect health is assigned a value of 1, and death a value of 0.

Early work by Tousignant et al.[109] in Quebec, Canada, in 1994 found that nasal CPAP treatment of 19 patients with moderate-to-severe OSA improved quality of life and was cost-effective. The mean utility before treatment was 0.63, and after treatment was 0.87. The annual treatment costs included CPAP supplies, rental and maintenance costs for CPAP devices, and one-night polysomnography for diagnosis. After treatment, they used Canadian life-expectancy tables, the change in utilities and life expectancy to calculate the gain in quality-adjusted life years (QALYs). Discounting costs at 5% to yield equivalent 'present-day dollars' in 1994, the cost per QALY gained was estimated at Canadian $3523 to $9809. After excluding three patients who positively skewed the results, the cost for incremental QALY rose to $18 737. Thus, the authors concluded that CPAP treatment was cost-effective. For comparison, the incremental cost per QALY saved for lung transplant recipients was estimated to be $176 817.[110]

Chervin et al.[111] performed a cost–utility study on three methods of diagnosing OSA using preference values obtained by Tousignant et al. or by introspection. A more recent study in Europe by Chakravorty et al.[112] found CPAP improved health status by 8 QALYs as compared to 4.7 QALYs in the lifestyle treatment group by using standard gamble. Utility increased from 0.32 to 0.55 with CPAP treatment, and from 0.31 to 0.35 only with lifestyle changes. Undoubtedly, future research into the health economic burden of under-diagnosis and cost-effectiveness of treatment of OSA is sorely needed.

Insomnia

Chronic insomnia is estimated to affect 10% (range 9–15%) of the population,[60] but between 30% and 50% of the general population are estimated to have insomnia of any duration or severity. Furthermore, the prevalence of insomnia symptoms 'generally increases with age, while the rates of sleep dissatisfaction and diagnoses have little variation with age'.[113]

In 1992, Balter and Uhlenhuth[114] reported that before treatment, insomniacs were more than four times as likely as controls to report a motor vehicle accident or other serious accidents within the past year. Léger et al.[115] found that workplace accidents were two to seven times more common among insomniacs than good sleepers, respectively.

The total direct costs for insomnia in the USA were estimated at between $10.9 and

15.4 billion in 1990 by Walsh and Engelhardt[117] and increased to $13.9 billion by 1995. The costs were separated into health care services and substances used for insomnia. Health care services included outpatient visits to physician, psychologist, social worker, sleep specialist, and mental health organization. Inpatient and nursing home care, when the primary reason for placement was the elders' sleep disturbances, were also included. Nursing home care was the major contributor to the total health care services cost of $13.9 billion in 1995. Substances used for insomnia included prescription medications, non-prescription medications, alcohol, and melatonin. Prescription medications and alcohol were the top contributors to the total costs of $1.9 billion. For indirect costs, Walsh and Engelhardt[116] estimated in 1990 that transportation to and from health care providers generated 10 million visits; the estimated additional expense was $20 million at a minimum average cost of $2.00 per visit.

Insomniacs often had increases in health utilization. Léger[117] cited work from Weyerer and Dilling in 1991,[118] who had reported that insomniacs had about twice as many outpatient physician visits as good sleepers (12.9 vs. 5.2) in one year. Insomniacs were also more likely to have been hospitalized compared with good sleepers (21.9% vs. 12.2%). Insomnia also generates a loss of productivity. In 1991, Leigh[119] surveyed 1308 workers in a cross-sectional study for workers employed for at least 20 hours weekly. The number of self-reported absences during the last 14 days were examined. The author analyzed 37 variables, and found that insomnia was the most predictive of absenteeism at work. Adults who were described as having seven or more nights of poor sleep per month missed 5.2 days of work per year more than persons who slept well in 1992. Stoller[120] estimated the loss of productivity to be $41.1 billion in 1998. Hopefully, more investigations into the various deleterious effects of insomnia will further clarify its health and economic consequences.

Circadian disorders

In 1991, Phillips et al.[68] reported the effects of shift work on police officers' work performance. After changing from rotating to permanent shifts, sleep quality and sleep hygiene improved, absentee hours decreased from 1400 hours for six months preceding the shift to 883 hours following this change. Drake et al.[121] also recently reported that shift workers had proportionally higher rates of medical morbidity and symptoms than their non-shift working peers. There were 360 people working rotating shifts, 174 people working nights, and 2036 working days. Individuals who met criteria for shift work sleep disorder had significantly higher rates of ulcers (OR = 4.18, 95% CI: 2.00–8.72), sleepiness-related accidents, absenteeism, depression, and missed family and social activities more frequently compared with those shift workers who did not meet these criteria. The authors further suggested the prevalence of shift work sleep disorder as being approximately 10% of the night and rotating shift work population. Obviously, future research will be helpful in confirming these provocative results.

From the Nurses' Health Study there have been suggestions that nurses who worked 15–30 years of shift work had a higher incidence of breast or colorectal cancer.[122,123] It is unclear if this relationship can be substantiated; further studies are ongoing.

Carskadon et al.[124] discussed adolescent sleep behavior in a presentation to the New York Academy of Science in 2004. They found that whereas certain aspects of the homeostatic system are unchanged from late childhood to young adulthood, there were changes in other features that permit later bedtimes in older adolescents through analysis of the circadian phase and period, melatonin secretory pattern, light sensitivity, and phase relationships. Apparently, this pattern was associated with increased risks for excessive sleepiness, difficulty with mood regulation, impaired academic performance, learning difficulties, school tardiness, absenteeism (from school), accidents and injuries.

Restless legs syndrome

Restless legs syndrome (RLS) is the subjective sensation of discomfort with an urge to move one's limb(s). Movement temporarily relieves the discomfort. Dr Ekbom first reported this syndrome in 1960 in association with iron deficiency anemia.[125] Despite its high prevalence in the general population and other often-cited comorbid conditions, currently there are no data to evaluate its economic impact.

Restless legs syndrome affects about 5–15% of the general population, about 11–20% of pregnant women,[126–128] 15–20% of uremic patients, and up to 30% of patients with rheumatoid arthritis.[129] Phillips et al.[130] found that 3% of participants aged 18 to 29, 10% of those aged 30 to 79, and 19% of those aged 80 or more were experiencing restless legs for five or more nights per month in 1996. The elderly population is proportionally affected; 10–35% of those over 65 years old are estimated to be affected by RLS.[131] In large kindreds, an autosomal dominant pattern of inheritance[129] and major susceptibility locus on chromosome 12q have been cited.[132]

Symptomatology has been reported, such as insomnia or fatigue;[133] 'reduced concentration and memory, decreased motivation and drive, and depression and anxiety', and poorer general and mental health have also been found.[130] However, its economic impact remains to be evaluated.

Periodic limb movement disorder

Similar to RLS, periodic limb movement disorder has gained recognition but has not yet been the subject of economic assessment. Periodic limb movement disorder 'is characterized by periodic episodes of repetitive and highly stereotyped limb movements that occur during sleep'.[126] It is reported to affect up to 34% of patients over age 60 years, and 1–15% of patients with insomnia.

Movements are associated with partial awakening or arousals. Patients with isolated periodic limb movements in sleep (PLMS) without RLS may be asymptomatic.

Most recently, Chervin et al.[134] found in 113 children aged 2–18 years that 26% had five or more PLMS per hour of sleep (PLMI ≥ 5). 'Restless legs, growing pains, sleep-maintenance insomnia, unrefreshing sleep, and morning headaches show moderate associations with polysomnographically-defined PLMS, but several other symptoms do not.' Future research will address whether PLMS contributes to the socioeconomic impact of sleep disruption in children and adults.

Narcolepsy

Narcolepsy is a rare neurological disorder with dramatic symptomatology. Prevalence of narcolepsy with cataplexy is one in 10 000 or 0.02% to 0.16% worldwide.[135] Patients typically present with complaints of excessive daytime sleepiness at an early age, before the onset of hypnogogic/hypnopompic hallucination, sleep paralysis, sleep attacks, or cataplexy. Furthermore, nocturnal sleep is also frequently fragmented. Of those patients that have experienced cataplexy – unexpected loss of muscle tone during wakefulness – driving can present a challenge. There are limited data linking motor vehicle accidents related to cataplexy or sleep attacks caused by narcolepsy before treatment.

The National Commission on Sleep Disorders Research published an estimated direct medical cost of narcolepsy as a minimum of $64.1 million in 1990.[101] An earlier study reported that over 75% of 180 narcoleptic individuals in Canada as compared to age- and sex-matched controls had occupational problems.[136] The narcolepsy group had statistically significant lower job performance, fewer promotions, lower earning capacity, more fear of, or having more actual, job loss, and had higher disability insurance as compared with controls. Sixty-six per cent of the narcoleptic patients fell asleep at the wheel, 67% had near or actual motor vehicle accidents caused by drowsiness or falling asleep at the wheel, 29% experienced cataplexy while driving, and 12% had sleep paralysis while driving. Sleepiness or sleep-induced work or home accidents, and smoking-related accidents were found in 49% of narcoleptics. In 1984, Broughton et al.[137] compared 60 patients with narcolepsy with cataplexy, against 60 patients with temporal lobe seizure or primary generalized epilepsy, but without major organic pathology, and another 60 age- and sex-matched controls. The authors discovered that narcoleptic patients had 'poorer driving records, higher accident rates from smoking, and greater problems in planning recreation' than patients with epilepsy. The continuous excessive daytime sleepiness that persisted between 'attacks' was noted to be the major contributor to psychosocial problems in narcoleptic patients, whereas epileptic patients were more 'alert' between seizures.

Findley et al.[43] compared 10 patients with narcolepsy before treatment against 10 age- and sex-matched volunteers using the Steer Clear™ system – a 30-minute computer program simulating monotonous highway driving conditions with 780 obstacles. Narcoleptic patients, similarly to untreated sleep apneic patients, had a statistically significant poorer performance as compared to controls. More recently, Leon-Munoz et al.[138] in Spain studied 35 patients diagnosed as having narcolepsy with cataplexy between 1994 and 1998, and found that the narcoleptic group had a significantly higher number of accidents compared with 25 normal controls. Because of the fear of losing their driver's license, some patients have chosen not to seek help, thus further compounding the risks to the individual and the public's safety.

Prior to the use of wakefulness-promoting agents, and in some pediatric patients, the maintenance of wakefulness was dependent on stimulant medications and antidepressants. The safety of such medications during reproductive years and the risk of driving accidents without taking them were left up to the recommendations and discussion between the prescribing practitioner and the patient. Irritability, anxiety, and erectile or ejaculatory dysfunction have been reported with these medications.[139] The costs of the new wakefulness-promoting agents – modafinil and gamma-hydroxybutyrate – despite partial medical insurance coverage, remain prohibitive to some patients and their families. Ideally, studies into this aspect of direct medical costs will elucidate one aspect of narcolepsy's economic impact.

CONCLUSIONS

Living in a fast-paced society imposes a high cost. Sleepiness induced by voluntary sleep loss has contributed greatly to the number of traffic and industrial accidents. The loss of life and decreased work productivity have created a large price tag. We begin to glimpse its 'trickling-down' effects among children by their use of caffeinated beverages, and through reports of insufficient night-time sleep by the parents/caregivers.

Moreover, various sleep disorders further disrupt nocturnal sleep. The aging of those born during baby booms will undoubtedly increase the propensity for insomnia, while the rate of obesity in adults and children will contribute to the prevalence of OSA. The degree of socioeconomic impact that RLS or PLMS may have remains to be seen, but these disorders certainly have created difficulties in cognitive function and behavioral issues for the adults and children affected, respectively. With the trend towards more insufficient sleep, society needs more education to comprehend the great burden that sleep loss carries, not merely deflecting its temporary effects with caffeine or other countermeasures.

REFERENCES

1. National Sleep Foundation. Sleep in America Poll. Washington, DC: NSF, 2000–2003.

2. National Sleep Foundation. Sleep in America Poll. Washington, DC: NSF, 2004.
3. Ohayon MM, Carskadon MA, Guilleminault C, Vitiello MV. Meta-analysis of quantitative sleep parameters from childhood to old age in healthy individuals: developing normative sleep values across the human lifespan. Sleep 2004; 27(7): 1255–73.
4. Iglowstein I, Jenni OG, Molinari L, Largo RH. Sleep duration from infancy to adolescence: reference values and generational trends. Pediatrics 2003; 111(2): 302–7.
5. Casey P, Huntsdale C, Angus G, Janes C. Memory in pregnancy. II: Implicit, incidental, explicit, semantic, short-term, working and prospective memory in primigravid, multigravid and postpartum women. J Psychosom Obstet Gynaecol 1999; 20(3): 158–64.
6. Dzaja A, Arber S, Hislop J, et al. Women's sleep in health and disease. J Psychiatr Res 2005; 39(1): 55–76.
7. Lee KA. Sleep and fatigue. Annu Rev Nurs Res 2001; 19: 249–73.
8. Lee KA, Gay CL. Sleep in late pregnancy predicts length of labor and type of delivery. Am J Obstet Gynecol 2004; 191(6): 2041–6.
9. Waters MA, Lee KA. Differences between primigravidae and multigravidae mothers in sleep disturbances, fatigue, and functional status. J Nurse Midwifery 1996; 41(5): 364–7.
10. Manber R, Armitage R. Sex, steroids, and sleep: a review. Sleep 1999; 22(5): 540–55.
11. Manber R, Kuo TF, Cataldo N, Colrain IM. The effects of hormone replacement therapy on sleep-disordered breathing in postmenopausal women: a pilot study. Sleep 2003; 26(2): 163–8.
12. Manconi M, Ferini-Strambi L. Restless legs syndrome among pregnant women. Sleep 2004; 27(2): 350.
13. Driver HS, Shapiro CM. A longitudinal study of sleep stages in young women during pregnancy and postpartum. Sleep 1992; 15(5): 449–53.
14. Reynolds CF, 3rd, Kupfer DJ, Taska LS, et al. Sleep of healthy seniors: a revisit. Sleep 1985; 8(1): 20–9.
15. Reynolds CF, 3rd, Monk TH, Hoch CC, et al. Electroencephalographic sleep in the healthy 'old old': a comparison with the 'young old' in visually scored and automated measures. J Gerontol 1991; 46(2): M39–46.
16. Redline S, Kirchner HL, Quan SF, et al. The effects of age, sex, ethnicity, and sleep-disordered breathing on sleep architecture. Arch Intern Med 2004; 164(4): 406–18.
17. Bonnet MH. Acute sleep deprivation. In: Kryger M, Roth, T, Dement W, eds. Principles and Practice of Sleep Medicine. 4th edn. Philadelphia, PA: Elsevier/Saunders, 2005; 51–66.
18. Hoddes E, Zarcone V, Smythe H, Phillips R, Dement WC. Quantification of sleepiness: a new approach. Psychophysiology 1973; 10(4): 431–6.
19. Akerstedt T, Gillberg M. Subjective and objective sleepiness in the active individual. Int J Neurosci 1990; 52(1–2): 29–37.
20. Melendres MC, Lutz JM, Rubin ED, Marcus CL. Daytime sleepiness and hyperactivity in children with suspected sleep-disordered breathing. Pediatrics 2004; 114(3): 768–75.
21. Johns M. Rethinking the assessment of sleepiness. Sleep Med Rev 1998; 2(1): 3–15.
22. Punjabi NM, Bandeen-Roche K, Young T. Predictors of objective sleep tendency in the general population. Sleep 2003; 26(6): 678–83.
23. Chen NH, Johns MW, Li HY, et al. Validation of a Chinese version of the Epworth sleepiness scale. Qual Life Res 2002; 11(8): 817–21.
24. Johns MW. Sleep propensity varies with behaviour and the situation in which it is measured: the concept of somnificity. J Sleep Res 2002; 11(1): 61–7.
25. Johns MW. Reply. J Sleep Res 2000; 9(4): 400–1.
26. Johns MW. Sensitivity and specificity of the multiple sleep latency test (MSLT), the maintenance of wakefulness test and the Epworth sleepiness scale: failure of the MSLT as a gold standard. J Sleep Res 2000; 9(1): 5–11.
27. Johns M, Hocking B. Daytime sleepiness and sleep habits of Australian workers. Sleep 1997; 20(10): 844–9.
28. Johns MW. Sleepiness in different situations measured by the Epworth Sleepiness Scale. Sleep 1994; 17(8): 703–10.
29. Johns M. Understanding insomnia. Aust Fam Physician 1993; 22(3): 318–24, 28.
30. Johns MW. Daytime sleepiness, snoring, and obstructive sleep apnea. The Epworth Sleepiness Scale. Chest 1993; 103(1): 30–6.
31. Johns MW. Reliability and factor analysis of the Epworth Sleepiness Scale. Sleep 1992; 15(4): 376–81.
32. Johns MW. A new method for measuring daytime sleepiness: the Epworth sleepiness scale. Sleep 1991; 14(6): 540–5.

33. Johns MW. Polysomnography at a sleep disorders unit in Melbourne. Med J Aust 1991; 155(5): 303–8.

34. Chervin RD, Aldrich MS. The Epworth Sleepiness Scale may not reflect objective measures of sleepiness or sleep apnea. Neurology 1999; 52(1): 125–31.

35. Chervin RD, Aldrich MS, Pickett R, Guilleminault C. Comparison of the results of the Epworth Sleepiness Scale and the Multiple Sleep Latency Test. J Psychosom Res 1997; 42(2): 145–55.

36. Kim H, Young, T. Subjective daytime sleepiness: dimensions and correlates in the general population. Sleep 2005; 28(5): 625–34.

37. Carskadon MA, Dement WC, Mitler MM, et al. Guidelines for the multiple sleep latency test (MSLT): a standard measure of sleepiness. Sleep 1986; 9(4): 519–24.

38. Banks S, Barnes M, Tarquinio N, et al. The maintenance of wakefulness test in normal healthy subjects. Sleep 2004; 27(4): 799–802.

39. Doghramji K, Mitler MM, Sangal RB, et al. A normative study of the maintenance of wakefulness test (MWT). Electroencephalogr Clin Neurophysiol 1997; 103(5): 554–62.

40. Littner MR, Kushida C, Wise M, et al. Practice parameters for clinical use of the multiple sleep latency test and the maintenance of wakefulness test. Sleep 2005; 28(1): 113–21.

41. Dinges DF, Pack F, Williams K, et al. Cumulative sleepiness, mood disturbance, and psychomotor vigilance performance decrements during a week of sleep restricted to 4–5 hours per night. Sleep 1997; 20(4): 267–7.

42. Findley LJ, Suratt PM, Dinges DF. Time-on-task decrements in 'steer clear' performance of patients with sleep apnea and narcolepsy. Sleep 1999; 22(6): 804–9.

43. Findley L, Unverzagt M, Guchu R, Fabrizio M, Buckner J, Suratt P. Vigilance and automobile accidents in patients with sleep apnea or narcolepsy. Chest 1995; 108(3): 619–24.

44. Merritt SL, Schnyders HC, Patel M, Basner RC, O'Neill W. Pupil staging and EEG measurement of sleepiness. Int J Psychophysiol 2004; 52(1): 97–112.

45. McLaren JW, Hauri PJ, Lin SC, Harris CD. Pupillometry in clinically sleepy patients. Sleep Med 2002; 3(4): 347–52.

46. Kraemer S, Danker-Hopfe H, Dorn H, et al. Time-of-day variations of indicators of attention: performance, physiologic parameters, and self-assessment of sleepiness. Biol Psychiatry 2000; 48(11): 1069–80.

47. Sanchez-Ortuno M, Moore, N, Taillard J, et al. Sleep duration and caffeine consumption in a French middle-aged working population. Sleep Med 2005; 6(3): 247–51.

48. Ware JE, Kosinski M. Interpreting SF–36 summary health measures: a response. Qual Life Res 2001; 10(5): 405–13; discussion 15–20.

49. Ware JE, Jr, Gandek B. Overview of the SF–36 Health Survey and the International Quality of Life Assessment (IQOLA) Project. J Clin Epidemiol 1998; 51(11): 903–12.

50. Ware JE, Jr, Keller SD, Gandek B, Brazier JE, Sullivan M. Evaluating translations of health status questionnaires. Methods from the IQOLA project. International Quality of Life Assessment. Int J Technol Assess Health Care 1995; 11(3): 525–51.

51. Weaver TE, Laizner AM, Evans LK, et al. An instrument to measure functional status outcomes for disorders of excessive sleepiness. Sleep 1997; 20(10): 835–43.

52. Weaver TE. Outcome measurement in sleep medicine practice and research. Part 1: assessment of symptoms, subjective and objective daytime sleepiness, health-related quality of life and functional status. Sleep Med Rev 2001; 5(2): 103–28.

53. Flemons WW, Reimer MA. Measurement properties of the Calgary sleep apnea quality of life index. Am J Respir Crit Care Med 2002; 165(2): 159–64.

54. Flemons WW, Reimer MA. Development of a disease-specific health-related quality of life questionnaire for sleep apnea. Am J Respir Crit Care Med 1998; 158(2): 494–503.

55. Flemons WW. Measuring health related quality of life in sleep apnea. Sleep 2000; 23(Suppl 4): S109–14.

56. Salkind MR. Beck depression inventory in general practice. J R Coll Gen Pract 1969; 18(88): 267–71.

57. Mathew RJ, Swihart AA, Weinman ML. Vegetative symptoms in anxiety and depression. Br J Psychiatry 1982; 141: 162–5.

58. Hamilton M. Development of a rating scale for primary depressive illness. Br J Soc Clin Psychol 1967; 6(4): 278–96.

59. Zung W. A rating instrument for anxiety disorders. Psychosomatics 1971; 12: 371–9.

60. Kryger M, Roth T, Dement W, eds. Principles and Practice of Sleep Medicine, 3rd edn. Philadelphia PA: WB Saunders, 2000.

61. Ohayon MM, Caulet M, Philip P, Guilleminault C, Priest RG. How sleep and mental disorders are related to complaints of daytime sleepiness. Arch Intern Med 1997; 157(22): 2645–52.

62. Howard ME, Desai AV, Grunstein RR, et al. Sleepiness, sleep-disordered breathing, and accident risk factors in commercial vehicle drivers. Am J Respir Crit Care Med 2004; 170(9): 1014–21.

63. McConnell CF, Bretz KM, Dwyer WO. Falling asleep at the wheel: a close look at 1269 fatal and serious injury-producing crashes. Behav Sleep Med 2003; 1(3): 171–83.

64. Lyznicki JM, Doege TC, Davis RM, Williams MA. Sleepiness, driving, and motor vehicle crashes. Council on Scientific Affairs, American Medical Association. JAMA 1998; 279(23): 1908–13.

65. Gander PH, Marshall NS, Harris RB, Reid P. Sleep, sleepiness and motor vehicle accidents: a national survey. Aust N Z J Public Health 2005; 29(1): 16–21.

66. Léger D. The cost of sleep related accidents: a report for the National Commission of Sleep Disorders Research. Sleep 1994; 17: 84–93.

67. Kuppermann M, Lubeck DP, Mazonson PD, et al. Sleep problems and their correlates in a working population. J Gen Intern Med 1995; 10(1): 25–32.

68. Shimizu T, Horie S, Nagata S, Marui E. Relationship between self-reported low productivity and overtime working. Occup Med (Lond) 2004; 54(1): 52–4.

69. Phillips B, Magan L, Gerhardstein C, Cecil B. Shift work, sleep quality, and worker health: a study of police officers. South Med J 1991; 84(10): 1176–84, 96.

70. Melamed S, Oksenberg A. Excessive daytime sleepiness and risk of occupational injuries in non-shift daytime workers. Sleep 2002; 25(3): 315–22.

71. Hublin C, Kaprio J, Partinen M, Koskenvuo M. Insufficient sleep – a population-based study in adults. Sleep 2001; 24(4): 392–400.

72. Kapur VK, Redline S, Nieto FJ, Young TB, Newman AB, Henderson JA. The relationship between chronically disrupted sleep and healthcare use. Sleep 2002; 25(3): 289–96.

73. Young T, Palta M, Dempsey J, et al. The occurrence of sleep-disordered breathing among middle-aged adults. N Engl J Med 1993; 328(17): 1230–5.

74. Ancoli-Israel S, Kripke DF, Klauber MR, et al. Morbidity, mortality and sleep-disordered breathing in community dwelling elderly. Sleep 1996; 19(4): 277–82.

75. Molho M, Shulimzon T, Benzaray S, Katz I. Importance of inspiratory load in the assessment of severity of airways obstruction and its correlation with CO_2 retention in chronic obstructive pulmonary disease. Am Rev Respir Dis 1993; 147(1): 45–9.

76. Baum GL, Zwas T, Katz I, Roth Y. Changes in mucociliary clearance during acute exacerbations of asthma. Am Rev Respir Dis 1992; 145(1): 237–8.

77. Katz I, Stradling J, Slutsky AS, Zamel N, Hoffstein V. Do patients with obstructive sleep apnea have thick necks? Am Rev Respir Dis 1990; 141(5 Pt 1): 1228–31.

78. Kripke DF. Mortality risk of major depression. Am J Psychiatry 1995; 152(6): 962.

79. Schmidt-Nowara WW, Coultas DB, Wiggins C, Skipper BE, Samet JM. Snoring in a Hispanic-American population. Risk factors and association with hypertension and other morbidity. Arch Intern Med 1990; 150(3): 597–601.

80. Bixler EO, Vgontzas AN, Lin HM, et al. Association of hypertension and sleep-disordered breathing. Arch Intern Med 2000; 160(15): 2289–95.

81. Nieto FJ, Young TB, Lind BK, et al. Association of sleep-disordered breathing, sleep apnea, and hypertension in a large community-based study. Sleep Heart Health Study. J Am Med Assoc 2000; 283(14): 1829–36.

82. Peppard PE, Young T, Palta M, Skatrud J. Prospective study of the association between sleep-disordered breathing and hypertension. N Engl J Med 2000; 342(19): 1378–84.

83. Partinen M, Jamieson A, Guilleminault C. Long-term outcome for obstructive sleep apnea syndrome patients. Mortality. Chest 1988; 94(6): 1200–4.

84. Edwards N, Blyton DM, Kirjavainen TT, Sullivan CE. Hemodynamic responses to obstructive respiratory events during sleep are augmented in women with preeclampsia. Am J Hypertens 2001; 14(11 Pt 1): 1090–5.

85. Connolly G, Razak AR, Hayanga A, et al. Inspiratory flow limitation during sleep in pre-eclampsia: comparison with normal pregnant

and nonpregnant women. Eur Respir J 2001; 18(4): 672–6.

86. Maasilta P, Bachour A, Teramo K, Polo O, Laitinen LA. Sleep-related disordered breathing during pregnancy in obese women. Chest 2001; 120(5): 1448–54.

87. Lefcourt LA, Rodis JF. Obstructive sleep apnea in pregnancy. Obstet Gynecol Surv 1996; 51(8): 503–6.

88. Kim HC, Young T, Matthews CG, et al. Sleep-disordered breathing and neuropsychological deficits. A population-based study. Am J Respir Crit Care Med 1997; 156(6): 1813–19.

89. Baran A, Richert AC. Obstructive sleep apnea and depression. CNS Spectrum 2003; 8(2): 120–34.

90. McMahon JP, Foresman BH, Chisholm RC. The influence of CPAP on the neurobehavioral performance of patients with obstructive sleep apnea hypopnea syndrome: a systematic review. WMJ 2003; 102(1): 36–43.

91. Means MK, Lichstein KL, Edinger JD, et al. Changes in depressive symptoms after continuous positive airway pressure treatment for obstructive sleep apnea. Sleep Breath 2003; 7(1): 31–42.

92. Akashiba T, Kawahara S, Akahoshi T, et al. Relationship between quality of life and mood or depression in patients with severe obstructive sleep apnea syndrome. Chest 2002; 122(3): 861–5.

93. Baldwin CM, Griffith KA, Nieto FJ, et al. The association of sleep-disordered breathing and sleep symptoms with quality of life in the Sleep Heart Health Study. Sleep 2001; 24(1): 96–105.

94. Wiegand L, Zwillich CW. Obstructive sleep apnea. Dis Mon 1994; 40(4): 197–252.

95. Stoohs RA, Guilleminault C, Itoi A, Dement WC. Traffic accidents in commercial long-haul truck drivers: the influence of sleep-disordered breathing and obesity. Sleep 1994; 17(7): 619–23.

96. Teran-Santos J, Jimenez-Gomez A, Cordero-Guevara J. The association between sleep apnea and the risk of traffic accidents. Cooperative Group Burgos-Santander. N Engl J Med 1999; 340(11): 847–51.

97. Barbe, PJ, Munoz A, et al. Automobile accidents in patients with sleep apnea syndrome. An epidemiological and mechanistic study. Am J Respir Crit Care Med 1998; 158(1): 18–22.

98. Masa JF, Rubio M, Findley LJ. Habitually sleepy drivers have a high frequency of automobile crashes associated with respiratory disorders during sleep. Am J Respir Crit Care Med 2000; 162(4 Pt 1): 1407–12.

99. George CF. Reduction in motor vehicle collisions following treatment of sleep apnoea with nasal CPAP. Thorax 2001; 56(7): 508–12.

100. Ulfberg J, Carter N, Edling C. Sleep-disordered breathing and occupational accidents. Scand J Work Environ Health 2000; 26(3): 237–42.

101. Report. NCoSDRRESaE. Bethesda, MD, 1993.

102. Ronald J, Delaive K, Roos L, Manfreda J, Bahammam A, Kryger MH. Health care utilization in the 10 years prior to diagnosis in obstructive sleep apnea syndrome patients. Sleep 1999; 22(2): 225–9.

103. Bahammam A, Delaive K, Ronald J, et al. Health care utilization in males with obstructive sleep apnea syndrome two years after diagnosis and treatment. Sleep 1999; 22(6): 740–7.

104. Kapur V, Blough DK, Sandblom RE, et al. The medical cost of undiagnosed sleep apnea. Sleep 1999; 22(6): 749–55.

105. Ohayon MM, Guilleminault C, Paiva T, et al. An international study on sleep disorders in the general population: methodological aspects of the use of the Sleep-EVAL system. Sleep 1997; 20(12): 1086–92.

106. Schechter MS. Technical report: diagnosis and management of childhood obstructive sleep apnea syndrome. Pediatrics 2002; 109(4): e69.

107. Gozal D. Sleep-disordered breathing and school performance in children. Pediatrics 1998; 102(3 Pt 1): 616–20.

108. Reuveni H, Simon T, Tal A, Elhayany A, Tarasiuk A. Health care services utilization in children with obstructive sleep apnea syndrome. Pediatrics 2002; 110(1 Pt 1): 68–72.

109. Tousignant P, Cosio MG, Levy RD, Groome PA. Quality adjusted life years added by treatment of obstructive sleep apnea. Sleep 1994; 17(1): 52–60.

110. Gross CR, Savik K, Bolman RM, 3rd, Hertz MI. Long-term health status and quality of life outcomes of lung transplant recipients. Chest 1995; 108(6): 1587–93.

111. Chervin RD, Murman DL, Malow BA, Totten V. Cost-utility of three approaches to the diagnosis of sleep apnea: polysomnography, home testing, and empirical therapy. Ann Intern Med 1999; 130(6): 496–505.

112. Chakravorty I, Cayton RM, Szczepura A. Health utilities in evaluating intervention in the sleep

apnoea/hypopnoea syndrome. Eur Respir J 2002; 20(5): 1233–8.

113. Ohayon MM, Zulley J, Guilleminault C, Smirne S, Priest RG. How age and daytime activities are related to insomnia in the general population: consequences for older people. J Am Geriatr Soc 2001; 49(4): 360–6.

114. Balter MB, Uhlenhuth EH. New epidemiologic findings about insomnia and its treatment. J Clin Psychiatry 1992; 53 Suppl: 34–9; discussion 40–2.

115. Léger D, Guilleminault C, Dreyfus JP, Delahaye C, Paillard M. Prevalence of insomnia in a survey of 12 778 adults in France. J Sleep Res 2000; 9(1): 35–42.

116. Walsh JK, Engelhardt CL. The direct economic costs of insomnia in the United States for 1995. Sleep 1999; 22(Suppl 2): S386–93.

117. Léger D. Public health and insomnia: economic impact. Sleep 2000; 23 Suppl 3: S69–76.

118. Weyerer S, Dilling H. Prevalence and treatment of insomnia in the community: results from the Upper Bavarian Field Study. Sleep 1991; 14(5): 392–8.

119. Leigh JP. Employee and job attributes as predictors of absateeism in a national sample of workers: the importance of health and dangerous working conditions. Soc Sci Med 1991; 33: 127–37.

120. Stoller MK. Economic effects of insomnia. Clin Ther 1994; 16(5): 873–97; discussion 54.

121. Drake CL, Roehrs T, Richardson G, Walsh JK, Roth T. Shift work sleep disorder: prevalence and consequences beyond that of symptomatic day workers. Sleep 2004; 27(8): 1453–62.

122. Schernhammer ES, Laden F, Speizer FE, et al. Night-shift work and risk of colorectal cancer in the nurses' health study. J Natl Cancer Inst 2003; 95(11): 825–8.

123. Schernhammer ES, Laden F, Speizer FE, et al. Rotating night shifts and risk of breast cancer in women participating in the nurses' health study. J Natl Cancer Inst 2001; 93(20): 1563–8.

124. Carskadon MA, Acebo C, Jenni OG. Regulation of adolescent sleep: implications for behavior. Ann N Y Acad Sci 2004; 1021: 276–91.

125. Ekbom KA. Restless legs syndrome. Neurology 1960; 10: 868–73.

126. Association ASD. The International Classification of Sleep Disorders: Revised Diagnostic and Coding Manual. Rochester, NY: American Sleep Disorders Association, 1997.

127. Goodman JD, Brodie C, Ayida GA. Restless leg syndrome in pregnancy. Br Med J 1988; 297(6656): 1101–2.

128. Lee KA, Zaffke ME, Baratte-Beebe K. Restless legs syndrome and sleep disturbance during pregnancy: the role of folate and iron. J Womens Health Gend Based Med 2001; 10(4): 335–41.

129. Allen RP, Earley CJ. Restless legs syndrome: a review of clinical and pathophysiologic features. J Clin Neurophysiol 2001; 18(2): 128–47.

130. Phillips B, Young T, Finn L, et al. Epidemiology of restless legs symptoms in adults. Arch Intern Med 2000; 160(14): 2137–41.

131. Milligan SA, Chesson AL. Restless legs syndrome in the older adult: diagnosis and management. Drugs Aging 2002; 19(10): 741–51.

132. Desautels A, Turecki G, Montplaisir J, et al. Identification of a major susceptibility locus for restless legs syndrome on chromosome 12q. Am J Hum Genet 2001; 69(6): 1266–70.

133. Earley CJ. Clinical practice. Restless legs syndrome. N Engl J Med 2003; 348(21): 2103–19.

134. Chervin RD, Hedger KM. Clinical prediction of periodic leg movements during sleep in children. Sleep Med 2001; 2(6): 501–10.

135. Ohayan MM, Priest RG, Zulley J, et al. Prevalence of narcolepsy symptomatology and diagnosis in the European general population. Neurology 2002; 58: 1826–33.

136. Broughton R, Ghanem Q, Hishikawa Y, et al. Life effects of narcolepsy in 180 patients from North America, Asia and Europe compared to matched controls. Can J Neurol Sci 1981; 8(4): 299–304.

137. Broughton RJ, Guberman A, Roberts J. Comparison of the psychosocial effects of epilepsy and narcolepsy/cataplexy: a controlled study. Epilepsia 1984; 25(4): 423–33.

138. Leon-Munoz L, de la Calzada MD, Guitart M. Accidents prevalence in a group of patients with the narcolepsy-cataplexy syndrome. Rev Neurol 2000; 30(6): 596–8.

139. Douglas NJ. The psychosocial aspects of narcolepsy. Neurology 1998; 50(2) (Suppl 1): S27–30.

CHAPTER 14

Pain and poor sleep

Gilles Lavigne and Christiane Manzini

WHAT IS PAIN?

The word pain comes from the Latin *poena*, meaning punishment.[1] According to a consensus from the International Association for the Study of Pain (IASP), pain is defined as 'an unpleasant sensory and emotional experience associated with actual or potential tissue damage, or described in terms of such damage'.[2] The integration of both sensory and emotional experiences related to pain is now well accepted.

The sensory experience, defined as nociception in neurophysiology, is the process by which an individual is informed of a condition that is potentially harmful to body integrity. Review of the neuroscience-related literature suggests that: (1) cellular and molecular mechanisms are involved in pain; (2) ascending and descending spinal and brain pathways play an important role in pain perception or its modulation (e.g., relief or attenuation); (3) specific sensory and emotional brain and cortical sites are activated in presence of pain.[1,3–5] The fact that conscious individuals report this sensory experience implies that pain is much more than just a sensory process (unlike nociception under general anesthesia) and that the emotional component promotes its expression.

Brain imaging studies have clearly demonstrated that both cortical sensory and affective areas are activated by pain.[6,7] The emotional experience and its unpleasant aspects depend on context and meaning of pain (e.g., pain episode immediately after a car accident or the one associated with the relapse of a cancer), age (e.g., older patients tend to cope better with chronic pain than middle-aged ones), past experience (e.g., childhood, parental modeling, previous trauma), religious or health beliefs, attitude (e.g., anxiety, catastrophizing), etc.

The integration of both sensory and emotional pain components may trigger aggressive or passive behaviour: individuals may adopt a sick role, involving excessive visits to health professionals, hospitalization, and absenteeism from work along with withdrawal from familial responsibilities. In the presence of chronic pain, it is common for all family members to be affected; for example, if one family member with chronic pain adopts a passive role, then other household members have to become more active in daily tasks and must cope with the mood alteration, depression, and other changes found in the person with pain disability.

The consequences of pain in patients' daily lives are of major concern in pain research. It is important to mention that more than 40% of chronic pain patients do not get adequate pain relief, around 50% report interference in their daily activities, and 70% feel that 'society' does not provide adequate support for their pain condition.[8–10] The consequences of pain include low daytime productivity, reduced capacity to execute familial or work tasks, increased risk of accident, suicide, and depression. All these burdens have direct and indirect consequences within society, and these consequences are increasing in prevalence as life expectancy and population aging increase. However, the paucity of published data makes it difficult to assess the cost of the interaction between pain and poor sleep. Pain relief or management does not seem to respond to popular expectation, and political actions have been taken to develop strategies for raising public awareness of the social impact and cost of chronic pain. Recently, the Senate of the United States of America (USA) declared the current decade to be one of 'pain management'. The Senate of Canada also is working on a bill to recognize the first week of November as Pain Awareness Week.

PREVALENCE OF CHRONIC PAIN ACROSS THE WORLD

The list of cited articles on chronic pain prevalence does not include all published papers but provides an overview of the magnitude of the pain 'epidemic' in communities under the so-called Western medical system. The estimated prevalence of chronic pain in the adult population is between 11% and 46% depending on the population surveyed, questionnaire used, and the goals of the studies.[8–15] For example, self-reports of daily chronic pain present for at least three months in the general population of Finland (n=4542 individuals surveyed by questionnaire) is 14.3%; based on symptoms present for at least once a month or several times a week or daily-continuously it is rated at 35.1%.[14] This study also showed that in the presence of daily pain the odds ratio (OR) of having poor self-rated health was also high (OR=11.8). In Denmark, the prevalence of overall non-malignant chronic pain is reported to be 19% in the population (n=10 066

individuals; questionnaire SF-36); the effect of aging on reports of pain was evident, with an OR of 3.9 if individuals were older than 67 years in comparison to individuals of 16–24 years old.[9] In Scotland (UK), 46.5% of the adult general population (n=3605 individuals; questionnaire) reported chronic pain, with the majority describing complaints related to lower back pain or arthritic pain; age, gender, housing tenure, and employment status were all identified as significant predictors.[11] In Australia, the prevalence of chronic pain in the general population is 20% in adult females and 17.1% in adult males (n=1000; telephonic interviews).[12] In Canada, the prevalence of non-cancer-related chronic pain is reported at 29% in the general population (n=2012 individuals; telephonic interviews); mean pain intensity was rated at 6.3 on a 0–10 scale with 80% of individuals reporting moderate-to-severe pain and a history of symptoms lasting for an average of 10.7 years.[8] According to a survey from the American Pain Society (1998), chronic pain persisted after five years in 50% of patients (www.ampainsoc.rg).

There is a paucity of publications on the epidemiology of chronic pain in relation to ethnicity. A survey of Canadians of various ethnicities (Statistics Canada survey; n=125 574) found that the prevalence of chronic pain is 18% for females and 14% for males.[10] Although no major difference was observed in chronic pain prevalence regarding ethnicity, Black-African Canadian males younger than 65 years showed a low prevalence (5%) of pain, while this prevalence was high for South Asian Canadians older than 65 years (55.7% for females and 38.2% for males) and aboriginal Canadians younger than 65 years (20.7% for females and 17.9% for males). A surprising publication directed toward cultural and language differences for cancer pain of patients from Beijing (China), Delhi (India), France, and the USA revealed that twice as many patients from Beijing and Delhi report severe cancer pain; also while 42% and 51% of patients from USA and France do report inadequate cancer pain relief, these numbers are at 67% and 79% in Beijing and Delhi, respectively.[16] Although analgesic medications seem to be less available in some countries due to legal control or drug availability in terms of cost and distribution, other factors such as beliefs, words used to describe pain and its meaning, mode of drug delivery, and racial 'prejudgment' can be partially responsible for such discrepancy. Interestingly, while 1% of Chinese and 54% of Scandinavians request local anesthetic for dental drilling pain, 90% of English Americans request local anesthetic; such pain is described as being expected and 'unpleasant' by Chinese patients, as being 'not so bad and not lasting long' by Scandinavians, and as being 'excruciating' by North Americans.[17,18] It is also surprising that certain racial discrepancies persist in some areas: African Americans receive less daily pain medication than Caucasian Americans;[19,20] back pain, migraine and headaches are two to four times more frequent in North America and Europe than in Asia or Africa.[21,22] Future studies across several ethnicities are necessary for better planning in health prevention and care regarding chronic pain at a local level (i.e., taking account of racial differences, languages, first generation immigrants) and at the global level (i.e., extending to developing countries).[21,23,24]

PREVALENCE OF PAIN AND SLEEP DISTURBANCES

The National Sleep Foundation (USA) has recognized the importance of the interaction between pain and sleep in a document entitled *Pain and Sleep* published on its website: www.sleepfoundation,org/publications/sleepa ndpain.cfm. The author (JR Goldberg) states that 'pain and sleep coincide and affect every aspect of our life'. According to a survey conducted by the National Sleep Foundation in 2000, 20% of the USA adult population reported that pain or physical discomfort has an effect on their sleep a few nights a week. People who suffer from pain are also concerned that they feel unrefreshed after sleep.

Several clinical studies (see Box 14.) report that between 50% and 90% of patients with pain (orofacial, lower back, headache, fibromyalgia, etc.) also complain that their sleep is of poor quality.[25–29] Other acute and chronic pain conditions associated with poor sleep are postoperative pain, skin burn-related pain, headache, irritable bowel syndrome, spinal cord injury, and breast cancer.[30–36]

Interestingly, the presence of orofacial pain increases the relative risk (RR) of poor sleep by 3.7 times, according to a cross-sectional population based study ($n=2504$ adult individuals) done in the UK.[37] A survey done in the USA ($n=1506$ community women and men aged between 55 and 84 years) found that 'bodily' pain is associated with a risk of insomnia complaints (difficulty falling asleep, waking during the night or too early, sensation of unrefreshing sleep), with an OR estimated at 1.9–2.7.[38] One of the most frequent comorbid conditions reported in chronic pain patients is insomnia, which has a prevalence two times higher in chronic pain patients than the general population without pain.[32,39] A cross-sectional study ($n=12\,643$ adult individuals) performed in Hungary revealed that chronic pain is present in 38% of the population, with 15% of the population complaining of concomitant insomnia. The prevalence of insomnia in these pain patients was three times higher than in those without pain.[40]

The concomitance of sleep disorders and pain may modify the subjective sensation related to sleep quality (e.g., whether it is refreshing), since 50% of insomnia patients with pain report that pain interferes with daily activities,[40] and since reports of daytime sleepiness (prevalence 7%, with an OR=1.73) increase in the presence of bodily pain.[38] Such findings in chronic pain patients need to be controlled for the presence of respiratory disturbances (e.g., snoring, upper airway resistance syndrome, sleep apnea), which may not be systematically assessed in large population studies.

Interestingly, bodily pain and snoring were associated with a small but significant OR of 1.4[38] and males with neck or orofacial pain presented with sleep apnea more frequently than females.[41] Although the association between fibromyalgia and sleep apnea is rather weak,[42] recordings of respiratory variables during sleep need to be made for pain patients presenting with poor sleep, in order to rule out slight respiratory disturbances that may have a deleterious effect upon the maintenance of daytime vigilance. Another concomitant sleep disorder is the periodic limb movement in sleep (PLMS), a condition frequently associated with the awake restless legs syndrome (RLS) that is present in 5–12% of the general population (see Chapter 13, this volume). The reports of bodily pain are associated with unpleasant feeling in the legs in 10% of the subgroup with an OR of 4.7.[38]

RISK FACTORS

Aging is another major variable that explains the rise in the prevalence of chronic pain. Close to 50% of older people of both genders suffer from chronic pain.[13,43] Based on a calculation of pain prevalence in older citizens projected to the year 2025, the prevalence of chronic pain may reach 70%, this being mainly due to the improvement of health care of the so-called baby boomers.[10,44] Interestingly, the OR of pain is 2.35 in the age range of 20–44 years old, 3.3 in the 45–64 age group, and it decreases to 2.77 after 65 years old.[10] The risk of difficulty in performing daily activities in older individuals reporting musculoskeletal pain was estimated with an OR of 2.93.[45] Conversely, older patients seem to cope better with the impact of chronic pain than younger active pain patients.[46] Similarly, following a night of sleep with sound to disrupt sleep continuity, older subjects performed a mathematical test much better than younger subjects who were also showing more mood alteration.[47]

Adolescents are not protected against sleep and pain problems. Sleep disturbance seems to be associated with more daytime sleepiness and longer nap time in juvenile rheumatoid arthritis patients.[48] Interestingly, it was found in a cohort of 86 teenagers and adolescents that although mood alteration and daytime sleepiness were aggravated it was again the depressive symptoms that were found to be the most robust predictor of sleep disturbances.[49]

Gender is an important covariable in assessing chronic pain prevalence.[8–12,50] The Canadian Community Health Survey, comprising 125 574 respondents, revealed that 18% of women and 14% of men report chronic pain.[10] Some types of chronic pain, such as pelvic pain and orofacial/temporomandibular pain, are twice as frequent in women: a RR of 1.36–2.81 and an OR of 4.7 were estimated for females who were more likely to report orofacial/temporomandibular pain than males.[24,41,51,52] Interestingly, women are in general more impaired by chronic pain and they tend to use more medications than men do. It was found that 93% of women with chronic pain use analgesics, and that antidepressants, codeine, and hypnotics are used three to four times more often by women with chronic pain.[10] Moreover, chronic pain patients of both genders tend to require more health services,[53] and women tend to show a higher body mass index, higher risk of depression, and more complaints related to reduced ability to perform daily tasks.[10,50]

Depressive symptoms are not rare in chronic pain patients, but it is not clear whether depression is a risk factor (precipitating or perpetuating persistent pain) or is secondary to the chronic state and disability related to pain. According to a small sample size study ($n = 137$), poor sleepers seem to have the highest orofacial pain intensity, greatest psychological distress and a poor perception of life control.[54] As reported above, depressive symptoms seem to explain approximately 30% of the variability between poor sleep complaints and pain, although others have suggested that daily pain intensity is more important.[28,50,55,56] Interestingly, a study done in 672 individuals reporting orofacial pain concluded that the presence of sleep disturbances is not a precipitating or perpetuating factor in pain but that female gender is an important factor.[51] A survey of 105 patients reporting chronic pain (e.g., low back pain, myofascial pain, causalgia) suggested that the onset of sleep problems was secondary to pain, in the absence of mood disturbance.[57] Therefore, mood disturbances or depressive symptoms do not exclusively explain the relationship between pain and poor sleep. However, a very large telephone interview study ($n = 18\,980$ individuals from UK, Germany, Italy, Portugal, and Spain) revealed that over the general population, 17% reported chronic pain with a physical condition for at least six months and that major depressive disorder was present in 4% of individuals interviewed.[15] Depressed mood was noted in 16.5% of the pain population and those suffering from major depressive disorder were four times more at risk of chronic pain (OR = 4). The same author reported that chronic pain is present in approximately half of patients with major depressive illness.[58] In that specific study, major depression as a disorder could be described as a secondary risk factor explaining the relation between chronic pain and poor sleep. This is further supported by the observation that patients with depression are also more at risk of presenting symptoms related to insomnia (OR = 2.44).[38] Self-perception of poor health status is another important variable that influences pain.[11,14,54]

Suicidal ideation in major depressive patients cannot be ignored and it is reported that patients with chronic pain are more at risk. Suicidal ideation is estimated at 13–24% in a population with chronic non-malignant pain; back or abdominal pain was associated with a higher risk of suicidal ideation if a familial history of suicide was present.[59,60] Six factors were associated with suicidal ideation: sleep onset insomnia, pain intensity, medication, pain interference with daily activities, affective distress and depressive symptoms; with severity of insomnia and intensity of pain being the most powerful discriminator. As reported above, pain prevalence is higher with age and depression is a frequent comorbidity with insomnia and bodily pain in elderly people aged over 65 years.[38] Consequently, those planning public health prevention and care programs for chronic pain patients need to consider depressive symptoms, age, suicidal history, and concomitant insomnia.

The effect of ethnicity in relation to variation in geographic origin, dietary habits, use of what Western societies label complementary medicine (e.g., acupuncture, medicinal herbs for pain or sleep problems), practicing meditation or praying on a regular basis, the role of religious leaders or shamans, etc. is rarely estimated and needs to be better understood if public health planning is directed to multicultural areas. For the successful management of neuropathic pain or fibromyalgia, the influences of comorbid disorders (e.g., anxiety, depression, poor sleep) need to be addressed in parallel with laboratory investigations or psychophysical measures (e.g., number of tender points, reduction in pain perception or tolerance threshold, mechanical or thermal dysesthesia, localized or widespread pain distribution) in order to achieve patient satisfaction and perceived success of treatment.[61,62]

Future epidemiological or experimental studies on the interaction between pain and poor sleep need to control for the potential influence of comorbid disorders (e.g., anxiety, diabetes, immune disorders, mental health disorders, sleep disorders), low income, educational status (if less than 10 years of education the OR = 1.9), marital status (divorced or separated, the OR = 1.5), type of work (e.g., physical or clerical), and napping habits, etc.[9,10,14,63]

Time course of relationship between pain and poor sleep

The time course of sleep disturbance and related complaints in patients with chronic pain seems to be bimodal.[64] Close to 90% of patients report that a 'novel' pain experience has preceded or coincided with awareness of a sleep problem, suggesting a linear progression.[26,27,57] However, when pain is chronic (more than three months) or constant and intense over a brief period (e.g., post-operative pain, hospitalization after a trauma or skin burn) most patients report a clear circular pattern or vicious cycle taking place: a night of poor sleep is followed by a day of increased pain and a day with intense pain is succeeded by sleep of poor quality.[36,56,65] The persistence of such a cycle may contribute to the deleterious effect of sleep fragmentation on daytime cognitive function.

It is not obvious that the circular pattern is an association of pure cause and effect that is totally self-explanatory. The role of concomitant anxiety, pain intensity, and depressive symptoms correlates with poor sleep reports: depression alone may explain up to 34% of the variance between variables in chronic pain patients suffering from headaches, back pain or neck aches.[55] Poor sleep reports in patients with chronic pain and fibromyalgia are also correlated with depression, but fatigue, daily sleep quality, and pain intensity seem to be inter-related: pain contributed to 4.7% of the variance in fatigue and sleep quality and pain for 6.5% in fatigue variance.[28,56] Conclusions from the two just-mentioned studies need to be interpreted with caution since only subjective outcomes were used to assess this interaction (e.g., no polygraphic data were recorded) and the population samples were small ($n=40$ and 122 patients, respectively). Moreover, since several analgesic medications may alter sleep continuity, it is important to control for the effect of analgesics on vigilance when assessing the cyclic relation between pain intensity during the daytime and perception of poor sleep quality.[66,67]

Fatigue is an important variable in the assessment of the interaction between pain and sleep.[64,68] Fatigue can result from boring activities, or lack of stimulation, can be secondary to medication or lack of exercise, or more importantly to lack of 'restorative' sleep. Experimental manipulations of pain perception following sleep fragmentation (e.g., brief

Table 14.1 Examples of impact and consequences of chronic pain and poor sleep

- Reduced family/daily activities
- Reduced social exchanges
- Reduced physical work or sports activities
- Poor health status and higher risk of comorbidity (e.g., depression, diabetes, insomnia)
- Reduced sexual activity – low libido
- Absenteeism
- Overuse of alcohol or drugs (e.g., cannabis, cocaine, and other narcotics)
- Risk of poverty
- Risk of depression, losing work, divorce, suicide, etc.
- Increase demand for health care with rise in direct and indirect costs for health prevention and care practices

alterations of sleep continuity) or sleep stage deprivation (e.g., the patient is not allowed to maintain a given sleep stage) have showed that pain and fatigue are inter-related.[69,70]

In summary, it can be concluded that approximately 5–30% of the interaction between pain and poor sleep can be explained by concomitant fatigue, depression or mood problems, low levels of physical exercise, and the prevalence of anxiety in the population.[26,28,31,54–56,71,72]

Public consequences of pain and poor sleep

The persistence of chronic pain is well known to induce an alteration in the ability to perform daily tasks (e.g., familial, social, recreational or work related; see Table 14.1) in at least half of patients.[8,10] This can be explained in part by a reduction in physical activity, impairment in cognitive function, and days on which patients cannot work or have to stay in bed.

Cognitive impairments, including alterations in memory or attention, are present in patients with chronic pain.[73–75] As described above, complaints of fatigue are common in chronic pain patients. Fatigue related to poor sleep and pain is more likely to be mental (e.g., the patient feels unable to think clearly and any intellectual task is very demanding) with a physical component (e.g., no more energy after a physical activity); it needs to be distinguished from fatigue related to boredom.[76,77] Fatigue complaints in chronic pain patients also need to be differentiated from 'chronic fatigue syndrome', which is an extreme condition present for at least six months.[77] Daily fatigue seems to influence pain, explaining 16% of the variance in poor sleep and pain.[56] As a consequence of poor sleep and fatigue in the presence of chronic pain, risk of daytime sleepiness is slightly higher (modest OR=1.73), but reports of daytime sleepiness need to be controlled for the influences of medications that may alter cognitive function (e.g., psychotropic medication), level of physical exercise, obesity, reports of mood problems and depression as described above.[10,29,38,72]

Moreover, as described above, it is mandatory to assess whether the pain is secondary or concomitant to specific and frequently underdiagnosed sleep disorders such as PLMS (prevalence between 5% and 12% of population, more than 40% over 50 years old) which also contributes to reduced sleep efficiency, although no clear deterioration of cognitive function is reported; sleep apnea (prevalence between 2% and 4% of population, more than 40% over 50 years old) which is recognized to be associated with daytime sleepiness and/or cognitive deterioration, as well as the presence of an upper airway resistance syndrome (no apnea or cessation of breathing but daytime sleepiness).[78,79]

Sleepiness and driving are also a concern, taking into consideration that most medications used by chronic pain patients may be associated with a lower level of vigilance (e.g., analgesics, anxiolytics, and antidepressants). Recent position papers have debated whether the use of psychotropic medications is a risk factor for transportation accidents.[80,81] Similar concerns have been raised for sleep medication; in tests of driving ability, benzodiazepine hypnotics and zopiclone were found to have residual effects that persisted from waking until noon in some individuals.[82] Interestingly, a risk factor assessment analysis of a cohort of Australian commercial drivers (n=2342 individuals) revealed that the use of narcotics was associated with an accident OR of 2.4, benzodiazepines with an OR of 1.91, and antihistaminics with an OR of 3.44.[83] Use of opioid medication in chronic pain patients is reported to be four times higher than in the general population (not surprising at first but some pain suffering individuals are driving every morning); antidepressants and anxiolytics are respectively used two and three times more frequently.[9] Other studies reported that antiinflammatory analgesics are used by 30–49% of chronic pain patients, opioid analgesics are used by 12–22%, antidepressants by 4–10%, anticonvulsant/anti-epileptic drugs by 5%, and anxiolytics by 3%.[8,9,63] In presence of a severe form of pain, the neuropathic pains (e.g., pain secondary to nerve pathology related to diabetes, AIDS, herpes zoster, mechanical nerve compression or entrapment, neuralgias, etc.), the analysis of medication use by those under contract with a private insurance firm in the USA (n=55 686) revealed different percentages: 53.9% used opioids, 21% benzodiazepines, 11–14% anti-epileptics or antidepressants, and 7% muscle relaxants.[84] To our knowledge, no systematic prospective study has been made in chronic pain patients with poor sleep quality and daytime sleepiness to assess the risk of driving accidents in comparison to pain patients without sleep or vigilance problems. Surprisingly, complementary and alternative medicines (vitamins, magnets, herbal remedies, chiropractic) were used by 43% of patients with peripheral neuropathies of whom one-quarter reported improvement in symptoms.[85] However, the additive effect of alternative and conventional medications on sleepiness or low vigilance risk in painful and sleep-disturbed patients needs to be assessed, for obvious safety reasons.

MEDICAL DEMAND

In terms of general medical demand, a pain-related problem motivates one patient in five to consult a family physician.[86] In the 2000–2001 period, according to a Canadian survey, three out of four patients with chronic pain visited a family general physician and approximately one in five chronic pain patients received care from a chiropractor, physiotherapist, and/or 'alternative' health care provider.[10] In Finland, chronic pain patients have two times more contacts with health care professionals than controls without pain, and health care system use is 25% higher.[9] An Australian study ($n = 17\,543$ individuals; telephone interviews) revealed that individuals with chronic pain were more frequent users of the health care system (incidence rate ratio of at least twofold) than patients with no pain and no disability.[53] Frequencies of primary care visits were 12–17 times higher, hospital admission 2.6 times higher and emergency visits 5.0 times higher in individuals with pain-related disability (interference with daily activities) than patients with pain and no disability. In Sweden, the incidence of patients using physical therapy is at 7.2% and the rate of using alternative care is at 5.9%.[87] According to a Statistics Canada survey, 20% of chronic pain patients visit a chiropractor, alternative, or physical therapist to obtain some pain relief; this rate is two to three times more frequent than that of individuals without pain.[10] For one-third of the 43% of patients using complementary and alternative medicines for peripheral neuropathies, as mentioned above, the motive was inadequate pain control by conventional health care.[85] It is important to reiterate that 40% of chronic pain patients do not feel that they receive adequate treatment for their pain condition and 70% feel that they do not receive adequate support from society.[9,10]

COST OF PAIN AND SLEEP INTERACTIONS

According to the literature, the direct costs of the interaction between sleep and pain are related to the costs of hospitalization/nursing homes, physician time, and therapies (e.g., pharmacology, cognitive behavioral or physical therapies plus over-the-counter or recreational drugs/alcohol used to alleviate the problem). Indirect costs include impact of the condition on quality of life, productivity/absenteeism, morbidity (e.g., secondary depression, the consequences of drug or alcohol abuse), and mortality.[88] General estimates of the cost of insomnia during the last decade rate indirect costs as two to six times higher than direct costs.[88]

Costs of chronic pain are partially known. A very general estimate from the USA suggested that chronic pain cost $100 billion in health care for 2001, probably mainly direct costs.[89] A recent analysis revealed that individuals with painful neuropathic disorders represent an estimated total health charge to a private USA health insurance company of $17 355 (based on year 2000) in comparison to $5715 for matched controls.[84] Comorbidities are not rare in such patients, some of whom also presented with fibromyalgia, osteoarthritis, coronary heart disease, diabetes, and depression that had a prevalence of two to six times that of matched controls. In 2001, the direct costs of health care over a six-month period for patients with fibromyalgia were estimated at CDN$2298 (about 50% the value of USA dollars).[90] Medications represented 33% of these direct costs, complementary and alternative medicine represented 17%, and diagnostic tests 15%, whereas indirect costs were estimated at CDN$5035.[90] Interestingly, one study reported that persistence of pain related to fibromyalgia or osteoarthritis reduced family income by approximately 70%.[91] Another study estimated direct and indirect costs of lower back pain in the USA to be $80 billion per year;[92] see also www.sleepfoundation.org/publications/sleepa

Box 14.1 Prevalence, percentage with poor sleep quality and estimate of direct costs[a] for various pain conditions associated with reports of poor sleep

- **Fibromyalgia** Prevalence = 2–8% with a dominance in females; 90% of patients report poor sleep quality; direct costs estimate (1990) = US$2274 per patient[24,29,98]
- **Osteoarthritis/Rheumatoid arthritis** Prevalence = 8.7–20%/1%; approximately 50% of patients report poor sleep quality with concomitant complaints of excessive daily fatigue; direct costs estimate (1993) = $777 million/$2.1 million[11,63,68,93]
- **Temporomandibular pain/orofacial pain** Prevalence = 3.6–12%, nearly twice as frequent in females; 50–70% of patients report poor sleep quality; estimate of direct costs accords with our experience, since these are the patients we see the most often: between CDN$1000 and CDN$30 000 per patient for consultation, medication, physiotherapy, oral devices, and in some cases dental rehabilitation[24,26,37,99,100]
- **Cervical or neck pain** Prevalence = 14.6% with gender distribution of 16% in females and 12% in males; unknown percentage with report of poor sleep quality; no data available that estimate direct costs, except 37% seem to present persistent pain over time[24,50]
- **Back pain** Prevalence = 15–37%; 50–89% with report of poor sleep quality; estimate of direct costs (1990) = $24.30 million, direct : indirect cost ratio = 1/9; in 1981, in Quebec, Canada, 7% of workers with back pain used 73% of worker medical costs and 76% of indemnity[11,24,28,92,101]
- **Abdominal pain (including gastric pain, heartburn, ulcers and irritable bowel syndrome, pelvic pain)** Prevalence = 8–20% for irritable bowel syndrome; 75–84% of patients show high rate of sleep arousal and waking but no direct report of poor sleep quality; estimate of direct costs (1996) = $881 billion[94,102,103]
- **Headache/migraine (prevalence of concomitant sleep apnea and upper airway resistance syndrome not controlled)** Median prevalence of headache = 69% in females and 46% in males, while for migraine = 15–17.6% in females and 6% in males; unknown percentage with report of poor sleep quality; no data that estimate direct costs, but highest prevalence is of workforce lost[24,27,28,96]
- **Cancer pain (with metastasis)** Prevalence depending on cancer type; 63% of patients report poor sleep quality; no data available that estimate direct costs[35]

[a]Not including disability (indirect costs); values are given in US dollars unless otherwise indicated

ndpain.cfm. Other studies providing additional information on the cost of chronic pain cite both the direct and indirect costs of rheumatoid arthritis as $992 billion (a 1983 estimation), and the direct cost of pelvic pain to be $881 billion (a 1996 estimation).[93,94]

To our knowledge, no systematic cost or cost-effectiveness analysis (e.g., cost per unit of health-related benefit) has been made of the interaction between pain and poor sleep. Box 14.1 describes the prevalence and direct costs of some chronic pain conditions known to have related complaints of poor sleep quality. Conservative estimates of the cost of chronic insomnia (frequently concomitant in chronic pain patients; see above sections) in the USA were in the range of $100 billion, while the costs of chronic pain were in the range of $100–125 billion.[88,89] Using a simplistic calculation that assumes two-thirds of patients with chronic pain also suffer from insomnia-related complaints, it could be extrapolated that the interaction between pain and sleep may represent $75 billion for the USA alone. The frequent presence of comorbidities makes such cost estimations difficult to arrive at, as does the cyclic interaction between pain and sleep; for a more accurate estimation of the costs related to insomnia, readers may consult other chapters in this volume. Future studies need to separate out the percentage of costs of insomnia and pain from their mutual interaction for accuracy in public health management strategies. Box 14.2 summarizes some management methods that may help reverse the vicious cycle of pain and poor sleep. However, the lack of controlled studies requires caution before generalizing the application of these methods in a public health program.

Finally, public awareness of the economic consequences of chronic pain is becoming a major concern. For example, in the UK back pain costs in terms of lost productivity are six times higher than direct health cost.[95] A study done in the USA on the cost of pain estimated that 13% of workforce productivity was lost due to headache (5.4%), back pain (3.2%), arthritis pain (2.0%) and other musculoskeletal pain (2.0%). The cost of lost productivity for blue- and white-collar workers in pain was estimated at $61 billion per year in the USA with a loss of up to four hours per week.[96] Furthermore, in Canada absenteeism in chronic pain patients was reported at 9.3 days per year (CI: 4.7–13.7) on which the chronic pain patient deems it impossible to work.[8] In Scandinaria on a short-term estimate, over a 14-day period, 0.8 days are lost every 2 weeks due to pain disability in comparison to 0.4 days in the general population.[9]

Availability and access to pain management across the planet

This section may sound surprising to some readers but our 'public health' review on pain and sleep interaction would have been ethically incomplete without reproducing some information available in literature. As reported above, patients with cancer pain from India and China present a higher prevalence of severe pain and of inadequate pain control.[16] According to the World Health Organization, in the year 2020 about 70% of new cancer cases will occur in developing countries.[97] This statement requires action since: (1) cancer pain is most effectively relieved by a mixture of medications including morphine and codeine; (2) North American (USA and Canada) and European countries which represent 19% of the world's population consume 82% of the 'legal' narcotics and 84% of world's morphine. Africa, with 7% of the world's population, consumes 1% of available narcotics or morphine, and Asia, with 60% of the world's population, consumes 7% of morphine or 12% of all narcotics.[97] It is obvious that an adequate approach to 'global' pain control will require that developing countries have access to analgesics, that regulations regarding illicit trafficking be enforced, that interventions to prevent addiction problems be developed, and that each country use analgesics according to its own cultural and religious values. We have to learn from each other: control and management of the overuse of medication in developed countries; and humanistic or different approaches (e.g., acupuncture, medicinal herbs) in developing countries.

In concluding this section, it is important to reiterate that improvement in pain management has been requested by 28% of the British and 40% of the Danish population with chronic pain,[9,11] and that only 36% of Canadians suffering from chronic pain reported that pain management was 'very' effective.[8] As revealed by a Canadian survey, the prevalence of chronic pain within a given country also varies according to ethnicity, with the highest prevalence being reported in aboriginal women under 65 years of age, and in Asian women over 65 years.[10] Again, pain management and control probably require geographically localized solutions according to culture, values, beliefs, economic wealth, etc.

Box 14.2 Methods or techniques for possible reversal of consequences of pain on sleep, including secondary fatigue or sleepiness[a]

- **Life and sleep hygiene advice** Relaxation techniques (e.g., abdominal respiration, mental imagery, yoga), initiation of a moderate fitness program, avoidance of intense exercise or heavy meals or alcohol in the evening, learning about managing life stress, etc.[64,104] (see www. sleepfoundation.org/publications/sleepandpain.cfm)

- **Patient complaints concerning sleeping partner disturbances** Advice to improve sleep:
  1 **ear plugs** if partner is snoring or tooth grinding;
  2 **twin beds** if partner is suffering from periodic movement;
  3 sleeping in a **separate room** at first sleep awakening or on a permanent basis if partner suffers from severe apnea, periodic leg movement, violent parasomnia, REM behavior disorder, frequent waking due to bladder problems, or is a late reader or TV watcher

- **Drugs and medication history** Identification of 'social' agents that may interfere with sleep quality: cocaine, ecstasy, nicotine, alcohol. Since many pain patients suffer from concomitant medical problems (e.g., depression, hypertension) and since some medications may alter waking performance (e.g., sleepiness/sedation, memory alteration), it is important to assess their effect on both sleep and daytime functioning (e.g., risk of work or transport accident). Pain management frequently includes use of medications such as non-steroidal anti-inflammatories, opioids, benzodiazepines, and antidepressants. Cardiovascular medications (e.g., beta-blockers, alpha-2-agonists), corticosteroids, antiparkinsonian and antiepileptic drugs have all been reported to trigger nightmares, exacerbate respiratory disturbances during sleep or insomnia, and induce daytime sleepiness. As an example, benzodiazepines and narcotics are reported to increase the risk of transport accident by 1.88 and 2.4 times, respectively[66,67,81,83,105]

- **Sleep disorders concomitant with pain**[b]
  1 *Insomnia.* Consider cognitive behavioral therapy to review deleterious life habits and develop new attitudes about sleep; consider medication that will facilitate sleep onset and continuity
  2 *Circadian rhythm alteration.* Consider sleep hygiene advice, light therapy, or medications that improve cycle rhythm (e.g., melatonin) or alertness (e.g., modafinil), although governmental regulatory agencies have yet to accept such indications for the latter
  3 *Periodic limb movement syndrome/restless leg syndrome.* Consider treatment with dopaminergic medication
  4 *Snoring or sleep apnea or upper airway resistance syndrome.* Consider continuous positive airway pressure (CPAP); oral device also named mandibular advancement device (MAD)
  5 *Sleep bruxism/tooth grinding.* About half of tooth grinders will complain of jaw muscle and joint pain with occasional morning headaches or cervical pain.[64] In patients with tooth grinding complaints and pain, life and sleep hygiene advice (including physical therapy and massage, hypnotherapy) are first recommended; use of medication is limited to short-term management (e.g., clonazepam) and a single dental arch oral device named an occlusal splint may help to reduce sound and further tooth damage. However, use of such devices may be at risk of exacerbating respiratory disturbance of patients with a clear diagnosis of sleep apnea.[106]

[a]Most of these lack systematic studies supporting their effectiveness of risk.
[b]Polygraphic recording is very useful to confirm diagnosis.

FUTURE DIRECTIONS IN RESEARCH AND MANAGEMENT

It is obvious that prospective and systematic studies need to be made regarding costs to health care of the interaction between chronic pain and poor sleep quality. The analysis will have to be corrected for concomitant conditions such as diabetes, obesity, cardiovascular problems, sleep disorders (e.g., sleep breathing disorders, PLMS, insomnia), depression and anxiety. Moreover, indirect costs related to absenteeism, low working performance, low familial activities and transportation or work accident risks also need to be included in the calculations. Five priorities are suggested: (1) assessment of risk factors of 'pain and poor sleep' interactions; (2) estimation of 'pain and poor sleep' consequences and/or impacts; (3) development of prevention programs; (4) development of guidelines about best management strategies (e.g., cognitive behavioral therapies vs. pain and sleep medications); (5) accessibility of pain or sleep prevention strategies and therapies to developing countries according to their values and respecting strategies already in place (e.g., lifestyle, medicinal products).

REFERENCES

1. Nagda J, Bajwa ZH. Definitions and classification of pain. In: Principles and Practice of Pain Medicine. New York: McGraw-Hill, 2004; 4: 51–4.
2. Merskey H, Bogduk N. Classification of Chronic Pain: Descriptions of Chronic Pain Syndromes and Definitions of Pain Terms. IASP, Task Force on Taxonomy, 2nd edn. Seattle, WA: IASP Press.
3. Price DD. Psychological and neural mechanisms of the affective dimension of pain. Science 2000; 288(5472): 1769–72.
4. Julius D, Basbaum AI. Molecular mechanisms of nociception. Nature 2001; 413: 203–10.
5. Scholtz J, Woolf CJ. Can we conquer pain? Nat Neurosci 2002; 5(1): 1062–7.
6. Casey Kl, Bushnell MC. Pain Imaging. Seattle, WA: IASP Press, 2000.
7. Peyron R, Laurent B, Garcia-Larrea L. Functional imaging of brain responses to pain. A review and meta-analysis. Neurophysiol Clin 2000; 30: 263–88.
8. Moulin DE, Clark AJ, Speechley M, Morley-Forster PK, Chronic pain in Canada – prevalence, treatment, impact and the role of opioid analgesia. Pain Res Manag 2002; 7: 179–84.
9. Eriksen J, Jensen MK, Sjogren P, Ekholm O, Rasmussen NK. Epidemiology of chronic non-malignant pain in Denmark. Pain 2003; 106: 221–8.
10. Meana M, Cho R, DesMeules M. Chronic pain: the extra burden on Canadian women. BMC Womens Health 2004; 4 (Suppl 1): S17.
11. Elliott AM, Smith BH, Penny KI, Smith WC, Chambers WA. The epidemiology of chronic pain in the community. Lancet 1999; 354: 1248–52.
12. Blyth FM, March LM, Brnabic AJ, et al. Chronic pain in Australia: a prevalence study. Pain 2001; 89: 127–34.
13. Harstall C, Ospina M. How prevalent is chronic pain? Pain Clinical updates; IASP 2003; 11: 1–4.
14. Mäntyselkä PT, Turunen JHO.; Ahonen RS, Kumpusalo EA. Chronic pain and poor self-rated health. J Am Med Assoc 2003; 290: 2435–42.
15. Ohayon MM, Schatzberg AF. Using chronic pain to predict depressive morbidity in the general population. Arch Gen Psychiatry 2003; 60: 39–47.
16. Cleeland CS, Serlin R, Nakamura Y, Mendoza T. Effects of culture and language on ratings of cancer pain and patterns of functional interference. In: Jensen JA, Wiesenfield-Hallin A eds, Progress in Pain Research and Management. Seattle, WA: IASP Press, 1997: 35–51.
17. Moore R, Brodsgaard I, Mao TK, Miller ML, Dworkin SF. Perceived need for local anesthesia in tooth drilling among AngloAmericans, Mandarin Chinese and Scandinavians. Anesth Prog 1998; 45: 22–28.
18. Moore R, Brodsgaard I, Mao TK, Miller ML, Dworkin SF. Acute pain and use of local anesthesia: tooth drilling and childbirth labor pain beliefs among AngloAmericans, Mandarin Chinese and Scandinavians. Anesth Prog 1998; 45: 29–37.

19. Ng B, Dimsdale JE, Rollnik JD, Shapiro H. The effect of ethnicity on prescriptions for patient-controlled analgesia for post-operative pain. Pain 1996; 66: 9–12.

20. Bernabei R, Gambassi G, Lapane K, et al. Management of pain in elderly patients with cancer. J Am Med Assoc 1998; 279: 1877–82.

21. Moore RB, Brodsgaard I. Cross-cultural investigations of pain. In: Crombie IK, ed. Epidemiology of Pain. Seattle, WA: IASP Press, 1999: 53–80.

22. Scher AI, Stewart WF, Lipton RB. Migraine and headache: a meta-analytic approach. In: Crombie IK, ed. Epidemiology of Pain. Seattle, WA: IASP Press, 1999: 159–70.

23. Green CR. Racial disparities in access to pain treatment. Pain Clinical Updates – International Association for the Study of Pain, 2004; 12(6).

24. Von Korff M, LeResche L. Epidemiology of Pain. In: Merskey H, Dubner R, eds. The Paths of Pain, 1975–2005. Seattle, WA: IASP Press, 2005: 339–52.

25. Dao TT, Lund JP, Lavigne GJ. Comparison of pain and quality of life in bruxers and patients with myofascial pain of the masticatory muscles. J Orofac Pain 1994; 8(4): 350–56.

26. Riley III JL, Benson MB, Gremillion HA, et al. Sleep disturbances in orofacial pain patients: pain-related or emotional distress? J Craniomandib Pract 2001; 19: 106–13.

27. Smith MT, Perlis ML, Smith MS, Giles DE, Carmody TP. Sleep quality and presleep arousal in chronic pain. J Behav Med 2000; 23: 1–13.

28. McCracken LM, Iverson GL. Disrupted sleep patterns and daily functioning in patients with chronic pain. Pain Res Manag 2002; 7: 75–9.

29. Okifuji A, Turk DC. Stress and psychophysiological dysregulation in patients with fibromyalgia syndrome. Appl Psychophysiol Biofeedback 2002; 27: 129–41.

30. Cohen M, Menefee LA, Doghramji K, Anderson WR, Frank ED. Sleep in chronic pain: problems and treatments. Int Rev Psychiat 2000; 12: 115–26.

31. Menefee LA, Cohen M, Anderson WR, et al. Sleep disturbance and nonmalignant chronic pain: a comprehensive review of the literature. Pain Med 2000; 1: 156–72.

32. Moldofsky H. Sleep and pain: clinical review. Sleep Med Rev 2001; 5: 387–98.

33. Widerstrom-Noga EG, Felipe-Cuervo E, Yezierski RP. Chronic pain after spinal injury: interference with sleep and daily activities. Arch Phys Med Rehabil 2001; 82: 1571–77.

34. Rains JC, Penzien DB. Chronic headache and sleep disturbance. Curr Pain Headache Rep 2002; 6: 498–504.

35. Koopman C, Nouriani B, Erickson V, et al. Sleep disturbances in women with metastatic breast cancer. Breast J 2002; 6: 362–70.

36. Raymond I, Nielsen TA, Lavigne GJ, Manzini C, Choinière M. Quality of sleep and its daily relationship to pain intensity in hospitalized adult burn patients. Pain 2001; 92: 381–8.

37. Macfarlane TV, Worthington HV. Association between orofacial pain and other symptoms: a population based study. Oral Biosci Med 2004; 1: 45–54.

38. Foley D, Ancoli-Israel S, Britz P, Walsh J. Sleep disturbances and chronic disease in older adults: results on the 2003 National Sleep Foundation Sleep in America Survey. J Psychosom Res 2004; 56: 497–502.

39. Sutton DA, Moldofsky H, Badley EM. Insomnia and health problems in Canadians. Sleep 2001; 24: 665–70.

40. Novak M, Mucsi I, Shapiro CM, Rethelyi J, Kopp MS. Increased utilization of health services by insomniacs—an epidemiological perspective. J Psychosom Res 2004; 56: 527–36.

41. Lobbezoo F, Visscher CM, Naeije M. Impaired health status, sleep disorders, and pain in the craniomandibular and cervical spinal regions. Eur J Pain 2004; 8: 23–30.

42. Dauvilliers Y, Touchon J. Sleep in fibromyalgia: review of clinical and polysomnographic data. Neurophysiol Clin 2001; 31: 18–33.

43. Scudds R, Ostbye T. Pain and pain-related interference with function in older Canadians: the Canadian study of health and aging. Disabil Rehabil 2001; 15: 654–64.

44. Schopflocher D, Borowski C, Harstall C, et al. Chronic Pain in Alberta: A Portrait from the 1996 National Population Health Survey and the 2001 Canadian Community Edmonton, Alberta: Health Survey. Health Surveillance, Alberta Health and Wellness, 2003.

45. Scudds RJ, Robertson McDJ. Empirical evidence of the association between the presence of musculoskeletal pain and physical disability in community-dwelling senior citizens. Pain 1998; 75: 229–35.

46. Cook AJ, Chastain DC. The classification of patients with chronic pain: age and sex differences. Pain Res Manag 2001; 6: 142–51.

47. Bonnet MH. The effect of sleep fragmentation on sleep and performance in younger and older subjects. Neurobiol Aging 1989; 10: 21–5.

48. Zamir G, Press J, Tal A, Tarasiuk A. Sleep fragmentation in children with juvenile rheumatoid arthritis. J Rheumatol 1998; 25: 1191–97.

49. Palermo TM, Kiska R. Subjective sleep disturbances in adolescents with chronic pain: relationship to daily functioning and quality of life. J Pain 2005; 6: 201–7.

50. Côté P, Cassidy JD, Carroll LJ, Kristman V. The annual incidence and course of neck pain in the general population: a population based cohort study. Pain 2004; 112: 267–73.

51. Kamisaka M, Yatani H, Kuboki T, Matsuka Y, Minakuchi H. Four-year longitudinal course of TMD symptoms in an adult population and the estimation of risk factors in relation to symptoms. J Orofac Pain 2000; 14: 224–32.

52. Macfarlane TV, Blinkhorn AS, Davies RM, Kincey J, Worthington HV. Predictors of outcome for orofacial pain in the general population: a four-year follow-up study. J Dent Res 2004; 83: 712–17.

53. Blyth FM, March LM, Brnabic AJ, Cousins MJ. Chronic pain and frequent use of health care. Pain 2004; 111: 51–8.

54. Yatani H, Studts J, Cordova M, Carlson CR, Okeson JP. Comparison of sleep quality and clinical and psychologic characteristics in patients with temporomandibular disorders. J Orofac Pain 2002; 16: 221–8.

55. Sayar K, Arikan M, Yontem T. Sleep quality in chronic pain patients. Can J Psychiatry 2002; 47: 844–8.

56. Nicassio PM, Moxham EG, Schuman CE, Gervirtz RN. The contribution of pain, reported sleep quality, and depressive symptoms to fatigue in fibromyalgia. Pain 2002; 100: 271–9.

57. Morin CM, Gibson D, Wade J. Self-reported sleep and mood disturbance in chronic pain patients. Clin J Pain 1998; 14: 311–14.

58. Ohayon MM. Specific characteristics of the pain/depression association in the general population. J Clin Psychiatry 2004; 65: 5–9.

59. Smith MT, Edwards RR, Robinson RC, Dworkin RH. Suicidal ideation, plans, and attempts in chronic pain patients: factors associated with increased risk. Pain 2004; 111: 201–8.

60. Smith MT, Perlis ML, Haythornthwaite JA. Suicidal ideation in outpatients with chronic musculoskeletal pain: an exploratory study of the role of sleep onset insomnia and pain intensity. Clin J Pain 2004; 20: 111–18.

61. Nicholson B, Verma S. Comorbidities in chronic neuropathic pain. Pain Med 2004; 5(Suppl 1): S9–S27.

62. Thieme K, Turk DC, Flor H. Comorbid depression and anxiety in fibromyalgia syndrome: relationship to somatic and psychosocial variables. Psychosom Med 2004; 66: 837–44.

63. Badley EM, Kasman NM. The impact of arthritis on Canadian women. BMC Womens Health 2004; 4: 1–10.

64. Lavigne GJ, McMillan D, Zucconi M. Pain and sleep. In: Kryger MH, Roth T, Dement WC, eds. Principles and Practice of Sleep Medicine, 4th edn. Philadelphia, PA: Elsevier/Saunders, 2005: 1246–55.

65. Affleck G, Urrows S, Tennen H, Higgins P, Abeles M. Sequential daily relations of sleep, pain intensity, and attention to pain among women with fibromyalgia. Pain 1996; 68: 363–68.

66. Schweitzer PK. Drugs that disturb sleep and wakefulness. In: Kryger MH, Roth T, Dement WC, eds. Principles and Practice of Sleep Medicine. Philadelphia, PA: Elsevier/Saunders, 2005: 499–518.

67. Raymond I, Ancoli-Israel S, Choiniere M. Sleep disturbances, pain and analgesia in adults hospitalized for burn injuries. Sleep Med 2004; 5: 551–59.

68. Mahowald MW, Mahowald SR, Bundlie SR, Ytterberg SR. Sleep fragmentation in rheumatoid arthritis. Arthritis Rheum 1989; 32: 974–83.

69. Moldofsky H, Scarisbrick P. Induction of neurasthenic musculoskeletal pain syndrome by selective sleep stage deprivation. Psychosom Med 1976; 38: 35–44.

70. Older SA, Battafarano DF, Danning CL, et al. The effects of delta wave sleep interruption on pain thresholds and fibromyalgia like symptoms in healthy subjects; correlations with insulin like growth factor I. J Rheumatol 1998; 25: 1180–6.

71. Smith RP, Veale D, Pepin JL, Levy PA. Obstructive sleep apnea and the autonomic nervous system. Sleep Med Rev 1998; 2: 69–92.

72. de Leeuw R, Studts JL, Carlson CR. Fatigue and fatigue-related symptoms in an orofacial pain

population. Oral Surg Oral Med Oral Pathol Oral Radiol Endod 2005; 99: 168–74.

73. Kewman DG, Vaishampayan N, Zald D, Han B. Cognitive impairment in musculoskeletal pain patients. Int J Psychiat Med 1991; 21: 253–62.

74. Landro NI, Stiles TC, Sletvold H. Memory functioning in patients with primary fibromyalgia and major depression and healthy controls. J Psychosom Res 1997; 42: 297–306.

75. Côté KA, Moldofsky H. Sleep, daytime symptoms, and cognitive performance in patients with fibromyalgia. J Rheumatol 1997; 24: 2014–23.

76. Mahowald ML, Mahowald MW. Nighttime sleep and daytime functioning (sleepiness and fatigue) in less well-defined chronic rheumatic diseases with particular reference to the 'alpha-delta NREM sleep anomaly'. Sleep Med 2000; 1(3): 195–207.

77. Moldofsky H, MacFarlane JG. Fibromyalgia and chronic fatigue syndromes. In: Kryger MH, Roth T, Dement WC, eds. Principles and Practice of Sleep Medicine. Philadelphia, PA: Elsevier/ Saunders, 2005: 1225–36.

78. Montplaisir J. Neurologic disorders. In: Kryger MH, Roth T, Dement WC, eds. Principles and Practice of Sleep Medicine. Philadelphia, PA: Elsevier/Saunders, 2005 Section 10: 761–888.

79. Engleman H, Joffe D. Neuropsychological function in obstructive sleep apnea. Sleep Med Rev 1999; 3: 59–78.

80. Chapman S. The effects of opioids on driving ability in patients with chronic pain. APS Bulletin 2001; 11: 5–9.

81. Alvarez FJ, del Rio MC. Medicinal drugs and driving: from research to clinical practice. Trends Pharmacol Sci 2002; 23(9): 441–3.

82. Vester JC, Veldhuijzen DS, Volkerts ER. Residual effects of sleep medication on driving ability. Sleep Med Rev 2004; 8: 309–25.

83. Howard ME, Desai AV, Grunstein RR, et al. Sleepiness, sleep-disordered breathing, and accident risk factors in commercial vehicle drivers. Am J Respir Crit Care Med 2004; 179(9): 927–28.

84. Berger A, Dukes EM, Oster G. Clinical characteristics and economic costs of patients with painful neuropathic disorders. J Pain 2004; 5: 143–9.

85. Brunelli B, Gorson KC. The use of complementary and alternative medicines by patients with peripheral neuropathy. J Neurol Sci 2004; 218: 59–66.

86. Gureje O, Von Korff M.; Simon GE, Gater, R. Persistent pain and well–being: a World Health Organization Study in Primary Care. J Am Med Assoc 1998; 280: 147–51.

87. Andersen OK, Sonnenborg FA, Arendt-Nielsen L. Modular organization of human leg withdrawal reflexes elicited by electrical stimulation of the foot sole. Muscle Nerve 1999; 22: 1520–30.

88. Martin SA, Aikens JE, Chervin RD. Toward cost effectiveness analysis in the diagnosis and treatment of insomnia. Sleep Med Rev 2004; 8: 63–72.

89. Berry PH, Chapman CR, Covington EC. Pain: current understanding of assessment, management and treatments (monograph). Oakbrook Terrace; Joint Commission on Accreditation of Healthcare Organizations, 2001.

90. Penrod JR, Bernatsky S, Adam V, et al. Health services costs and their determinants in women with fibromyalgia. J Rheumatol 2004; 31: 1391–8.

91. Martinez JE, Ferraz MB, Sato EI, Atra E. Fibromyalgia versus rheumatoid arthritis: a longitudinal comparison of the quality of life. J Rheumatol 1995; 22: 270–4.

92. Wiesmann J, Deyo R. Back pain: epidemiologic data. APS Bulletin 1993; 14: 23.

93. Wolfe F. Rheumatoid arthritis and osteoarthritis. APS Bulletin 1994; 15: 22.

94. Mathias SD, Kuppermann M, Liberman RF, Lipschutz RC, Steege JF. Chronic pelvic pain: prevalence, health-related quality of life, and economic correlates. Obstet Gynecol 1996; 87: 321–7.

95. Maniadakis N, Gray A. The economic burden of back pain in the UK. Pain 2000; 84(1): 95–103.

96. Stewart WF, Ricci JA, Chee E, Morganstein D, Lipton R. Lost productive time and cost due to common pain conditions in the US workforce. J Am Med Assoc 2003; 290: 2443–54.

97. Ghodse H. Pain, anxiety and insomnia - a global perspective on the relief of suffering: comparative review. Br J Psychiatry 2003; 183: 15–21.

98. Bennett R. Management and outcomes of different treatment modalities in fibromyalgia. In: Carr DB, Novak G, Rathmell GP, Reuben SS, eds. The Spectrum of Pain. New York: McMahon Publishing Group, 2004: 86–102.

99. Goulet JP, Lavigne GJ, Lund JP. Jaw pain prevalence among French-speaking Canadians in

Québec and related symptoms of temporo-mandibular disorders. J Dent Res 1995; 74: 1738–44.

100. Dao TTT, Reynolds WJ, Tenenbaum HC. Comorbidity between myofascial pain of the masticatory muscles and fibromyalgia. J Orofacial Pain 1997; 11: 232–41.

101. Abenhaim L, Suissa S. Importance and economic burden of occupational back pain: a study of 2500 cases representative of Quebec. J Occup Med 1987; 29: 670–74.

102. Rotem AY, Sperber AD, Krugliak P, et al. Polysomnographic and actigraphic evidence of sleep fragmentation in patients with irritable bowel syndrome. Sleep 2003; 26: 747–52.

103. Haim A, Pillar G, Pecht A, et al. Sleep patterns in children and adolescents with functional recurrent abdominal pain: objective versus subjective assessment. Acta Paediatr 2004; 93: 677–80.

104. Morin CM. Psychological and behavioral treatments for primary insomnia. In: Kryger HM, Roth T, Dement WC, eds. Principles and practice of Sleep Medicine. Philadelphia, PA: Elsevier/Saunders, 2005: 726–37.

105. Moore P, Dimsdale JE. Opioids, sleep, and cancer-related fatigue. Med Hypoth 2002; 58: 77–82.

106. Gagnon Y, Mayer P, Morisson F, Rompré PH, Lavigne GJ. Aggravation of sleep apnea by the use of occlusal splint in apneic patients: a pilot study. Int J Prosthodont 2004; 17: 447–53.

CHAPTER 15

Sleep apnea and stroke

Henry Yaggi and Vahid Mohsenin

Stroke ranks as the second leading cause of death world wide, and it is the leading cause of disability among adults.[1] Therefore, understanding underlying pathophysiology, promoting preventative behaviors, and developing novel therapeutic approaches for stroke is of crucial importance. Understanding the link between obstructive sleep apnea and stroke may represent one such novel approach. Recent studies indicate that sleep apnea may serve as an independent risk factor for the development of stroke and therapy for sleep apnea may help to reduce cardiovascular and cerebrovascular risk.

The primary objective of this chapter is to explore the relationship between sleep apnea and stroke by critically reviewing the current literature. First, epidemiologic studies will be analyzed with respect to issues regarding the strength of the association, and the consistency of the association using different study designs and different populations. Next, the biologic plausibility of the relationship will be explored by reviewing studies that examine the pathophysiology of sleep apnea and stroke. Subsequently, studies exploring the therapeutic impact of sleep apnea on stroke and cardiovascular risk will be reviewed. Finally, public health implications will be discussed.

SLEEP-DISORDERED BREATHING AND STROKE

Snoring and stroke

Early epidemiologic studies that examined the relationship between sleep-disordered breathing and cerebrovascular disease used self-reported snoring as the primary exposure variable. The majority of these studies clearly show an association between snoring and stroke. They also demonstrate that the strength of this association is similar to traditional risk factors for stroke such as hypertension, smoking, atrial fibrillation, and hypercholesterolemia. Furthermore, even when adjusted for confounding risk factors such as obesity, hypertension, age, and gender, there remained an independent association between snoring and stroke. The designs of these initial studies were predominantly case-control or cross-sectional[2-9] and subject to recall bias. An additional limitation was their ability to establish the temporal relationship between stroke and sleep apnea, because snoring and sleep apnea can be a consequence of stroke.[10]

More convincing evidence comes from several large prospective studies, which corroborate these case-control and cross-sectional studies. In an early cohort study exclusively of men, using a Finnish nationwide registry, there was a two-fold increase in the relative risk for the combined outcome of stroke and ischemic heart disease in habitual snorers compared to non-snorers.[3] A smaller but still significant positive association (relative risk = 1.33) between regular snoring and the combined cardiovascular outcome of stroke and ischemic heart disease was seen in women in the Nurses Health Study.[9]

Sleep apnea and stroke

Overnight polysomnography is considered the gold standard diagnostic test to evaluate the presence of sleep apnea. A number of cross-sectional and case-control studies[11–16] have used overnight polysomnography in order to define sleep apnea more precisely in an attempt to sort out whether it is the minority of patients with sleep apnea who account for the apparent increased risk of snoring with stroke (Table 15.1). These studies were largely performed in patients with pre-existing stroke, and consistently demonstrate a high prevalence of sleep apnea in stroke (60–90%), significantly higher than that seen in the general population of North American adults (3–28%).[17]

One study demonstrating the association between sleep-disordered breathing and cerebrovascular disease comes from the cross-sectional results of Sleep Heart Health Study.[16] This community based study explored the association between sleep-disordered breathing and prevalent self-reported cardiovascular disease, (myocardial infarction, angina, coronary revascularization procedures, heart failure, or stroke) in a large cohort of 6,424 individuals who underwent unattended overnight polysomnography at home. With respect to stroke, there was a significant association (odds ratio = 1.58; 95% confidence interval 1.02–2.46) between patients with an apnea-hypopnea index (AHI) > 11.0 and prevalent cerebrovascular events increasing to odds ratio of 1.80 for patients with more moderate to severe sleep apnea. Indeed, in a trend analysis, increasing severity of sleep apnea was associated with increasing odds for cardiovascular disease and stroke (Figure 15.1).

An inarguable criterion for causal inference is that exposure must precede the onset of the disease. Though in general, case-control and cross-sectional studies are efficient study designs for evaluating strength of association, they have a significant limitation in their ability to establish the temporal course in a cause-and-effect relationship. Such study designs might reflect reverse causal pathways, whereby sleep-disordered breathing has been the consequence rather than the cause of stroke. Indeed, several case reports of sleep apnea after bulbar stroke have been reported in the literature.[10,18,19] Furthermore, the pharyngeal muscles may be affected in hemispheric stroke as dysphagia has been demonstrated in 30% to 40% of patients admitted to the hospital with unilateral hemispheric stroke.[20] However, in the absence of a sleep study demonstrating sleep apnea preceding the stroke, it is difficult to be certain that sleep apnea is a consequence of the stroke. The direction of this arrow of causation can ultimately only be definitively determined by analysis of incident cerebrovascular disease events.

Recently, prospective observational cohort studies have clarified this temporal relationship and have demonstrated that sleep apnea increases the risk for stroke,[21,22] stroke and all-cause-mortality,[23] and fatal and nonfatal cardiovascular events.[24] Arzt et al peformed cross-sectional and longitudinal analyses on 1,475 and 1,189 subjects, respectively, from the general population. In the cross-sectional analyses, subjects with an AHI ≥ 20 had increased odds for stroke (odds ratio = 4.33; 95% confidence interval, 1.32–14.24; $P = 0.02$) compared with those without sleep-disordered breathing (AHI < 5) after adjustment for known confounding factors. In the prospective analysis, sleep-disordered breathing with an AHI ≥ 20 was associated with an increased risk of suffering a first ever stroke over the next four years (unadjusted odds

Table 15.1 Selected studies of sleep apnea and stroke using polysomnography

Study	Study Design	n(patients)/ n(controls)	Mean Rdi	Study Population	Confounding Assessment	Prevalence Sleep apnea in Stroke (%)
Mohsenin[11]	Case-control	10/10	52	Predominantly hemispheric stroke in a rehabilitation unit	Age, BMI, hypertension, smoking	80% with RDI ≥20
Lavie[32]	Descriptive	47 (19 underwent PSG)	NA	Rehabilitation patients recently hospitalized for stroke	NA	32% had ≥10 desaturation events/hr based on computerized overnight oximetry
Dyken[12]	Case-control	24/19	26	Recently hospitalized for stroke	Age, gender	71% with RDI ≥10
Bassetti[13,14]	Case-control	128/25 (80 underwent PSG)	28	Inpatients with stroke and TIA	Age, BMI, diabetes, severity of stroke	63% with RDI ≥10
Para[15]	Descriptive	161	21	Inpatients with stroke and TIA	NA	71% with RDI ≥10 *('Acute Phase') 61% with RDI ≥10 ('stable phase')
Shahar[16]	Cross-sectional (Sleep Heart Health Study)	6,424	NA (see text)	Assembled from several ongoing population based studies of CVD in the United States	Age, race, gender, smoking, diabetes, hypertension, BMI, cholesterol	NA (see text) *RR of stroke comparing lowest quartile to highest quartile = 1.58 with 95% CI (1.02–2.46)

RDI indicates respiratory disturbance index which is the # of apneas + hyporpneas /hour of sleep; BMI indicates body mass index, PSG indicates polysomnography; NA indicates not applicable; TIA indicates transient ischemic attack; * 'acute phase' after admission and 'stable phase' indicates >3 months later; RR indicates relative risk.

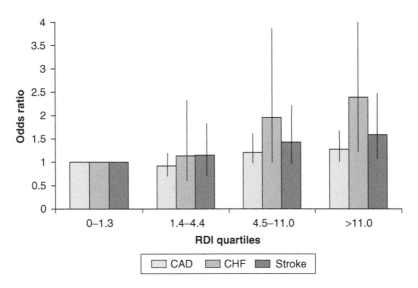

Figure 15.1 Adjusted relative odds ratios of coronary artery disease (CAD, $P=0.004$), congestive heart failure (CHF, $P=0.002$) and stroke ($P=0.03$) as a function of severity of sleep apnea expressed as quartiles of respiratory disturbance index (RDI). The P values are for the linear trend across quartiles I through IV based on a parsimonious model, which included age, race, sex, smoking status, self-reported diabetes, total cholesterol, and high-density lipoprotein cholesterol. The bars denote 95% confidence intervals. Adapted from.[16]

ratio = 4.31; 95% confidence interval, 1.31–14.15; $P=0.02$). However, after adjustment for age, sex, and body mass index, the odds ratio was still elevated, but was no longer significant (3.08; 95% confidence interval, 0.74–12.81; $P=0.12$). In part this may be due to the limited total number of stroke events in the cohort (14 participants suffered a first ever stroke event).

Our work revealed that after excluding prevalent stroke, sleep apnea was associated with the composite endpoint of transient ischemic attack (TIA), stroke, or all cause mortality (hazard ratio = 2.24; 95% confidence interval 1.30–3.86; $P=0.004$). After adjustment for age, gender, race, smoking status, alcohol consumption, body mass index, diabetes mellitus, hyperlipidemia, atrial fibrillation, and hypertension (which may itself be on the causal pathway), sleep apnea retained a statistically significant association

with stroke or death (hazard ratio = 1.97; 95% confidence interval 1.12–3.48; $P=0.01$). In a trend analysis, increasing severity of sleep apnea at baseline was associated with an increased risk for the development of the composite endpoint ($P=0.005$).[23] Those patients in the highest severity quartile of the cohort (AHI > 36) had a greater than three-fold increased risk for the devlopment of stroke or death. A similar magnitude of risk has recently been described in a population based cohort of elderly patients where severe sleep apnea (AHI ≥ 30) more than doubled the risk of ischemic stroke, even after adjustment for traditional cerebrovascular risk factors (hazard ratio = 2.52; 95% confidence interval 1.04–6.01).[22] Therefore, the assocation between sleep apnea and stroke is of the same order of magnitude as other traditional cardiovascular risk factors, which has been consistently observed using different study design and

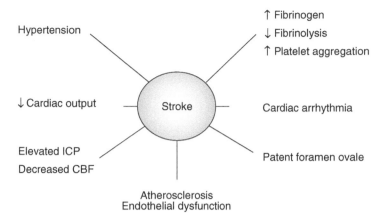

Figure 15.2 Mechanisms underlying the complications of obstructive sleep apnea.

in different populations. Furthermore, the risk of stroke appears to increase with increasing severity of sleep apnea. Taken together, these data point towards sleep apnea as a novel and independent cerebrovascular risk factor. This implies that there are mechanisms unique to sleep apnea that confer cerebrovascular risk which are subsequently discussed below.

PATHOPHYSIOLOGIC MECHANISMS OF STROKE IN SLEEP APNEA

There are likely multiple mechanisms whereby sleep apnea may lead to the development of stroke. During sleep apnea, repetitive episodes of airway occlusion result in hypoxemia, hypercapnia, significant changes in intrathoracic pressure, and arousals from sleep. Consequently, this elicits inflammatory, autonomic, hemodynamic, coagulopathic, and metabolic processes that serve as plausible mechanisms whereby sleep apnea may lead to stroke (Figure 15.2).

Inflammation

Systemic inflammation plays an important role in the development of atherosclerosis. Indeed,

C-reactive protein (CRP), an important marker of inflammation, is also a strong predictor of future atherosclerotic events.[25] CRP levels have been shown to be increased in patients with sleep apnea compared to obesity matched controls. CRP levels rise with increasing severity of sleep apnea and decrease with CPAP treatment.[26]

The pathogenesis of inflammation and atherosclerosis in sleep apnea has not been entirely elucidated, but intermittent hypoxia followed by re-oxygenation (common to sleep apnea) appears to play a key role. A higher frequency of repetitive oxygen desaturations has been correlated with increasing severity of atherosclerosis.[27] In a cell culture model, repetitive episodes of hypoxia and re-oxygenation resulted in selective activation of vascular inflammatory pathways (mediated by transcription factor nuclear factor kappa B (NFκB) over adaptive hypoxia inducible factor-1 (HIF-1)-dependent pathways. This suggests different molecular responses to intermittent hypoxia than to sustained hypoxia, which may in part explain the different cardiovascular outcomes in conditions with sustained hypoxia as a predominant feature as compared to sleep apnea.

Experimental evidence has also linked hypoxia with atherosclerosis through other pathways of oxidative stress. It is suggested that intermittent hypoxia promotes the formation of reactive oxygen species (ROS), particularly during the re-oxygenation period, which can be deleterious to cells (e.g., endothelial cells, leukocytes, and platelets). These cells express adhesion molecules (ICAM-1, VCAM-1, IL-8, and MCP-1) and pro-inflammatory cytokines that may lead to endothelial injury and dysfunction and consequently to atherosclerosis.[28–33]

Nocturnal sympathetic activation

Sympathetic overactivity in the pathogenesis of cardiovascular and cerebrovascular complications in obstructive sleep apnea has been suggested for several years and evidence continues to accumulate. Early reports found increased plasma and urinary catecholamine levels in patients with sleep apnea[34] and a fall of these levels after treatment with tracheostomy.[35] Others employed more direct measures of sympathetic nerve activity through the use of a tungsten microelectrode in the peroneal nerve. This methodology demonstrated increased sympathetic nerve activity following acute apneic events.[36] Superimposed on these bursts of sympathetic activation are 'surges' of blood pressure of up to 240 mm Hg at apnea termination (Figure 15.3). These acute blood pressure elevations during apnea appear to be driven by changes in baroreceptor sensitivity during sleep and chemoreceptor responses to progressive hypoxia.[37] Considering that humans typically spend one third of their lives sleeping, these nocturnal increases in blood pressure might in themselves contribute to hypertensive cardiovascular and cerebrovascular consequences. Indeed, patients with sleep apnea commonly do not have the normal nocturnal fall or 'dipping' in blood pressure.[38,39] Among patients with hypertension, those who exhibit a diminished nocturnal decline in blood pressure 'non-dippers',[40] have been reported to have more cardiovascular target organ damage than dippers[41,42] including silent cerebrovascular damage.[43] Three longitudinal studies conducted in patients with hypertension have confirmed that a diminished nocturnal decline in blood pressure predicted cardiovascular

events[44,45] including a worse stroke prognosis.[46] Moreover, diminished nocturnal decline of blood pressure is a risk factor for cardiovascular mortality independent of overall blood pressure load during a 24 hour period, with 5% decrease in nocturnal dipping being associated with a 20% increase in cardiovascular mortality.[47] Furthermore, the normal morning circadian pattern peak occurrence of stroke and vascular events[48] appears to be inverted in patients with sleep apnea. Patients with obstructive sleep apnea have a peak in sudden cardiac death during the sleeping hours from midnight to 6.00 a.m.[49]

Sleep apnea as a cause of diurnal hypertension

In addition to acute blood pressure swings at night, epidemiologic evidence strongly supports that sustained diurnal hypertension can arise from obstructive apnea. Lugaressi et al, described a strong correlation between snoring and hypertension, even when controlling for body weight.[50] More recently, from the Sleep Heart Health Study,[51] sleep apnea was associated with prevalent hypertension even after controlling for potential confounders such as age, gender, body mass index (BMI and other measures of adiposity), alcohol, and smoking. The relative risk for the highest category of respiratory disturbance index (RDI >30 events per hour) compared with the lowest category (<1.5 events per hr) was 1.37 (95% confidence interval, 1.03–1.83). Overall, the odds of hypertension appeared to increase with increases in RDI in a dose-response fashion. Furthermore, in the prospective study of the Wisconsin Sleep Cohort the presence of sleep apnea at baseline was accompanied by a substantially increased risk for future hypertension at four-year follow-up.[52] Even after adjusting for baseline hypertension status, age, gender, BMI, waist and neck circumference, weekly alcohol and cigarette use, the risk was elevated with an odds ratio of 2.89 (95% confidence interval 1.46–5.64) for subjects with an RDI >15 compared to those without apnea. Indeed, the most recent report, Seventh

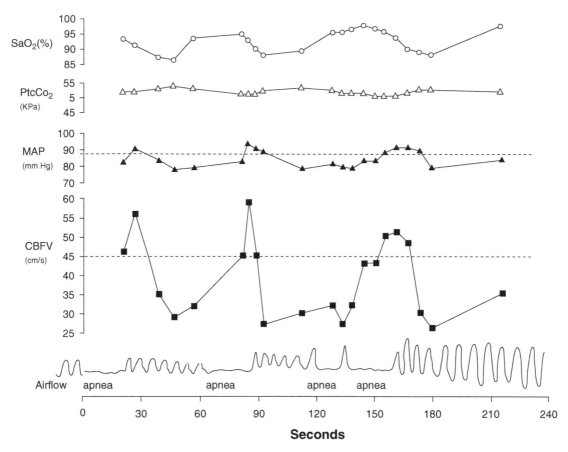

Figure 15.3 Simultaneous recordings of arterial oxygen saturation (SaO_2), transcutaneous arterial PCO_2 ($P_{tc}CO_2$), mean arterial blood pressure (MAP), cerebral blood flow velocity (CBFV) and respiratory airflow during sleep in a patient with obstructive sleep apnea. The recording shows prolonged periods of low CBFV compared to baseline (dashed line) during the obstructive apnea with a steep rise at the end of the apnea paralleling rises in MAP. Adapted from.[60]

Report of the Joint Committee on Prevention, Detection, Evaluation, and Treatment of High Blood Pressure (JCN 7) recognizes the etiologic role of sleep apnea as an identifiable cause of hypertension.[53]

Cardiac arrhythmia

Cardiac arrhythmia is a known cause of stroke. Sleep apnea is associated with cardiac arrhythmias, conduction abnormalities such as second-degree atrioventricular block,[54] and potentially life threatening arrhythmias such as ventricular tachycardia.[55] Sleep apnea has also been specifically associated with atrial fibrillation.[56–58] In a population of 81 patients with stable heart failure, atrial fibrillation was approximately four times higher in heart failure patients with sleep apnea than in those without.[56] The authors speculated that the increased right heart afterload due to hypoxic vasoconstriction and pulmonary hypertension might have been responsible in part for this excess frequency of atrial fibrillation. Indeed, sleep apnea is significantly more prevalent in patients with atrial fibrillation than in high-risk patients with multiple other cardiovascular diseases. Moreover, patients with untreated sleep apnea have a higher recurrence of atrial fibrillation after cardioversion than patients without sleep apnea.[57] This association with atrial fibrillation and the risk of cardioembolic stroke with this arrhythmia, provides another potential mechanism whereby sleep apnea increases the risk for stroke.

Mechanical load: cerebral hemodynamics, shunting through a patent foramen ovale

Marked changes in cerebral blood flow and intracranial pressure occur during individual episodes of obstructive sleep apnea. Several studies have attempted to gain insight into changes in cerebral blood flow by measuring middle cerebral artery blood flow velocities non-invasively, using transcranial Doppler ultrasonography in direct relation to individual obstructive apneic events.[59–62] Most of these studies consistently showed an increase in cerebral blood flow velocity during the apnea, with a steep rise at the end of the apnea paralleling rises in systemic mean arterial pressure, followed by a subsequent decrease of almost 25% below baseline after apnea termination. It has been suggested that these apnea induced cerebral blood flow velocity changes occur despite cerebral autoregulation, which must have been overridden by such rapid and high amplitude systemic arterial blood pressure changes.

Several physiologic mechanisms may be responsible for the changes of cerebral blood flow during sleep apnea. Large negative intrathoracic pressures during obstructive apneas (as low as -80 cm H_2O pressure have been reported)[63] result in increased central venous volume. At the termination of apnea, intracranial pressure rises rapidly because of increased central venous volume and the absence of valves in the veins between the brain and the heart. In

addition, as noted previously, large blood pressure surges occur at the termination of the apnea, which may affect cerebral perfusion pressure thus increasing intracranial pressure. Finally, apneas are associated with hypoxic and hypercapnic cerebral vasodilation causing a further increase of the intracranial blood volume. The mechanical effects of increased intracranial pressure with impedance to cerebral blood flow as well as concomitant hypoxemia may predispose to cerebral ischemia.[64]

In subjects with ischemic stroke, the prevalence of patent foramen ovale (PFO) is approximately 20–54%.[65] It is thought that a PFO can potentially give rise to ischemic stroke by means of paradoxical embolism.

Transient right sided pressure elevations occur during obstructive sleep apneas permitting right to left shunting through PFO. In a study by Beelke et al., 10 patients with sleep apnea and PFO (but only detectable during Valsalva maneuver) underwent transcranial Doppler ultrasonography with injection of agitated saline solution. Right to left shunting was present in 9 out of 10 subjects and only appeared during obstructive apneas lasting greater than 17 seconds. No right to left shunting was detected during normal breathing and during wakefulness.[66] This finding is important, in view of the increased prevalence of PFO in patients with sleep apnea.[67]

Abnormal coagulation

Sleep apnea may act through multiple mechanisms to predispose to acute thrombosis and thus cardiovascular and cerebrovascular events. Platelets play a key role in ischemic cerebrovascular disease and increases in platelet aggregability and activation have been demonstrated in patients with sleep apnea,[68–73] which improves with CPAP.[68,73] The mechanism for increased platelet reactivity in patients with sleep apnea is quite possibly the cyclic hypoxemia, hypercapnia, and catecholamine surges that are part of sleep apnea and have also been reported to cause platelet activation.[34,35,74] In one study, the arousal index was the independent factor best associated with baseline platelet activation supporting a pathophysiologic paradigm that of sleep arousal precipitating increased neural activation leading to increased platelet activation.[75] The observation that CPAP reduces platelet activation supports this same paradigm and suggests that treatment intervention for sleep apnea may be cardioprotective. Whether such a benefit of CPAP would be additive to the effects of antiplatelet therapy is not known.

Elevated plasma fibrinogen levels are believed to be associated with increased risk of stroke and other cardiovascular events.[76–81] Plasma fibrinogen is an acute-phase protein that is synthesized in the liver and is intrinsically involved in coagulation enhancing thrombosis and atherosclerosis by effects on platelet aggregation, blood vessel wall, and endothelial cell injury.[82,83] Patients with sleep apnea have been shown to have increased morning levels of fibrinogen,[84] therefore elevated fibrinogen levels may be one mechanism linking to stroke. Further evidence of the association between sleep apnea and increased fibrinogen levels and stroke comes from a cross-sectional study of 113 stroke patients undergoing neurologic rehabilitation. Fibrinogen level was positively correlated to RDI and length of respiratory events and negatively correlated to minimal and average minimal oxygen saturation measured polysomnographically.[85]

Metabolic dysregulation

There is significant overlap between sleep apnea and the cluster of cardiovascular risk factors that constitutes the metabolic syndrome. In fact, there is accumulating evidence to suggest that sleep loss (in the form of sleep restriction or disrupted sleep from sleep disordered breathing) may worsen these metabolic abnormalities. Sleep curtailment has been linked to impaired carbohydrate tolerance and insulin resistance,[86] type 2 diabetes,[87] decreased leptin levels, elevated

ghrelin levels, and increased hunger and appetite, which may lead to obesity.[88] In addition, a number of reports have found the presence of insulin resistance, impaired glucose tolerance, and dyslipidemia independent of body weight.[89] It remains to be determined whether sleep apnea is independently linked to the development of type 2 diabetes and whether treatment with CPAP may reduce this risk.

THERAPY FOR SLEEP APNEA AND IMPACT ON CEREBROVASCULAR RISK

Ethical considerations

Compared with control, CPAP (the main medical therapy for sleep apnea) shows significant improvements in objective and subjective measures of sleepiness, quality of life, and cognitive function.[90] CPAP has also been demonstrated to improve left ventricular function in patients with congestive heart failure and sleep apnea,[91] reduce twenty four hour systolic blood pressure,[92–94] and decrease automobile accidents.[95] Thus, ethical considerations have been raised with respect to the conducting of long-term controlled trials in which symptomatic patients with sleep apnea are randomly assigned to not receiving treatment. To date, no published prospective randomized controlled trials have demonstrated that the treatment of sleep apnea decreases the risk of stroke, in terms of either primary or secondary prevention. However, several longitudinal observational cohort studies have attempted to evaluate the impact of therapy on cardiovascular outcomes in patients with sleep apnea.

Long-term observational studies

An early study that gives some insight into the impact of treatment of sleep apnea on the risk of myocardial infarction and stroke was a retrospective cohort study of patients who were diagnosed with sleep apnea with polysomnography in the 1970s, prior to the availability of CPAP. At this time, the only known definitive therapy for sleep apnea consisted of tracheostomy.[96] Here, seven years of follow-up was provided on 198 patients, of which 71 patients received tracheostomy (considered 'effective treatment') and 127 received 'conservative treatment' consisting of recommended weight loss (the only alternative). Any new hypertension, myocardial infarction or stroke occurring since the original polysomnography was considered the main vascular morbidity outcome. Despite the fact that at study entry the tracheostomy group included more patients with a history of hypertension, myocardial infarction or stroke, it was the conservatively treated group which developed considerably more vascular morbidity.

More recently, prospective observational cohorts designed to examine the impact of treatment on long-term cardiovascular outcomes in patients with sleep apnea have demonstrated that CPAP therapy may reduce mortality in severe sleep apnea,[97] and protect against death from cardiovascular disease.[98] In a study conducted by Marin et al,[24] the incidence of fatal and nonfatal cardiovascular events was highest in patients with severe untreated sleep apnea. Patients who received and complied with CPAP (who largely had severe sleep apnea) had a significantly reduced cardiovascular risk, suggesting that long-term therapy with CPAP may reduce risk of fatal and nonfatal cardiovascular events. However, all of the above studies were long-term observational cohorts and not randomized controlled trials, and the observed risk reductions may also be that those patients who used CPAP were also complying with other medical therapy and otherwise leading healthier lifestyles.

Short-term randomized controlled trials with CPAP

With respect to cardiovascular outcomes, short-term (up to 3 months) randomized controlled trials have been published looking at arterial blood pressure as the outcome. Though the studies vary with respect to the magnitude of blood pressure reduction, overall there appears to be a clinically important blood pressure reduction in both 24 hour systolic and diastolic pressures, similar in magnitude to the use of antihypertensive therapy. The characteristics of the patients selected for these trials give clues to those most and least likely to gain any blood pressure lowering benefits. In general, those more likely to experience benefit have more severe and symptomatic sleep apnea, are hypertensive or on hypertensive therapy at baseline, receive more effective therapy for sleep apnea (longer use), and have more frequent oxygen desaturations.[92–94] Those less likely to experience benefit are normotensive at baseline, asymptomatic, and have more mild sleep apnea.[99,100] A recent systematic literature review conducted by the Cochrane Collaboration[90] found that mean 24 hour systolic and diastolic pressures were significantly lower on CPAP (−7.24 mm Hg systolic, −3.07 mm Hg diastolic). When extrapolated to antihypertensive epidemiologic data, such blood pressure lowering effects would be predicted to reduce stroke risk by 35% and coronary heart disease event risk by 20%.[94,101]

CPAP treatment in stroke

The question then arises whether CPAP treatment in stroke patients with sleep apnea might improve functional outcomes, prognosis, and reduce the risk of recurrent vascular events. There is a significant need for further research in this area, but a few preliminary studies have begun to address these questions and raise important methodologic and logistical issues.

Regarding functional status, a recent randomized controlled trial[102] of patients 2–3 weeks post stroke with severe sleep apnea showed no benefit from 8 weeks of CPAP in physical function assessed at 8 weeks and 6 months. Patients were randomized to receive autotitrating CPAP versus conservative treatment. The investigators caution that a clinically significant benefit from CPAP cannot be ruled out, due to the poor compliance with CPAP in this study (1.4 hours per night).

Indeed, the reported compliance with CPAP in stroke varies widely,[73,103–105] with some reporting compliance rates of 50–70%[103,104] similar to that in the general sleep apnea population, where others report a significantly lower compliance (10–15%).[73,105] This variation is likely to reflect differences in patient selection, environment in which the treatment is given, the CPAP system used, and the amount and type of support and training. Difficulties with CPAP adherence in stroke include the common problems of mask fit, tolerance, and upper airway symptoms compounded by the functional and cognitive disability of stroke such as facial palsy, paralysis, and confusion.[102] Aphasia, severity of motor disability, and depression predict decreased compliance,[102,104] suggesting that compliance may be improved in future studies by focusing on less depressed, and less cognitively and functionally impaired patients, but this may limit generalizability. However, given the high prevalence of sleep apnea in stroke (60–90%),[11–16] even CPAP compliance rates of 30–50% could potentially benefit up to one third of all stroke patients. Given the same high prevalence of sleep apnea in TIA[14] some have suggested that patients with TIA would be a population likely to benefit from CPAP[106] by reducing the risk of recurrent vascular events. As obstructive apneas result in recurrent hypoxemia and cerebral blood flow fluctuations that could damage the area of the acute ischemic penumbra, whether treatment of sleep apnea in the setting of acute stroke results in reduced stroke severity and progression. (it as to remains another important unanswered question).

No randomized controlled trials have been published regarding the secondary prophylaxis of CPAP with respect to recurrent stroke, though a recent observational cohort[107] suggests a potential benefit. In this 18-month prospective study of patients with sleep apnea (AHI ≥20) two–months post–stroke, patients who tolerated CPAP (used the device for at least 4 hours per night during at least 70% of follow-up nights) had a significantly reduced risk of recurrent vascular events. As with other observational cohort studies examining the impact of treatment,[24,97,98] compliance with CPAP may also indicate compliance with other healthier lifestyle habits.

Controlled trials examining the impact of CPAP on stroke severity in acute stroke and recurrent vascular events in 'stable' stroke (secondary prophylaxis) are greatly needed. Such studies will need to address the important methodologic and logistical issues including determining the optimal timing of the initiation of CPAP treatment post–stroke. Regarding treatment in acute stroke, is an 'all-sleeptime' or simply a 'nocturnal-sleeptime' the preferable dosing strategy? Is use of CPAP safe in acute stroke? What strategies can be used to maximize adherence in stroke patients with cognitive and functional disability? Regarding longer-term secondary prophylaxis trials, what treatment allocation schemes will provide robust comparison groups, while simultaneously maintaining ethical standards in not randomizing symptomatic patients with known sleep apnea to receiving no treatment?

Summary and public health implications

Multiple prospective observational cohort studies have demonstrated that obstructive sleep apnea significantly increases the risk of stroke, independent of confounding cerebrovascular risk factors. This implies that there are mechanisms mediated by sleep apnea that confer cerebrovascular risk. The current literature suggests that such mechanisms include: intermittent hypoxia and reoxygenation leading to oxidative stress, systemic inflammation, and atherosclerosis; nocturnal sympathetic activation; diurnal hypertension; cardiac arrythmia (including atrial fibrillation); changes in cerebrol blood flow associated with individual apneas; shunting through PFO; abnormal coagulation; and metabolic dysregulation in the form of insulin resistance and glucose intolerance.

The increasing prevalence of sleep disordered breathing in the population associated with the increasing prevalence of obesity suggests that the population attributable risk percent (the percentage of the total risk of stroke due to sleep apnea) is high, making this an important public health issue. This is particularly true given that sleep apnea is a potentially modifiable risk factor. Indeed recent guidelines from the American Heart Association and American Stroke Association Stroke Council regarding the primary prevention of ischemic stroke recommend 'questioning bed partners and patients, particularly those with abdominal obesity and hypertension, about symptoms of sleep disordered breathing and referring to a sleep specialist as appropriate.'[108]

Short-term randomized controlled trials of CPAP in hypertension and long-term observational cohort studies with follow-up of cerebrovascular and cardiovascular outcomes suggests a clinically significant stroke risk reduction associated with the use of CPAP. However, there are currently no prospective randomized studies demonstrating the efficacy of treating sleep apnea in reducing stroke. Such studies are critical prior to instituting large-scale sleep apnea screening guidelines. Furthermore, evidence suggests that clinical trials assessing the effectiveness of CPAP in improving stroke outcome are warranted from a cost-effectiveness standpoint.[109] In the meantime, clinicians should have a low threshold for evaluating symptoms in their patients consistent with sleep disordered breathing.

REFERENCES

1. Murray C, Lopex A. Mortality by cause for eight regions of the world: Global Burden of Disease Study. Lancet 1997; 349: 1269–76.

2. Partinen M, Palomaki H. Snoring and cerebral infarction. Lancet 1985; 2: 1325–6.

3. Koskenvuo M, Kaprio J, Telakivi T, et al. Snoring as a risk factor for ischaemic heart disease and stroke in men. Br Med J (Clin Res Ed) 1987; 294: 16–9.

4. Spriggs D, French J, Murdy J, Curless R, et al. Snoring increases the risk of stroke and adversely affects prognosis. Q J Med 1992; 83: 555–62.

5. Palomaki H. Snoring and the risk of ischemic brain infarction. Stroke 1991; 22: 1021–5.

6. Smirne S, Palazzi S, Zucconi M, et al. Habitual snoring as a risk factor for acute vascular disease. Eur Respir J 1993; 6: 1357–61.

7. Jennum P, Schultz-Larsen K, Davidsen M, Christensen NJ. Snoring and risk of stroke and ischaemic heart disease in a 70-year-old population. A 6-year follow-up study. Int J Epidemiol 1994; 23: 1159–64.

8. Neau J, Meurice J, Paquereau J, et al. Habitual snoring as a risk factor for brain infarction. Acta Neurol Scand 1995; 92: 63–8.

9. Hu F, Willet W, Manson J, et al. Snoring and the risk of cardiovascular disease in women. J Am Coll Cardiol 2000; 35: 308–13.

10. Askenasy J, Goldhammer I. Sleep apnea as a feature of bulbar stroke. Stroke 1988; 19: 637–9.

11. Mohsenin V, Valor R. Sleep apnea in patients with hemispheric stroke. Arch Phys Med Rehabil 1995; 76: 71–6.

12. Dyken M, Somers V, Yamada T, et al. Investigating the relationship between stroke and obstructive sleep apnea. Stroke 1996; 27: 401–7.

13. Bassetti C, Aldrich M. Sleep apnea in acute cerebrovascular diseases: final report on 128 patients. Sleep 1999; 22: 217–23.

14. Bassetti C, Aldrich M, Chervin R, Quint D. Sleep apnea in patients with transient ischemic attack and stroke: a prospective study of 59 patients. Neurology 1996; 47: 1167–73.

15. Parra O, Arboix A, Bechich S, et al. Time course of sleep-related breathing disorders in first-ever stroke or transient ischemic attack. Am J Respir Crit Care Med 2000; 161: 375–80.

16. Shahar E, Whitney C, Redline S, et al. Sleep-disordered breathing and cardiovascular disease: cross-sectional results of the Sleep Heart Health Study. Am J Respir Crit Care Med 2001; 163: 19–25.

17. Young T, Peppard P, Gottlieb D. Epidemiology of obstructive sleep apnea: a population health

perspective. Am J Respir Crit Care Med 2002; 165: 1217–39.

18. Chaudhary B, Elguindi A, King D. Obstructive sleep apnea after lateral medullary syndrome. South Med J 1982; 75: 65–7.

19. Waller P, Bhopal R. Is snoring a cause of vascular disease? An epidemiological review. Lancet 1989; 1: 143–6.

20. Barer D. The natural history and functional consequences of dysphagia after hemispheric stroke. J Neurol Neurosurg Psychiatry 1989; 52: 236–41.

21. Arzt M, Young T, Finn L, et al. Association of sleep-disordered breathing and the occurrence of stroke. Am J Respir Crit Care Med 2005; 172: 1447–51.

22. Munoz R, Duran-Cantolla J, Martinez-Vila E, et al. Severe sleep apnea and risk of ischemic stroke in the elderly. Stroke 2006; 37: 2317–21.

23. Yaggi H, Concato J, Kernan W, et al. Obstructive sleep apnea as a risk factor for stroke and death. New Engl J Med 2005; 353: 2034–41.

24. Marin JM, Carrizo SJ, Vicente E, Agusti AG. Long-term cardiovascular outcomes in men with obstructive sleep apnoea-hypopnoea with or without treatment with continuous positive airway pressure: an observational study. Lancet 2005; 365(9464): 1046–53.

25. Ridker PM, Hennekens CH, Buring JE, Rifai N. C-reactive protein and other markers of inflammation in the prediction of cardiovascular disease in women. N Engl J Med 2000; 342: 836–43.

26. Yokoe T, Minoguchi K, Matsuo H, et al. Elevated levels of C-reactive protein and interleukin-6 in patients with obstructive sleep apnea syndrome are decreased by nasal continuous positive airway pressure. Circulation 2003; 107: 1129–34.

27. Hayashi M, Fujimoto K, Urushibata K, et al. Nocturnal oxygen desaturation correlates with the severity of coronary atherosclerosis in coronary artery disease. Chest 2003; 124: 936–41.

28. Dyugovskaya L, Lavie P, Lavie L. Increased adhesion molecule expression and production of reactive oxygen species in leukocytes of sleep apnea patients. Am J Respir Crit Care Med 2002; 165: 934–9.

29. El-Solh A, Mador M, Sikka P, et al. Adhesion molecules in patients with coronary artery disease and moderate to severe obstructive sleep apnea. Chest 2002; 121: 1541–7.

30. Ohga E, Nagase T, Tomita T, et al. Increased levels of circulating I-CAM-1, VCAM-1, and L-selectin in obstructive sleep apnea syndrome. J Appl Physiol 1999; 87: 10–4.

31. Lavie L. Obstructive sleep apnoea syndrome: an oxidative stress disorder. Sleep Med Rev 2003; 7: 35–51.

32. Lavie L, Dyugovskaya L, Lavie P. Sleep apnea related intermittent hypoxia and atherogenesis: adhesion molecules and monocytes/endothelial cells interactions. Atherosclerosis 2005; 183: 183–4.

33. Lavie L. Sleep-disordered breathing and cerebrovascular disease: a mechanistic approach. Neurol Clin 2005; 23: 1059–75.

34. Dimsdale J, Coy T, Ziegler M, et al. The effect of sleep apnea on plasma and urinary catecholamines. Sleep 1995; 18: 377–81.

35. Fletcher E, Miller J, Schaaf J. Urinary catecholamines before and after tracheostomy in patients with obstructive sleep apnea and hypertension. Sleep 1987; 10: 35–44.

36. Somers V, Dyken M, Clary M, Abboud F. Sympathetic neural mechanisms in obstructive sleep apnea. J Clin Invest 1995; 96: 1897–904.

37. O'Donnell C, King E, Schwartz A, et al. Relationship between blood pressure and airway obstruction during sleep in the dog. J Appl Physiol 1994; 77: 1819–28.

38. Akashiba T, Minemura H, Yamamoto H, et al. Nasal continuous positive airway pressure changes blood pressure "non-dippers" to "dippers" in patients with obstructive sleep apnea. Sleep 1999; 22: 849–53.

39. Ancoli-Israel S, Stepnowsky C, Dimsdale J, et al. The effect of race and sleep-disordered breathing on nocturnal BP "dipping": analysis in an older population. Chest 2002; 122: 1148–55.

40. O'Brien E, Sheridan J, O'Malley K. Dippers and non-dippers. Lancet 1988; 2(8607): 397.

41. Bianchi S, Bigazzi R, Baldari G, et al. Diurnal variations of blood pressure and microalbuminuria in essential hypertension. Am J Hypertens 1994; 7: 23–9.

42. Verdecchia P, Schillaci G, Guerrieri M. Circadian blood pressure changes and left ventricular hypertrophy. Circulation 1990; 81: 528–36.

43. Shimada K, Kawamoto A, Matsubayashi K, Ozawa T. Silent cerebrovascular disease in the elderly. Correlation with ambulatory pressure. Hypertension 1990; 16: 692–9.

44. Verdecchia P, Porcellati C, Schillaci G, et al. Ambulatory blood pressure. An independent

predictor of prognosis in essential hypertension. Hypertension 1994; 24: 793–801.

45. Staessen JA, Thijs L, Fagard R, et al. Predicting cardiovascular risk using conventional vs ambulatory blood pressure in older patients with systolic hypertension. Systolic Hypertension in Europe Trial Investigators. JAMA 1999; 282: 539–46.

46. Kario K, Pickering TG, Matsuo T, et al. Stroke prognosis and abnormal nocturnal blood pressure falls in older hypertensives. Hypertension 2001; 38: 852–7.

47. Ohkubo T, Hozawa A, Yamaguchi J, et al. Prognostic significance of the nocturnal decline in blood pressure in individuals with and without high 24-h blood pressure: the Ohasama study. J Hypertens 2002; 20: 2183–9.

48. Marler JR, Price TR, Clark GL, et al. Morning increase in onset of ischemic stroke. Stroke 1989; 20: 473–6.

49. Gami AS, Howard DE, Olson EJ, Somers VK. Day-night pattern of sudden death in obstructive sleep apnea. N Engl J Med 2005; 352: 1206–14.

50. Lugaresi E, Cirignotta F, Coccagna G, Piana C. Some epidemiologic data on snoring and cardiocirculatory disturbances. Sleep 1980; 3: 221–4.

51. Neito F, Young T, Lind B, et al. Association of sleep-disordered breathing, sleep anea, and hypertension in a large community based study. JAMA 2000; 283: 1829–36.

52. Peppard P, Young T, Palta M, Skatrud J. Prospective study of the association between sleep-disordered breathing and hypertension. N Engl J Med 2000; 342: 1378–84.

53. Chobanian AV, Bakris GL, Black HR, et al. The Seventh Report of the Joint National Committee on Prevention, Detection, Evaluation, and Treatment of High Blood Pressure: the JNC 7 report. JAMA 2003; 289: 2560–72.

54. Zwillich C, Devlin T, White D, et al. Bradycardia during sleep apnea. Characteristics and mechanism. J Clin Invest 1982; 69: 1286–92.

55. Fichter J, Bauer D, Arampatzis S, et al. Sleep-related breathing disorders are associated with ventricular arrhythmias in patients with an implantable cardioverter defibrillator. Chest 2002; 122: 558–61.

56. Javaheri S, Parker T, Liming J, et al. Sleep apnea in 81 ambulatory male patients with stable heart failure: types and their prevalences, consequences, and presentations. Circulation 1998; 97: 2154–9.

57. Kanagala R, Murali N, Friedman P, et al. Obstructive sleep apnea and the recurrence of atrial fibrillation. Circulation 2003; 107: 2589–94.

58. Gami AS, Pressman G, Caples SM, et al. Association of atrial fibrillation and obstructive sleep apnea. Circulation 2004; 110: 364–7.

59. Siebler M, Nachtmann A. Cerebral hemodynamics in obstructive sleep apnea. Chest 1993; 103: 1118–9.

60. Balfors E, Franklin K. Impairment in cerebral perfusion during obstructive sleep apneas. Am J Respir Crit Care Med 1994; 150: 1587–91.

61. Klingelhofer J, Hajak G, Matzander G, et al. Dynamics of cerebral blood flow velocities during normal human sleep. Clin Neurol Neurosurg 1995; 97: 142–8.

62. Netzer N, Werner P, Jochums I, et al. Blood flow of the middle cerebral artery with sleep-disordered breathing: correlation with obstructive hypopneas. Stroke 1998; 29: 87–93.

63. Shiomi T, Guilleminault C, Stoohs R, Schnittger I. Leftward shift of the intraventricular septum and pulsus paradoxus in obstructive sleep apnea syndrome. Chest 1991; 100: 894–902.

64. Franklin K. Cerebral haemodynamics in obstructive sleep apnoea and Cheyne-Stokes respiration. Sleep Med Rev 2002; 6: 429–41.

65. Lechat P, Mas J, Lascault G, et al. Prevalence of patent foramen ovale in patients with stroke. N Engl J Med 1988; 318: 1148–52.

66. Beelke M, Angeli S, Del Sette M, et al. Obstructive sleep apnea can be provocative for right-to-left shunting through a patent foramen ovale. Sleep 2002; 25: 856–62.

67. Shanoudy H, Soliman A, Raggi P, et al. Prevalence of patent foramen ovale and its contribution to hypoxemia in patients with obstructive sleep apnea. Chest 1998; 113: 91–6.

68. Bokinsky G, Miller M, Ault K, et al. Spontaneous platelet activation and aggregation during obstructive sleep apnea and its response to therapy with nasal continuous positive airway pressure: a preliminary investigation. Chest 1995; 108: 625–30.

69. Eisensehr I, Ehrenberg BL, Noachtar S, et al. Platelet activation, epinephrine, and blood pressure in obstructive sleep apnea syndrome. Neurology 1998; 51: 188–95.

70. Sanner BM, Konermann M, Tepel M, et al. Platelet function in patients with obstructive sleep apnoea syndrome. Eur Resp J 2000; 16: 648–52.

71. Geiser T, Buck F, Meyer BJ, et al. In vivo platelet activation is increased during sleep in patients with obstructive sleep apnea syndrome. Respiration 2002; 69: 229–34.

72. von Kanel R, Dimsdale JE. Hemostatic alterations in patients with obstructive sleep apnea and the implications for cardiovascular disease. Chest 2003; 124: 1956–67.

73. Hui DS, Ko FW, Fok JP, et al. The effects of nasal continuous positive airway pressure on platelet activation in obstructive sleep apnea syndrome. Chest 2004; 125: 1768–75.

74. Wedzicha J, Syndercombe-Court D, Tan K. Increased platelet aggregate formation in patients with chronic airflow obstruction and hypoxemia. Thorax 1991; 46: 504–7.

75. Olson LJ, Olson EJ, Somers VK. Obstructive sleep apnea and platelet activation: another potential link between sleep-disordered breathing and cardiovascular disease. Chest 2004; 126: 339–41.

76. Di Minno G, Mancini M. Measuring plasma fibrinogen to predict stroke and myocardial infarction. Ateriosclerosis 1990; 10: 1–7.

77. Kannel W, Wolf P, Castelli W, D'Agostino R. Fibrinogen and risk of cardiovascular disease: The Framingham Study. JAMA 1987; 258: 1183–6.

78. Meade T, North W, Chakrabarti R, et al. Haemostatic function and cardiovascular death: early results of a prospective study. Lancet 1980: 1050–4.

79. Resch K, Ernst E, Matrai A, Paulsen H. Fibrinogen and viscosity as risk factors for subsequent cardiovascular events in stroke survivors. Ann Intern Med 1992; 117: 371–5.

80. Toss H, Lindhaul B, Siegbahn A, Wallentin L. Prognostic influence of increased fibrinogen and C-reactive protein levels in unstable coronary artery disease. Frisc Study Group. Fragmin during Instability in Coronary Artery Disease. Circulation 1997; 96: 4204–10.

81. Wilhelmsen L, Svardsudd K, Kristoffer K, Larsson B, Wellin L, Tiblin G. Fibrinogen as a risk factor stroke and myocardial infarction. N Engl J Med 1984; 311: 501–5.

82. Eber B, Schumacher M. Fibrinogen: its role in the hemostatic in atherosclerosis. Semin Thromb Hemost 1993; 19: 104–7.

83. Smith E, Keen G, Grant A, Stirk C. Fate of fibrinogen in human arterial inima. Arteriosclerosis 1990; 10: 263–75.

84. Chin K, Ohi M, Kita H, et al. Effects of NCPAP therapy on fibrinogen levels in obstructive sleep apnea syndrome. Am J Respir Crit Care Med 1996; 153: 1972–6.

85. Wessendorf T, Thilmann A, Wang Y, et al. Fibrinogen levels and obstructive sleep apnea in ischemic stroke. Am J Respir Crit Care Med 2000; 162: 2039–42.

86. Spiegel K, Leproult R, Van Cauter E. Impact of sleep debt on metabolic and endocrine function. Lancet 1999; 354: 1435–9.

87. Yaggi HK, Araujo AB, McKinlay JB. Sleep duration as a risk factor for the development of type 2 diabetes. Diabetes Care 2006; 29: 657–61.

88. Spiegel K, Tasali E, Penev P, Van Cauter E. Brief communication: Sleep curtailment in healthy young men is associated with decreased leptin levels, elevated ghrelin levels, and increased hunger and appetite. Ann Intern Med 2004; 141: 846–50.

89. Ip MS, Lam B, Ng MM, et al. Obstructive sleep apnea is independently associated with insulin resistance. Am J Respir Crit Care Med 2002; 165: 670–6.

90. Giles T, Lasserson T, Smith B, et al. Continuous positive airways pressure for obstructive sleep apnoea in adults. Cochrane Database Syst Rev 2006; 3: CD001106.

91. Kaneko Y, Floras J, Usui K, et al. Cardiovascular effects of continuous positive airway pressure in patients with heart failure and obstructive sleep apnea. N Engl J Med 2003; 348: 1233–41.

92. Becker H, Jerrentrup A, Ploch T, et al. Effect of nasal continuous positive airway pressure treatment on blood pressure in patients with obstructive sleep apnea. Circulation 2003; 107: 68–73.

93. Faccenda J, Mackay T, Boon N, Douglas N. Randomized placebo-controlled trial of continuous positive airway pressure on blood pressure in the sleep apnea-hypopnea syndrome. Am J Respir Crit Care Med 2001; 163: 344–8.

94. Pepperell J, Ramdassingh-Dow S, Crosthwaite N, et al. Ambulatory blood pressure after therapeutic and subtherapeutic nasal continuous positive airway pressure for obstructive sleep apnoea: a randomised parallel trial. Lancet 2002; 359: 204–10.

95. Findley L, Smith C, Hooper J, et al. Treatment with nasal CPAP decreases automobile accidents in patients with sleep apnea. Am J Respir Crit Care Med 2000; 161: 857–9.

96. Partinen M, Guilleminault C. Daytime sleepiness and vascular morbidity at seven-year follow-up in obstructive sleep apnea patients. Chest 1990; 97: 27–32.

97. Marti S, Sampol G, Munoz X, et al. Mortality in severe sleep apnoea/hypopnoea syndrome patients: impact of treatment. Eur Respir J 2002; 20: 1511–8.

98. Doherty LS, Kiely JL, Swan V, McNicholas WT. Long-term effects of nasal continuous positive airway pressure therapy on cardiovascular outcomes in sleep apnea syndrome. Chest 2005; 127: 2076–84.

99. Barbe F, Mayoralas LR, Duran J, et al. Treatment with continuous positive airway pressure is not effective in patients with sleep apnea but no daytime sleepiness: a randomized, controlled trial. Ann Intern Med 2001; 134: 1015–23.

100. Monasterio C, Vidal S, Duran J, et al. Effectiveness of continuous positive airway pressure in mild sleep apnea-hypopnea syndrome. Am J Respir Crit Care Med 2001; 164: 939–43.

101. MacMahon S, Peto R, Cutler J, et al. Blood pressure, stroke, and coronary heart disease. Part 1, Prolonged differences in blood pressure: prospective observational studies corrected for the regression dilution bias. Lancet 1990; 335(8692): 765–74.

102. Hsu CY, Vennelle M, Li HY, et al. Sleep disordered breathing after stroke. A randomized controlled trial of continuous positive airway pressure. J Neurol Neurosurg Psychiatry 2006.

103. Sandberg O, Franklin KA, Bucht G, et al. Nasal continuous positive airway pressure in stroke patients with sleep apnoea: a randomized treatment study. Eur Respir J 2001; 18: 630–4.

104. Wessendorf T, Wang Y, Thilmann A, et al. Treatment of obstructive sleep apnoea with nasal continuous positive airway pressure in stroke. Eur Respir J 2001; 18: 623–9.

105. Bassetti CL, Milanova M, Gugger M. Sleep-disordered breathing and acute ischemic stroke: diagnosis, risk factors, treatment, evolution, and long-term clinical outcome. Stroke 2006; 37: 967–72.

106. Parra O. Sleep-disordered breathing and stroke: is there a rationale for treatment? [letter comment]. European Respiratory Journal 2001; 18: 619–22.

107. Martinez-Garcia MA, Galiano-Blancart R, Roman-Sanchez P, et al. Continuous positive airway pressure treatment in sleep apnea prevents new vascular events after ischemic stroke. Chest 2005; 128: 2123–9.

108. Goldstein LB, Adams R, Alberts MJ, et al. Primary prevention of ischemic stroke: a guideline from the American Heart Association/American Stroke Association Stroke Council. Circulation 2006; 113: e873–923.

109. Brown DL, Chervin RD, Hickenbottom SL, et al. Screening for obstructive sleep apnea in stroke patients: a cost-effectiveness analysis. Stroke 2005; 36: 1291–3.

CHAPTER 16

Narcolepsy and idiopathic hypersomnia

Michel Billiard

Narcolepsy and idiopathic hypersomnia are two important sleep disorders included in the category 'hypersomnia not due to a sleep related breathing disorder' of the *International Classification of Sleep Disorders.*[1] These disorders are not highly prevalent and sleeping too much is still often considered with amusement. However, each one impacts many life parameters including education, work, memory, driving, recreational activities, interpersonal relationships, sexual function, personality, and physical condition. Owing to distinct clinical features, the impact of each disorder might not be exactly the same, but in comparison with the number of studies concerning the impact of narcolepsy,[2–8] there is only one study concerning the impact of idiopathic hypersomnia,[9] and a tendency to mix up the life effects of both disorders. In this chapter we first consider narcolepsy, including epidemiology, clinical features, laboratory tests, course and life effects, and then idiopathic hypersomnia under the same headings.

NARCOLEPSY

Epidemiology

Narcolepsy affects 0.02–0.04% of the population.[10–12] Both sexes are affected, with a slight predominance of males. The age of onset is from childhood to the fifties, with a peak in the second decade. Diagnosis of the condition is often delayed by several years.

Clinical features

Narcolepsy includes two phenotypes: narcolepsy with cataplexy, and narcolepsy without cataplexy.[1] Narcolepsy with cataplexy is characterized by excessive daytime sleepiness and cataplexy, also with auxiliary symptoms referred to as hypnogogic hallucinations, sleep paralysis and disturbed nocturnal sleep, whereas narcolepsy without cataplexy is characterized by the same symptoms except cataplexy.

Excessive daytime sleepiness occurs in waves, at intervals that vary from patient to patient. At times excessive daytime sleepiness can be overcome, but it often leads to irresistible sleep episodes. The duration of these sleep episodes varies, depending on the situation in which the patient finds himself. They always restore normal alertness for a period ranging from one to several hours. This fact is of considerable diagnostic value and the number of hours during which the patient does not feel sleepy after a sleep episode reflects the degree of severity of the disease. Excessive daytime sleepiness may also lead to automatic behavior;

that is, performing a series of actions such as putting away objects in unlikely places, driving a vehicle to an unintended destination, or pronouncing words out of context.

Cataplexy is distinct from excessive daytime sleepiness and irresistible sleep episodes. It is pathognomonic of the disease. It consists of an abrupt drop of muscle tone in reaction to emotional factors, which are most often positive such as a fit of laughter, receiving a compliment, humour expressed by the individual, the sight of a prey for the hunter, perception of a fish biting at the hook for the angler, a well-caught ball at tennis; less often the factors are negative such as anger or frustration. Cataplexy worsens with poor sleep and fatigue. All striated muscles may be affected, except the extraocular and respiratory musculature, leading to the progressive slackening of the whole body. Cataplexy may be also limited to facial muscles or to the upper or lower limbs, leading to dysarthria, facial rictus, dropping objects, or unblocking the knees. Cataplexy is short lived, lasting between seconds and one or two minutes, rarely more. Frequency may vary widely, from one or less per year to several per day. A neurological examination carried out at the exact moment of the event reveals the deep tendon reflexes to be abolished, with occasional Babinski sign.

Other clinical features are deemed accessory as they are not indispensable for diagnosis. Hallucinations, whether hypnogogic (at the onset of sleep) or hypnopompic (on awakening), are mental imagery that may be so real as to be mistaken for something that actually happened. Visual imagery is predominant, but it can also be auditory, tactile, or kinetic. The feeling that a threatening person is at the door or in the bedroom itself or that the subject is flying through space is frequently reported. The accompanying effect is often fear to the extent that the patient may develop a veritable dread of going to bed and resort to reassuring strategies such as keeping a weapon within reach or having a dog sleep in the same room. These hallucinations are experienced by 40–60% of narcoleptic patients. Sleep paralysis is a transient inability to move the limbs and the head during the transition from wakefulness to sleep or vice versa, at a moment when the person is still conscious, and is often accompanied by hypnogogic hallucinations, making it even more frightening. It differs from cataplexy with respect to its timing, the absence of emotional trigger, and its duration up to 10 minutes. It occurs in approximately 30–50% of narcoleptic patients.

Disturbed nocturnal sleep is also a frequent feature of narcolepsy. Patients fall asleep quickly but have repeated awakenings during the night. Parasomnias such as sleep talking or rapid eye movement (REM) sleep behavior disorder are common. Interestingly, there is no relation between the poor sleep quality and the excessive daytime sleepiness.[13] It is noteworthy that narcoleptic patients tend to have an increased body mass index,[14] which may be associated with obstructive sleep apneas.

Course

The general course of narcolepsy varies considerably among individuals. The pattern tends to be for excessive daytime sleepiness and irresistible sleep episodes to persist throughout life, even if improvement is commonly observed with advancing age. A progressive increase in the mean sleep latency on the multiple sleep latency test (MSLT) has been reported as a function of age.[15] Cataplexy often improves with advancing age. In rare cases it disappears, but in most patients it becomes less frequent due to emotional control. Nocturnal sleep tends to worsen with age.

Laboratory tests

Narcolepsy with cataplexy is primarily diagnosed on the basis of the patient's history. However, the diagnosis of narcolepsy should, whenever possible be confirmed by nocturnal polysomnography followed by MSLT. A sleep onset REM period (SOREMP) during nocturnal sleep is observed in about 50% of cases and is highly specific. An increased amount of stage 1 sleep and repeated awakenings are frequently observed. MSLT mean sleep latency is less than or equal to eight minutes and two or more SOREMPs are found in most patients.[1]

HLA typing almost always shows the presence of HLA DQB1*0602. However, this test is not diagnostic for narcolepsy, as about 25% of Caucasians, 12% of Japanese and 38% of African Americans are positive for the same antigen. HLA typing may only be useful to exclude narcolepsy in selected cases.

Measuring cerebrospinal fluid (CSF) hypocretin-1 is highly specific for the diagnosis of narcolepsy with cataplexy.[16] Low CSF hypocretin-1 levels (less than or equal to 110 pg/ml) are found in over 90% of patients with narcolepsy with cataplexy. Currently, this measurement is performed in only a few laboratories and should be asked for in a few selected indications only: when the MSLT cannot be used (associated medications, inability to follow MSLT directions); in patients with possible cataplexy who also have obstructive sleep apnea syndrome; and in young children who are not able to undergo an MSLT.

Narcolepsy without cataplexy cannot be diagnosed on purely clinical basis. Positive diagnosis requires an MSLT demonstrating a mean sleep latency less than or equal to eight minutes and two or more sleep onset REM episodes. Only 10% of cases are reported to have CSF hypocretin-1 levels less than 110 pg/ml.[16]

Life effects

Education

It is not possible from the available literature to distinguish problems of learning based on age, childhood, adolescence, and early adulthood. However, there is little doubt that sleepiness impacts learning ability. Table 16.1 shows the impact of narcolepsy on education through three different studies.[3,4,6] As can be seen, the impact of narcolepsy symptoms was comparable in the three studies except for embarrassement, which was much more prevalent in the study

by Alaia,[6] reflecting the frequent poor self-esteem and social isolation of these patients. Nevertheless there is no significant difference between narcoleptics and controls in the proportion of subjects who reach secondary school or high school; as for university education, the less frequent attainment by narcoleptic patients almost reaches significance.[3]

Work

Various studies have evaluated the effects of narcolepsy symptoms on work. According to a study by Broughton et al.[3] in which the impact of narcolepsy symptoms in 180 patients was compared to the impact of sleepiness in 180 controls, the following effects were recorded: reduced job performance (78.4% in the narcoleptic sample vs. 8.7% in the controls), fear of job loss (49.3% vs. 0.0%), decreased earnings (46.6% vs. 1.2%), prevented promotion (38.5% vs. 0.0%), job dismissal (21.1% vs. 0.0%), disability insurance (10.6% vs. 0.0%). Subsequently, Kales et al.[4] found that work problems were reported by 92% of 50 narcoleptics, with 80% falling asleep at work on at least several occasions, 24% having to quit their jobs, and 18% having been fired because of their condition. According to Alaia[6] nearly 85% of 102 narcoleptic subjects felt that their symptoms had reduced their job performance and 15% had become permanently disabled by their disease. Goswami et al.[5] indicated that among 68 subjects who returned a structured questionnaire, 11 (16%) were unemployed, seeking work, and nine (13%) were unemployed, unable to work. Finally, in a series of 49 subjects with narcolepsy, a significant problem at work was an increase in work-related accidents, which occurred in 15%.[8]

Memory

Reported poor school and work performance have led to research looking for some memory deficit. Broughton et al.[3] reported that 88 narcoleptic subjects (48.9%) found that their memory had worsened after the onset of the

227

Table 16.1 Impact of narcolepsy on education in three different studies

	Broughton et al. (1981)[3]		Kales et al. (1992)[4]	Alaia (1992)[6]
	Narcoleptics (180)	Controls (180)	Narcoleptics (50)	Narcoleptics (102)
Age range	15–71	15–71	18–72	28–80
Life effects	Narcolepsy symptoms	Sleepiness	Narcolepsy symptoms	Narcolepsy symptoms
Symptoms began before formal education was completed	76 (42.2%)	5 (3.0%)	—	63 (61.8%)
Symptoms caused poor marks	39 (51.3%)	1 (0.55%)	29 (58%)	64 (62.7%)
Interpersonal problems with teachers	26 (34.2%)	1 (0.55%)	18 (36%)	49 (48%)
Embarrassment	24 (31.5%)	1 (0.55%)	—	83 (81.3%)
Problems led to quit school	—	—	9 (18%)	—

disease, while 17 controls (9.4%) noted poor memory due to sleepiness. Smith et al.,[17] in a survey of 700 narcoleptic subjects, found that 38% reported moderate or severe memory problems, while 39% had problems with forgetfulness, 40% with concentration, and 26% with general learning.

Based on these data several studies have attempted an objective evaluation of memory function in narcoleptic subjects. Aguirre et al.[18] compared attention, concentration, short-term and long-term memory in narcoleptic and control subjects and did not find objective differences between the two groups. Rogers and Rosenberg[19] investigated patient self-reports of memory deficits by comparing the scores of 30 narcoleptic subjects and 30 controls, but did not find any significant difference in the various tests of memory. Thus one may conclude that a consistent proportion of narcoleptic subjects experience subjective impressions of memory dysfunction that are not transferred to objective differences. Several explanations for this discrepancy have been suggested. Even if narcoleptics perform memory tests at normal levels under challenging conditions, as soon as they return to ordinary conditions, recurrent episodes of drowsiness return and impair attention and short-term memory mechanisms.[18] Routine memory tasks may have limited external validity in relation to everyday memory performance.[20] Furthermore, narcoleptic subjects may have lower self-efficacy for memory performance than controls. This lowered self-efficacy is expressed through increased anxiety about memory function, decreased evaluation of memory capacity, and increased perception of memory decline in relation to the comparison groups.[21]

Driving

The effects of excessive daytime sleepiness and other narcolepsy symptoms on driving are of obvious concern. Broughton et al.[3] found that out of 180 narcoleptic subjects 87 drove, while out of 180 controls 113 drove. Fifty-seven narcoleptic subjects (65.5% of the drivers) fell asleep while driving against seven controls (6.2% of the drivers), 25 (28.7%) had cataplexy, 16 (11.5%) had sleep paralysis, 58 (66.7%) had had frequent near-accidents against no controls (0%), and 32 (36.8%) had had accidents against six controls (5.3%). However, the figures concerning cataplexy and sleep paralysis appear fairly high. In a more recent study using a similar questionnaire, only six out of 35 narcoleptics (17%) reported cataplectic attacks or sleep paralysis episodes while driving, more in agreement with clinical experience.[22] In another study[23] the proportion of individuals with sleepiness-related motor vehicle accidents and near-accidents was compared in obstructive sleep apnea subjects (181), narcoleptic subjects (25), subjects with excessive daytime sleepiness due to other causes (35) and a control group (35). The proportion of narcoleptic subjects with motor vehicle accidents was 52%, compared to 29% of subjects with excessive daytime sleepiness due to other causes, 19% of obstructive sleep apnea subjects and 11% of controls. The proportion of narcoleptic subjects with near-accidents in motor vehicles was 72%, compared to 66% of obstructive sleep apnea subjects, 60% of subjects with excessive daytime sleepiness due to other causes, and 51% of controls. However, these two studies were based on self-reports by the patients and could be biased by the patients' subjectivity. In another study, Alaia[6] interviewed 95 drivers with narcolepsy of whom 78% reported sleepiness while driving, 29% accidents due to their symptoms, and 74.2% near-accidents.

Therefore, driving is a critical issue in patients with excessive daytime sleepiness, particularly in those with narcolepsy, hence the need to identify those patients at risk for motor vehicle accidents. Several studies using driving simulators[24–26] have shown that such patients had worse performance than controls; however it seems difficult, based on any one of these tests, to predict those patients at risk for driving accidents. A review of regulations and guidelines for commercial and non-commercial drivers with sleep apnea and narcolepsy in North America, Europe and Australia has been published.[27]

Recreational activities

A majority of narcoleptic patients report that their symptoms interfere with their recreational activities, such as watching entertainment (90%), playing cards (40.5%), swimming (7.2%), dancing (4.4%);[3] enjoyment of recreational activities (70.6%), pursuit of favorite leisure activities,[6] cinema (81%), meeting friends (59%), playing sports (48%), taking holidays (44%).[8] Given different population samples and questionnaires, these results are difficult to compare. The findings nevertheless suggest strongly that narcolepsy has a definite impact on this important part of life.

Interpersonal relationships

A majority of patients report deterioration of interpersonal relationships due to irresistible sleep episodes or cataplexy during conversation.[3,4,8] According to Broughton et al.,[3] 65.6% of people are understanding and tolerant of symptoms of their narcoleptic relatives or friends, while 34% are not. Sleepiness may be interpreted as laziness, boredom, or drunkenness. An intentional decrease in contacts with people to avoid the embarrassment of an irresistible sleep episode was reported by 56% of narcoleptic subjects[4] and a cessation of contacts by 30%.[8] In another study, 36% of patients indicated a control of emotions when with others to ward off a possible attack of cataplexy.[4]

Persons with narcolepsy often suffer from difficulties in marital relationship. Kales et al.[4] reported marital and family problems in 72% of patients, tension in the family in 42%, and separation or divorce in 20%.

Sexual life

Sexual dysfunction is of concern for many narcoleptic patients. According to Broughton,[3] 17 of 112 male respondents (15.2%) revealed impotence, generally attributed to medication, to the point that males with narcolepsy occasionally discontinued their antidepressant medication.[28–29] Kales et al.[4] reported difficulty with sex in 26% of narcoleptics against 8% of normals, women being mainly responsible for this difference, and Alaia[6] reported a decrease in sexual drive in 36.1% of subjects.

Personality

Narcolepsy impacts the psychological well-being of individuals. In the study by Kales et al.[4] no psychiatric diagnosis was established in 24 out of 50 patients, while 15 received a diagnosis of depressive disorder and 11 were given a diagnosis of personality disorder. The personality disorder diagnoses included obsessive–compulsive, histrionic, schizoid, and borderline personalities. Based on Minnesota multiphasic personality inventory (MMPI) findings, with higher mean values for narcoleptics than for controls on seven of the eight clinical scales ($p < .01$), it was suggested that narcoleptic subjects have more psychopathology than control subjects do. However, this would be an effect rather than a cause of narcolepsy. Indeed the wide diversity of MMPI code patterns and the presence of unusual codes in the sample were in favor of the secondary nature of the narcoleptic psychopathology. In line with this conclusion is the review of 130 subjects with narcolepsy carried out by Zarcone and Fuchs.[30] No one personality type was associated with narcoleptic symptomatology and the authors concluded that patients should be considered as having a neurological disease that may cause emotional disturbances, not as having a primary psychopathological disorder.

Physical condition

As already noted narcoleptic patients have a tendency toward increased body mass index with all the possible consequences of being overweight, including obstructive sleep apnea syndrome. Also, a cataplectic attack may lead to total body collapse with the risk, although not major, of serious injuries such as skull or other bone fractures.

Narcolepsy in comparison with other diseases

Narcolepsy has a profound negative impact on the patient's daily life. This has led to comparison between the life effects of narcolepsy and epilepsy, another neurological condition characterized by episodic events of another nature.[31] Strikingly, the conclusion of the study was that the life effects of narcolepsy with cataplexy were more marked and pervasive than those of epilepsy, at least when the latter is associated with absence of major organic cerebral pathology. Similarly, in a study comparing the impact of narcolepsy and other illness groups on psychological health and role behaviors, it was found that narcoleptics reported more adjustment problems in comparison with cardiac disease, a mixed group of cancers, and diabetes.[32]

IDIOPATHIC HYPERSOMNIA

Epidemiology

Due to long-standing nosological uncertainty and the relative rarity of the condition, prevalence studies have not been performed so far. However, some predictions can be made. Studies of both narcoleptic and idiopathic hypersomnia subjects in various sleep disorders center populations have been carried out, which have supported the general conclusion that the ratio of idiopathic hypersomnia to narcolepsy is somewhere between 10% and 20%. There is apparently no gender predominance; the age of onset varies from childhood to young adulthood with very few cases occurring after the age of 25 years.[33]

Clinical features

Idiopathic hypersomnia includes two distinct phenotypes, referred to as idiopathic hypersomnia with long sleep time and idiopathic hypersomnia without long sleep time.[1] Idiopathic hypersomnia with long sleep time is remarkable for three symptoms: a complaint of constant or recurrent daily excessive daytime sleepiness and unwanted naps, longer and less irresistible than in narcolepsy, and non-refreshing irrespective of their duration; night sleep is sound, uninterrupted by awakenings but abnormally prolonged; morning awakening is delayed and laborious. Patients do not awaken to the ringing of a clock or a telephone, and often rely on their spouse or a family member to wake them up. Even then, patients may remain confused, unable to react adequately to external stimuli, a state referred to as 'sleep drunkenness'. In that sense, idiopathic hypersomnia with long sleep may be portrayed as an inability to wake up, in contrast with narcolepsy characterized by an abnormal drive to fall asleep.

In comparison, idiopathic hypersomnia without long sleep stands as isolated excessive daytime sleepiness.

The physical examination is normal in either case.

Course

Once established the disorder is stable in severity and is long lasting. Any spontaneous disappearance of the symptoms is grounds for casting doubt on the initial diagnosis.

Laboratory tests

The basis for a diagnosis of idiopathic hypersomnia with long sleep time is mostly clinical, whereas that of idiopathic hypersomnia without long sleep time relies entirely on polysomnographic evaluation.

Polysomnographic monitoring of nocturnal sleep demonstrates normal sleep, except for its prolonged duration in the case of idiopathic hypersomnia with long sleep time. NREM sleep and REM sleep are in normal proportions. Sleep efficiency is commonly said to be above 90%. There is no SOREMP. Obstructive sleep apneas and periodic limb movements in sleep should theoretically be absent, but may be acceptable in the case of an early onset of idiopathic hypersomnia and of their late occurrence. Several authors have suggested the need for monitoring esophageal pressure during sleep to rule out mild sleep-disordered breathing that may fragment sleep and induce excessive daytime sleepiness.

The MSLT demonstrates a mean sleep latency of less than 10 minutes, which might be longer than in the case of narcolepsy in the form with long sleep time and in the same range as in narcolepsy in the form without long sleep time. In the case of idiopathic hypersomnia with long sleep time, the MSLT seems somewhat irrelevant. Awakening the patient in the morning for the purpose of carrying out the first MSLT session precludes documenting the abnormally prolonged night sleep, and the MSLT sessions preclude recording of prolonged non-refreshing daytime sleep episode(s), which are of major diagnostic value. Thus other procedures are of potential interest: 24-hour polysomnography on an ad-lib sleep/wake protocol, in order to document the major sleep episode (more than 10 hours) and daytime sleep episode(s) (at least one nap of more than one hour), which still awaits standardization and validation; and one-week actigraphy.

Cognitive evoked potential (P 300) performed in the evening and in the morning, immediately after awakening and later, is of particular interest in the assessment of sleep inertia.[34] Computed tomography (CT) and/or magnetic resonance imaging (MRI) of the brain should be performed if there is a clinical suspicion of an underlying brain lesion. Psychometric/psychiatric evaluation is mandatory to exclude hypersomnia associated with a psychiatric disorder.

Life effects

In comparison with narcolepsy, life effects of idiopathic hypersomnia, either with long sleep time or without, have been much less investigated, this being possibly due to less well-defined phenotypes and lower prevalence. The only available study to date is by Broughton et al.[9] using the same questionnaire as used in a previous study in narcoleptic subjects.[2] The subjects were 30 patients with idiopathic hypersomnia (without distinction at that time of the form with long sleep time and the form without long sleep time), 30 controls and 24 subjects with narcolepsy (22 with cataplexy and two without). Interpersonal relationships and marital problems have not been investigated.

Education

Idiopathic hypersomnia clearly impacts school performance. When compared to controls, affected individuals reported having poor marks (0% vs. 48%) and problems with teachers (0% vs. 24%), findings which are not significantly different from those seen in narcoleptic patients.

Work

Compared to controls, subjects with idiopathic hypersomnia felt that their condition had impaired their performance (97% vs. 0%), had prevented them from receiving promotions (50% vs. 0%), had reduced their earnings (53% vs. 0%), and had increased their fears of job dismissal (33% vs. 0%). These five work features, however, were not significantly different from those of narcoleptic subjects.

Memory

Patients' complaints about memory impairment were about as frequent as those of narcoleptics (50% vs. 46%). The memory deficit was mainly for recent events, again resembling the frequency of complaints in narcolepsy. In contrast with cognitive deficits associated with narcolepsy, an objective evaluation of memory dysfunction has not been carried out in people with idiopathic hypersomnia.

Driving

Compared to controls, patients reported significantly more problems with driving, but had fewer problems in this area than narcoleptic subjects. This was particularly clear for the degree to which excessive daytime sleepiness was judged to produce frequent near-accidents in idiopathic hypersomnia subjects (25%), more commonly than in controls (0%) but less frequently than in narcoleptic subjects (100%), probably in relation with the more paroxysmal and imperative nature of sleepiness in the latter group.

Recreational activities

Patients with idiopathic hypersomnia reported having significantly fewer recreational interests than did controls (33% vs. 60%). This level, however, was not significantly different from that of narcoleptics (46%).

Sexual life

Impotence in males was more frequent in hypersomniac patients than in controls (22% vs. 6%), but was not significantly different in incidence from narcoleptics (14%).

Personality

Idiopathic hypersomnia patients noted a change in their personality more frequently than controls (27% vs. 0%), but the figure was not significantly different from that in narcoleptic subjects (33%).

In view of these results one could think that the consequences of idiopathic hypersomnia are similar to those of narcolepsy with the exception of near-accidents being less frequent than in narcolepsy. This might be due to the limitation of a questionnaire specifically prepared for narcoleptic subjects and to the fact of not distinguishing idiopathic hypersomnia with long sleep time and idiopathic hypersomnia without long sleep time. Indeed, clinical experience shows that some effects are specific to idiopathic hypersomnia with long sleep time. First, these patients report arriving late to work, receiving remarks from their employer and often being dismissed as a consequence. Second, the lengthy time these patients spend in bed is usually not tolerated by the spouse nor family members over the long term and frequently leads to marital problems. Third, in contrast to narcoleptic subjects, hypersomniacs do not benefit from night sleep or naps, to the extent that they usually never feel refreshed. Finally, excessive daytime sleepiness is most often amenable to stimulant medications, whereas difficulty in awakening is not, hence hypersomniac patients have a continuing difficulty in being on time for work, even with relevant treatment.

CONCLUSION

Life effects of narcolepsy and idiopathic hypersomnia are of great concern for the patients affected with these conditions. Based on clinical experience rather than on specific questionnaires, this chapter underlines some of the consequences which might be specific to idiopathic hypersomnia with long sleep time. Unfortunately, the symptoms of these often go undiagnosed for years, which often compounds their deleterious effects. Indeed, precocious treatment may prevent, or at least limit, the impact that these conditions have on the lives of the affected patients.

REFERENCES

1. American Academy of Sleep Medicine. International Classification of Sleep Disorders, 2nd edn: Diagnostic and Coding Manual. Westchester, IL: American Academy of Sleep Medicine, 2005.

2. Broughton R, Ghanem Q. The impact of compound narcolepsy on the life of the patient. In: Guilleminault C, Dement WC, Passouant P, eds. Narcolepsy. New York: Spectrum, 1976: 201–19.

3. Broughton R, Ghanem Q, Hishikawa Y, et al. Life effects of narcolepsy in 180 patients from North America, Asia and Europe compared to matched controls. Can J Neurol Sci 1981; 8: 299–304.

4. Kales A, Soldatos CR, Bixler EO, et al. Narcolepsy-cataplexy. II. Psychosocial consequences and associated psychopathology. Arch Neurol 1992; 39: 169–71.

5. Goswami M, Pollak CP, Cohen FL, et al. eds. Psychosocial Aspects of Narcolepsy. New York: Haworth Press, 1992.

6. Alaia SL. Life effects of narcolepsy: measures of negative impact, social support, and psychological well-being. Loss Grief Care 1992; 5: 1–22.

7. Broughton WA, Broughton RJ. Psychosocial impact of narcolepsy. Sleep 1994; 17: S45–9.

8. Teixeira VG, Faccenda JF, Douglas NJ. Functional status in patients with narcolepsy. Sleep Med 2004; 5: 477–83.

9. Broughton R, Nevsimalova S, Roth B. The socioeconomic effects of idiopathic hypersomnia – comparison with controls and with compound narcoleptics. In: Popoviciu L, Asgian B, Badiu G, eds. Sleep 1978. Basel: Karger, 1980: 229–33.

10. Hublin C, Kaprio J, Partinen M, et al. The prevalence of narcolepsy: an epidemiological study of the Finnish twin cohort. Ann Neurol 1994; 35: 709–16.

11. Silber MH, Krahn LE, Olson EJ, Pankratz VS. The epidemiology of narcolepsy in Olmsted County, Minnesota: a population-based study. Sleep 2002; 25: 197–202.

12. Ohayon MM, Priest RG, Zulley J, Smirne S, Paiva T. Prevalence of narcolepsy symptomatology and diagnosis in European general population. Neurology 2002; 58: 1826–33.

13. Broughton R, Dunham W, Weisskopf M, et al. Night sleep does not predict day sleep in narcolepsy. Electroencephalogr Clin Neurophysiol 1994; 91: 67–70.

14. Schuld A, Helebrand J, Geller F, Pollmächer T. Increased body-mass index in patients with narcolepsy. Lancet 2000; 355: 1274–5.

15. Dauvilliers Y, Gosselin A, Paquet J, et al. Effect of age on MSLT results in patients with narcolepsy–cataplexy. Neurology 2004; 62: 436–50.

16. Mignot E, Lammers GJ, Ripley B, et al. The role of cerebrospianl fluid hypocretin measurement in the diagnosis of narcolepsy and other hypersomnias. Arch Neurol 2002; 59: 1553–62.

17. Smith KM, Merrit SL, Cohen FL. Can we predict cognitive impairment in persons with narcolepsy? Loss, Grief Care 1992; 5: 103–13.

18. Aguirre M, Broughton R, Stuss D. Does memory impairment exist in narcolepsy–cataplexy? J Clin Exp Neuropsychol 1985; 7: 14–24.

19. Rogers AE, Rosenberg RS. Tests of memory in narcoleptics. Sleep 1990; 13: 42–52.

20. Hood B, Bruck D. Sleepiness and performance in narcolepsy. J Sleep Res 1996; 5: 128–34.

21. Hood B, Bruck D. Metamemory in narcolepsy. J Sleep Res 1997; 6: 205–10.

22. Leon-Munoz L, de la Calzada MD, Guitart M. Prevalencia de accidentes en un grupo de pacientes afectos de sindrome de narcolepsia-cataplejia. Rev Neurol 2000; 30: 596–8.

23. Aldrich MS. Automobile accidents in patients with sleep disorders. Sleep 1989; 12: 487–94.

24. Findley L, Unverzagt M, Guchu R, et al. Vigilance and automobile accidents in patients with sleep apnea or narcolepsy. Chest 1995; 108: 619–24.

25. Findley LJ, Suratt PM, Dinges DF. Time-on-task decrements in 'steer clear' performance of patients with sleep apnea and narcolepsy. Sleep 1999; 22: 804–9.

26. George CFP, Boudreau AC, Smiley A. Comparison of simulated driving performance in narcolepsy and sleep apnea patients. Sleep 1996; 19: 711–17.

27. Pakola SJ, Dinges DF, Pack AI. Driving and sleepiness. Review of regulations and guidelines for commercial and noncommercial drivers with sleep apnea and narcolepsy. Sleep 1995; 18: 787–96.

28. Karacan I. Erectile dysfunction in narcoleptic patients. Sleep 1986; 9: 227–31.

29. Karacan I, Gokcebay N, Hirshkowitz M, et al. Sexual dysfunction in men with narcolepsy. Loss Grief Care 1992; 5: 81–90.

30. Zarcone VP, Fuchs HE. Psychiatric disorders and narcolepsy. In: Guilleminault C, Dement WC, Passouant P. eds. Narcolepsy. New York: Spectrum, 1976: 231–56.

31. Broughton R, Guberman A, Roberts J. Comparison of psychosocial effects of epilepsy and of narcolepsy-cataplexy: a controlled study. Epilepsia 1984; 25: 423–33.

32. Bruck D. The impact of narcolepsy on psychological health and role behaviors: negative effects and comparisons with other illness groups. Sleep Med 2001; 2: 437–46.

33. Billiard M, Dauvilliers Y. Idiopathic hypersomnia. Sleep Med Rev 2001; 5: 351–60.

34. Billiard, Rondouin G, Espa F, Dauvilliers Y, Besset A. Pathophysiology of idiopathic hypersomnia. Rev Neurol (Paris) 2001; 157: 5S101–6.

Index

Note to index: Page numbers in italic refer to tables and illustrations

A
abdominal pain, direct costs *201*
absenteeism
  daytime sleepiness 180
  insomnia 143, *146–7*
acaricides 89
accident risks 115–21
  daytime sleepiness 179
    measurements for population 179
  driving and sleep deprivation 20, 106, 116–17
  drugs and medications 119, 144–5, 199–200
  economic impact 119, 179
  excessive sleepiness *131*, 132–3
  insomnia 144–5, 157
  legislation to promote driver safety 131
  medicolegal issues, defendant claims
    'awake' 130–2
  narcolepsy 186
  noted examples 106–7, 116
  occupational/work-related 144, 181
    in shift working 106–7, 116
  sleep-disordered breathing (SDB)
    118–19, 181
  see also daytime sleepiness; driving;
    economic impact
adenoidectomy, impact on QoL in children
  with SDB *51–2*
age/aging 3, 21–2, 59–65
  chronic pain, prevalence 196
  circadian clock 61–2

and health 3, 12
insomnia 11, 59–60, *60–1*
  cognitive behavior therapy 29
  healthiest older population vs total
    older population *61*
peri/postmenopausal state 62
population growth of older
  Americans *60*
research directions 63–4
sleep-disordered breathing 6–7
sleep duration 6, 21–2
  excessive 31
sleep problems 59–60
  excessive daytime sleepiness and
    cognitive decline 63
  prevalences *60*
sleep–wake cycle and
  metabolism 60–1
suprachiasmatic nucleus (SCN)
  pathways 60–1
air
  humidity and ventilation 88–9
  ions 89
alcohol, treatment for insomnia 141
alertness level test (ALT), daytime
  sleepiness 178
allergies, house dust mite 89–90
allostatic load 102
antidepressants, REM sleep behavior
  disorder 125–6

anxiety disorder
  comorbidity with insomnia 142, 145, 158
  rating scales 178
apnea/hypopnea *see* sleep-disordered
    breathing (SDB)
apnea/hypopnea index (AHI) 53, 118, 210
aromatherapy 85–6
attention deficit hyperactivity disorder
    (ADHD) 43–4
automatism
  as defense 124–5, 128, 132
  and driving 128
  legal aspects 126–7
    alcohol consumptions 127
  sane/insane 124
autonomic responses
  activity during sleep 77
  noise levels 71

B
back pain 90–1
  direct costs *201*
beds
  mattresses 89–95
  pillows 94–5
  room disposition 95
  size 93
'brain music', EEG and PSG 82
Brooklyn study
  characteristics of participants *27*
  race 26–7
    Caribbean Americans and US-born
        Blacks 30–1
    and sleep-disordered breathing 29–30
    sleep disorders *27*
    within-group differences 30–1
  reliance on sleep medicine 29–30, *30*

C
caffeine
  consumption by children *176*
  consumption studies 178
Calgary Sleep Apnea QoL Index for OSA 178
cancer pain, direct costs *201*
cardiovascular deaths, sleep-disordered
    breathing 25

caregivers, and race differences in
    reappraisal 28
cataplexy, clinical features 230
cerebral blood flow, and PFO shunts 216
cervical or neck pain, direct costs *201*
Chernobyl nuclear disaster 106–7, 116
Child Health Questionnaire (CHQ-PF50) 50
children 39–58
  2–5 years 40–1
  5–10 years 41–3
  adolescence 39–40
  attention deficit hyperactivity disorder
      (ADHD) 43–4
  caffeine consumption 175, *176*
  daytime sleepiness 40, 42
    excessive daytime somnolence (EDS) 44–5
  health-related quality of life (HRQL)
      evaluation 49–53
  and music 79–80
    earphones 80
    lullaby 80
  obstructive sleep apnea (OSA) 182–3
  research, future directions 45–6
  sleep-disordered breathing 49–58
    impact of tonsillectomy and
        adenoidectomy on QoL *51–2*
    school performance 53–7, *54–6*
  sleep duration from infancy to
      adolescence *177*
  sleep restriction and ADHD 44
  sleep–wake patterns 43–5
  see also infants
Children's Depressive Inventory 50
circadian clock
  aging 61–2
  length of period 62, 77
  light intensity 62, 85
  suprachiasmatic nucleus (SCN)
      pathways 60–1
  temperature and sleep 87
circadian disorders 133, 184–5, 203
  animal model 61
  disturbance pattern in recent times 77–8
  dyssynchrony, melatonin treatment 63
  economics 184–5
  effects, adolescents 184–5

seasonal affective disorder (SAD) 83–4
    in shift working 107, 184
Cleveland Family Study 8
coagulation, abnormal in sleep-disordered
        breathing (SDB) 216–17
cognitive behavior therapy
    insomnia 29, 164–5
    multifaceted 165
computers 95, 96
confusional arousal 125
congestive heart failure
    comorbidity with insomnia 145
    and sleep apnea *212*
continuous positive airway pressure (CPAP)
        therapy 118–19
    ethical considerations 217
    long-term observational studies 217–18
    short-term randomized controlled trials 218
    for sleep-disordered breathing (SDB)
        182–3, 217–20
    stroke patients with sleep apnea 218–19
coping strategy, sleep complaint
        reporting 28–31
'core sleep' vs 'optional sleep' 31
coronary artery disease, and sleep apnea *212*
culture *see* race; socioeconomic status (SES)

D
daytime sleepiness 40, 42, 176–80
    age, and cognition 63
    excessive daytime somnolence (EDS) 175–6
        causes *131*
        children 44
        and cognitive decline in aged 63
        legal aspects 131–2
        vs hypersomnia 237
        see also narcolepsy
    and insomnia 142
    manifest vs physiological sleep
        tendency 42
    measurements for individuals 176–8
        alertness level test (ALT) 178
        driving performance (Steer Clear)
            178, 186
        maintenance of wakefulness test
            (MWT) 178

multiple sleep latency test (MSLT) 177
        psychomotor vigilance task (PVT) 178
        sleep duration from infancy to
            adolescence *177*
        sleepiness scales 177
    measurements for population 178–80
        accident costs 179
        loss of productivity 179–80
        major accidents 179
        motor vehicle accidents 179
    multiple sleep latency test (MSLT)
        40, 44, 45, 118, 177–8, 230
    see also hypersomnia
demographic factors 1–20
    age 3, 21–2
    gender 2, 5, 7–8, 11–12
    marital status 3
    socioeconomic status and education 3
    see also epidemiology
depression
    Children's Depressive Inventory 50
    comorbidity with insomnia
        142, 145, 158
    pain 196–7
    rating scales 178
    and sleep disorder 24, 25
developing world, availability/access to
        pain management 202
dissociative states 128
driving
    automatism 124–8, 132
    excessive sleepiness *131*
    hypnotics effects 144
    insomnia 144–5
    legislation to promote driver safety 131
    medicolegal issues, defendant claims
        'awake' 130–2
    narcolepsy 232–3
    sleep deprivation 20, 106, 115–21
        long distance driving association
            116–17
    sleep-related breathing disorders 118–19
    Steer Clear measurement of daytime
        sleepiness 178, 186
    taxis, no legislation to promote driver
        safety 131

use of drugs and medications for pain
199–200
see also accident risks
drug-facilitated sexual assault 129
drug-related sleep 133
automatism, sane/insane 124, 132
drugs and medications
accident risks 119, 144–5, 199–200
cost of pain and sleep interactions 203
temazepam 129, 144
duration of sleep *see* sleep duration

E
economic impacts
accident risks 119, 179
see also accident risks; driving
circadian disorders 184–5
common sleep disorders 180–6
costs of insomnia 148–9, 159–63, 183–4
cost of pain and sleep interactions 200–3
daytime sleepiness 176–80
accident costs 119, 179
loss of productivity 179–80
insomnia 148–9, 159–63, 183–4
narcolepsy 185–6
obstructive sleep apnea (OSA) 180–3
sleep loss 175–6
sleep-related accidents 119, 179
education, *see also* socioeconomic
status (SES)
electric and magnetic fields 73
electroencephalogram (EEG)
'brain music' 82
during music therapy 81–2
recorded micro-sleep 117
RLVMF pattern 39
emotion, index of self-regulation (ISE) 28
environmental factors *see* sleep
environment
epidemiology
demographic factors 1–20
hypersomnia 234
insomnia 140–1, 156
narcolepsy 229
epilepsy 126
Epworth Sleepiness Scale (ESS) 177

European Union
highway deaths, goal 115
legislation to promote driver safety
119–20, 131
excessive daytime somnolence (EDS)
see daytime sleepiness
Exxon Valdez disaster 106, 116

F
fatigue
legal aspects 133
pain perception 198
and sleepiness 116
Feng Shui 95
fetal experience, heart rate 82
fibrinogen, abnormal in sleep-disordered
breathing (SDB) 217
fibromyalgia 196, 198, 200–1
flunitrazepam 129
flying, and sleep deprivation 106
futon beds 92

G
gender
and health 2, 11–12
sleep-disordered breathing 7–8
sleep duration 5, 22
general adaptation syndrome (GAS) 101

H
headache/migraine, direct costs *201*
health demographic factors 1–20
age 3, 21–2
gender 2, 11–12
marital status 3
race 2–3, 12
research, conceptual framework *2*
sleep-disordered breathing 6–7
sleep duration 4–5
health utilization, economic measures 180
health-related quality of life (HRQL)
evaluation
children 49–5
insomniacs 149–51, 157
heart rate
fetal experience 82

and musical rhythms 82–3
  ethnomusic 82
  ill patients 83
  NREM/REM sleep 77
  odor/olfaction 86
house dust mite 89–90
humidity and ventilation 88–9
hypersomnia 234–7
  clinical features 235
  course 235
  epidemiology 234
  laboratory tests 235
  life effects 236–7
    driving 236
    education 236
    memory 236
    personality 236–7
    recreational activities 236
    sexual life 236
    work 236
  vs EDS 237
  see also daytime sleepiness
hypertension, and sleep-disordered
    breathing 25
hypnotics, drug-related accidents 144–5
hypocretin, involvement in sleep–wake
    cycle 61, 231
hypothalamo-pituitary-adrenocortical
    axis 102

I
idiopathic hypersomnia *see* hypersomnia
indecent exposure, legal aspects 128
index of self-regulation of emotion
    (ISE) 28
infants
  and maternal heart rate 82
  NREM/REM sleep, and temperature 87
  sleep duration from infancy to
    adolescence *177*
  see also children
insomnia 137–54, 155–74, 183–4
  and absenteeism 143, *146–7*
  accident risk 144–5, 157, 183–4
  age and aging 11, 59–60
  classification systems 155

comorbidities 142, 145, *146–7*, 158
costs 148–9, 159–63, 183–4
  breakdown *161*
  direct/indirect costs *160*, 161–2
  public health consequences 140–52,
    155–74
  research findings 159–63
defined 137, 155–6
diagnosis 137–40
  research diagnostic criteria 137–8
epidemiology 140–1
prevalence and risk factors *60*, 156
health status
  functional impairment 157–8
  health care use 145, *146–7*, 158–9
  healthiest older population vs total
    older population *61*
ISE scores 28
medicolegal issues 132
natural history 142
  primary/secondary 138–9
  transient/chronic 139
New Zealand adults 23
quality of life 149–51, 157
  HD-16 scale 150, *151*
and race 23–5
  response bias 27–8
repressive coping 28–31
research recommendations 169–70
severity 139–40
Sleep in America Poll (1998), DIS,
    DMS and EMA 20
stress markers 103
treatment 63, 141–2, 163–9
  cognitive therapy 29, 164–5
  late-life 29
  low-cost self-help interventions
    158–9, 166–9, *167–8*
  multifaceted cognitive therapy 165
  paradoxical intention 165
  psychological interventions 163–6
  relaxation techniques 163
  sleep hygiene 165
  sleep restriction 31, 164
  stimulus control 163–4
Wisconsin Sleep Cohort variables *7*

International Association for the Study of Pain (IASP) 193
intervertebral discs 91

J
Japan Collaborative Cohort Study on Evaluation of Cancer Risk, sleep duration 21

K
Karolinska Sleepiness Scale 177
Klein–Levin syndrome 128, 133

L
legal issues *see* medicolegal issues
light intensity 83–5
    and circadian clock 62, 85
    and melatonin 84, 85
    seasonal affective disorder (SAD) 83–4
low-cost self-help interventions, treatment of insomnia 158–9, 166–9, *167–8*
lullaby 80
lumbar lordosis 91, 92–3

M
magnetic fields 94–5
maintenance of wakefulness test (MWT) 178
manifest sleep tendency, defined 42
marital status
    health 3, 12
    sleep-disordered breathing 8–9
    sleep duration 6
mattresses 89–95
    anti-allergenic covers 89–90
    elasticity 92
    firm/soft support 92–3
    house dust mite 89–90
    humidity factors 88–9
    hysteresis 92
    materials 91–2
    stability 92
medication, reliance on 29–30, *30*
medicolegal issues 123–35
    claimant claims 'asleep' 129
    common sleep-related situations *123*
    defendant claims 'abnormal awareness' 128–9

defendant claims 'asleep' 124–8
defendant claims 'awake' 130–2
indecent exposure 128
sleep disorder claimed due to an accident 132–3
melanopsin 84
melatonin 84, 85
    circadian clock and light intensity 62
    treatment for circadian dysynchrony 63
mental health, and insomnia 142, 145, *146–7*, 158
metabolic syndrome, in sleep-disordered breathing (SDB) 217
micro-sleep, EEG recorded 117
modafinil, enhancement of alertness 108
multiple sleep latency tests (MSLT) 40, 44, 45, 118, 177–8, 230
    daytime sleepiness 178
music/music therapy 79–83
    'brain music' therapy 82
    ill patients 81
    mechanical devices 83
    psychophysiological effects 81–2
    rhythms and ethnomusic 82–3
    young children 79–80

N
narcolepsy 118, 126, 129, 133, 185–6, 229–34
    clinical features 229–30
        cataplexy 230
    course 230
    economics 185–6
    effects of medications and antidepressants 186
    epidemiology 229
    excessive daytime somnolence (EDS), *see also* daytime sleepiness
    hypocretin 61, 231
    laboratory tests 230–1
    life effects 231–4
        driving 232–3
        education 231, *232*
        interpersonal relationships 233

memory 231–2
personality 234
physical condition 234
recreational activities 233
sexual dysfunction 234
work 231
motor vehicle accidents 186
notification to DVLA 132
occupational problems 185–6
'Steer Clear' simulating highway driving
conditions 178, 186
National Health and Nutrition Examination
Survey 25–6
National Sleep Foundation (USA)
Pain and Sleep 195
see also Sleep in America Poll
New Zealand adults, insomnia 23
noise levels 69–73, 78–9
adaptation to 79
autonomic responses 71
awakenings 70
day levels, sleep efficiency 78
effects of noise-disturbed sleep on
health 72–3
laboratory vs field studies 72
long term habituation 72
physiologic sensitivity 71
secondary effects of noise exposure
during sleep 71–2
shortening sleep periods 70
sleep stage modifications 70
WHO recommendations 71
nonrestorative sleep 22
Sleep-EVAL system 22
normal sleep 176
NREM sleep see sleep stages
Nurses Health Study, sleep duration 21

O
obesity
association with short sleep 61
sleep apnea 220
sleep curtailment 217
weight loss as therapy for apnea 218
obstructive airway disease, comorbidity with
insomnia 145

obstructive sleep apnea (OSA) 180–3
Calgary Sleep Apnea QoL Index
for OSA 178
co-morbidities 180
continuous positive airway pressure (CPAP)
therapy 182–3
economics 180–3
costs of health care utilization 181
estimates of medical costs 181–2
health economic evaluations 183
pediatric 182–3
quality-adjusted life years (QALYs)
calculation 183
traffic and occupational accidents 181
see also sleep-disordered breathing (SDB)
Obstructive Sleep Apnea-18 HRQL survey
(OSD-18) 49–53
occupational risks, OSA 181
odor/olfaction 85–6
physiology 86
'optional sleep' vs 'core sleep' 31
orofacial pain, direct costs 201
osteoarthritis/rheumatoid arthritis,
direct costs 201

P
pain 193–208
chronic pain 196–7
cognitive impairments and fatigue 198–9
and poor sleep 197–200, 198
world prevalence 194–5
cost of pain and sleep interactions 200–3
drugs and medication history 203
patient complaints of sleep partner
disturbance 203
sleep disorders concomitant
with pain 203
sleep hygiene 203
world availability/access to pain
management 202
definition 193–4
depressive symptoms 196–7
medical demand 200
pain and poor sleep, time course of
relationship 197–8
prevalence and sleep disturbances 195–6

racial differences 195
research and management, future
    directions 204
risk factors 196–200
treatment, reversal of consequences
    on sleep *203*
paradoxical intention, insomnia 165
parasympathetic activity during sleep 77
patent foramen ovale (PFO) in OSA 216
Pediatric Sleep Questionnaire 53, *54*
PedsQL scores 50
periodic limb movements in sleep (PLMS)
    185, 196, 203
permethrin 90
physiological sleep tendency, defined 42
pillows 94–5
polysomnography
    'brain music' 82
    children
        ADHD 43
        sleep–wake patterns 44–5
    legal aspects 126–7, 133
    sleep apnea 210, *211*
    stress and 103, 105
post-traumatic hypersomnia 132–3
post-traumatic stress disorder 103, 125
posture and immobility 90
productivity loss, daytime sleepiness
    impacts 179–80
prostate disease, comorbidity with
    insomnia 145
psychological interventions, insomnia 163–5
psychomotor vigilance task (PVT),
    measurement of daytime sleepiness 178

Q
quality of life
    children 49–53
    insomniacs 149–51, 157
quality-adjusted life years (QALYs) calculation
    in OSA 183

R
race
    and age 3
    Brooklyn study 26–31

differences in pain perception 195
differences in reappraisal reported by
    caregivers 28
and health 2–3, 12
insomnia 23–5
    New Zealand adults 23
    respiratory disturbance index (RDI) 24
    sleep-disordered breathing 8, 12, 29–30
    sleep duration 5, 12, 22, 25–7
        European and American 23
    sleep paralysis 25
rape 127–8, 129
rapid eye movement (REM) sleep
    children 39–41
    thermoregulation and sleep stages 68–70
relaxation techniques, insomnia 163
REM sleep *see* sleep stages
REM sleep behavior disorder 125–6
    features of violence in *127*
repressive coping 28–31
respiratory disturbance index (RDI) 24, *212*
restless legs syndrome (RLS) 23, 185, 196
retina, and light intensity 84
road traffic accidents *see* accident risks; driving

S
seasonal affective disorder (SAD) 83–4
    and air ionizers 89
self-help, low-cost interventions for insomnia
    158–9, 166–9
sexsomnia 128
sexual assault/rape 127–8, 129
    drug-facilitated 129
sexual dysfunction 234
shift working 101–14
    accident risks 106–7, 116
    circadian rhythm disturbance 107, 184
    insufficient sleep as risk 130–1
    long-term effects 105
    polysomnography 105
    public health issues 101–14
    shift work sleep disorder (DSM IV
        and ICSD) 107–8
    sleep latency 105
    stress 104–8
    subjective alertness 105–7

short sleep periods
  association with obesity 61
  noise levels 70
Sleep in America Poll (1998) 20–2
  DIS, DMS and EMA 20, 22
  and sleep-disordered breathing in Blacks
    29–30
Sleep in America Poll (2000), sleep
    duration 175
Sleep in America Poll (2004), children's
    caffeine consumption 175, *176*
sleep apnea *see* sleep-disordered breathing
  (SDB)
sleep bruxism 203
sleep deprivation 4, 88
  consequences 20–1
sleep-disordered breathing (SDB) 6–7
  accidents
    apneas due to accident 133
    risk 25, 118–19
  apnea/hypopnea index (AHI) 53, 118, 210
  causes 25
  and cerebrovascular disease 210, *212*
  children 49–58
    school performance 53–7, *54–6*
  complications, mechanisms
    underlying *213*
  driving accidents 118–19
  gender 7–8
  genetics 24
  marriage 8–9
  pathophysiologic mechanisms 213–17
    abnormal coagulation 216–17
    cardiac arrhythmia 215–16
    diurnal hypertension 214–15
    inflammation 213–14
    nocturnal sympathetic activation 214
    shunting through PFO 216
  peri/postmenopausal state 62
  polysomnography, sleep apnea 210, *211*
  race 8, 12, 24–5
  respiratory disturbance index (RDI)
    24, 53
  severity spectrum 6
  socioeconomic status (SES) 8
  and stroke 209–24

therapy 217–20
  CPAP 118–19, 217–20
  weight loss 218
Wisconsin Sleep Cohort variables *7*
sleep disorders (other)
  automatism 124–8, 132
  cataplexy 230
  DIS, DMS and EMA 20, 22, *27*
  disorder is claimed due to an accident 132–3
  epilepsy 126
  Klein–Levin syndrome 133
  narcolepsy 118, 126, 129, 132, 133
  periodic limb movements 133
  post-traumatic hypersomnia 132–3
  sleep walking 124–7
  see also daytime sleepiness; insomnia;
    narcolepsy; sleep-disordered breathing
sleep duration 4–6, 19–39
  > 8h, mortality prediction 26
  age 6, 21–2
    from infancy to adolescence *177*
  decline 19–20, 31
  definitions 4
  excessive, older people 31
  factors affecting 21–3
  gender 5, 22
  health 4–5
  marital status 6
  modal duration 19
  and mortality 26
  and noise levels 70
  race 5, 12, 22, 25–7
  Sleep in America Poll (1998) 20–2
  Sleep in America Poll (2000) 175
  socioeconomic status/education 5–6
  specific mortality risks 21
  see also insomnia
sleep environment 67–75, 77–99
  air, humidity and ventilation 88–9
  ambient temperature 67–75, 86–8
  bed/mattress 90–5
  bed/room disposition 95
  electric and magnetic fields 73
  house dust mite 89–90
  light 83–5
  odor/olfaction 85–6

sound 78–83
  ambient noise 69–73
  temperature 86–8
Sleep-EVAL system, nonrestorative
    sleep 22
sleep hygiene
  pain and sleep interactions 203
  and treatment of insomnia 165
sleep latency
  multiple sleep latency test (MSLT)
      40, 44, 45, 118, 177–8, 230
  shift working 105
sleep loss 175–6
  children's caffeine consumption 175, *176*
  economics 175–6
  excessive daytime somnolence
      (EDS) 175–6
  normal sleep 176
sleep movements 90
sleep paralysis, race 25
sleep pattern, changes in recent
    times 77–8
sleep restriction 164
  children 44
  and obesity 217
  therapy for insomnia 31, 164
sleep spindles 79
sleep stages
  modification by noise levels 70
  NREM/REM sleep
    heart rate 77
    and sleep violence 124
    temperature 87
  rapid eye movement (REM) sleep
    children 39–41
    and temperature 68–70, 87
  REM sleep behavior disorder 125–6, *127*
  slow wave sleep (SWS)
    and age 176
    and thermoregulation 68–70
sleep terrors 125
sleep violence
  features *124*, *127*
  NREM/REM sleep 124
  REM sleep behavior disorder *127*

sleep walking 124–5
sleep–wake patterns
  children, polysomnography 44–5
  involvement of hypocretin 61
  suprachiasmatic nucleus (SCN) pathways
      60–1
sleepiness *see* daytime sleepiness
slow wave sleep (SWS)
  and age 176
  and thermoregulation 68–70
snoring, and stroke 209–10
socioeconomic status (SES)
  education 3
  evidence for association with sleep
      disorders *11*
  and health risks 12
  sleep-disordered breathing 8
  sleep duration 5–6
sodium oxybate 129
somnambulism (sleep walking) 124–5
sound 78–83
  infrasound 79
  music 79–83
  noise levels 69–73, 78–9
spine *see* vertebral column
Stanford Sleepiness Scale (SSS) 177
status dissociatus 126
stress 101–14
  allostatic load 102
  burnout increase 104
  connection with sleep 102–3
  markers of insomnia 103
  model: general adaptation
      syndrome 101
  shift working 104–8
    accident risks 106–7
    long-term effects 105
    polysomnography 105
    subjective alertness 105–7
stroke 209–24
  and severity of sleep apnea *212*
  sleep apnea and 210–20
    polysomnography *211*
  snoring and 209–10
suicidal ideation, pain 197

suprachiasmatic nucleus (SCN) pathways,
    sleep–wake cycle 60–1
sweating 68, 87
sympathetic activation
    during sleep 77
    pathophysiology of sleep-disordered
        breathing (SDB) 214
sympathetic adrenal medullary system
    activation 102

T
taxi drivers, no legislation to promote
    driver safety 131
temazepam 129, 144
temperature 67–75
    effects of large variations on sleep
        characteristics 69
    and sleep 86–8
    thermoneutrality and thermal
        comfort zone 67–8
    thermoregulation and sleep stages 68–9
        rapid eye movement (REM) sleep
            68–70
        slow wave sleep (SWS) 68–70
temperomandibular/orofacial pain,
    direct costs 201
Three Mile Island nuclear accident
    107, 116
tinnitus 79
Tonsil and Adenoid Health Status
    Instrument 49–53

tonsillectomy and adenoidectomy
    impact on QoL in children with
        SDB 51–2
    post T&A results 57
traffic accidents see accident risks; driving
train driving, and sleep deprivation 106
transient ischaemic attack 212
TVs 95, 96

V
ventilation 88–9
vertebral column
    intervertebral discs 91
    lordosis 91, 92–3
vigilance 42–3
violence see sleep violence

W
water beds 92
weight loss, for sleep apnea 218
Wisconsin Sleep Cohort
    insomnia/apnea 7, 11
    sociodemographic variables 7

Y
yin/yang 95

Z
zaleplon 145
zolpidem 144, 150
zopiclone 145, 150

T - #0608 - 071024 - C0 - 246/189/12 - PB - 9780367389727 - Gloss Lamination